CARDIOVASCULAR MEDICINE

CARDIOVASCULAR MEDICINE

New Therapeutic Drugs Approved by the US FDA (2013–2017)

Y. ROBERT LI, MD, MPH, PhD

Professor of Pharmacology
Chair of Department of Pharmacology, Campbell University SOM
Buies Creek, North Carolina 27506, USA

Adjunct Professor of Biomedical Engineering and Sciences
Virginia Tech–Wake Forest University School of Biomedical Engineering and Sciences
Blacksburg, Virginia 24061, USA

Adjunct Professor of Biomedical Sciences and Pathobiology
Department of Biomedical Sciences and Pathobiology, Virginia Polytechnic Institute and State University
Blacksburg, Virginia 24061, USA

Adjunct Professor of Biology
Department of Biology, University of North Carolina
Greensboro, North Carolina 27412, USA

CELL MED PRESS, AIMSCI Inc.

CARDIOVASCULAR MEDICINE   ISBN: 978-1-68056-004-6

Cell Med Press also publishes this book in digital formats. For more information on the products of Cell Med Press, please visit the website at aimsci.com/cmp or cellmedpress.org.

This book is printed on acid-free paper.

Printed in the United States of America

Cover design: Rachel E. Li

CONTENTS IN BRIEF

CONTENTS

PREFACE

"The heart has always held a special fascination for humans: it has been the seat of the soul; the home of emotions; and the pump that, when beating, symbolizes life, and when silent, signifies death" [Peterson ED, Gaziano JM. *JAMA* 2011; 306(19):2158]. Perhaps no other organ in the human body has been so closely scrutinized. Hence, the management of cardiovascular diseases (CVDs), especially with the use of medications, has always been a focus of modern medicine. In this context, CVDs remain the leading cause of death globally, though the mortality associated with these diseases in developed countries has been significantly reduced over the past decades owing to the availability of effective treatment approaches, particularly new therapeutic drugs approved by the United States Food and Drug Administration (US FDA). Thus, defecting CVDs relies, at least partly, on the continued development of newer and more effective cardiovascular drugs.

While there are multiple influential books devoted to cardiovascular therapeutics, a book that focuses on the most recently US FDA-approved novel drugs for CVDs would facilitate the learning of cutting-edge knowledge on using these new tools for more effective management of CVDs and promotion of human health. Accordingly, the aim of this book is to provide a comprehensive coverage of the new cardiovascular therapeutic drugs approved by the US FDA over the past five years (2013–2017), focusing on their molecular pharmacology and evidence-based clinical efficacy as well as the forefront new discoveries. As outlined below, the book contains five units with a total of 12 chapters.

Unit I: Chapters 1–3
Unit II   Chapters 4 and 5
Unit III   Chapters 6 and 7
Unit IV   Chapters 8–10
Unit V   Chapters 11 and 12

Unit I is on dyslipidemias, and consists of three chapters (Chapters 1–3). Chapter 1 provides an over-view on the various forms of dyslipidemias and the underlying molecular genetics, as well as the available drugs for their treatment. This sets a stage for the subsequent coverage of the new US FDA-approved lipid-lowering drugs in Chapters 2 and 3. In this regard, Chapter 2 considers two new drugs for treating hypercholesterolemia, namely, mipomersen (an antisense against apolipoprotein B-100) and Liptruzet (a fixed-dose combination of ezetimibe and atorvastatin), which were approved in 2013 and 2015, respectively. Chapter 3 covers Epanova, an omega-3 fatty acid-based drug for treating severe hypertriglyceridemia. Epanova was approved in 2014.

Unit II is on systemic hypertension, and includes two chapters (Chapters 4 and 5). Chapter 4 introduces several general aspects of hypertension, including definition, classification, epidemiology, and molecular pathophysiology, and outlines the various classes of antihypertensive drugs. Chapter 5 covers two new fixed-dose combination drugs for treating hypertension, namely, Prestalia (perindopril/amlodipine) and Byvalson (nebivolol/valsartan), and they were approved in 2015 and 2016, respectively.

Unit III is on pulmonary hypertension, and composed of two chapters (Chapters 6 and 7). Chapter 6 overviews the different groups of pulmonary hypertension as well as the commonly used drugs including both non-vasodilating agents and vasodilating drugs. Chapter 7 examines the three new US FDA-approved drugs for treating pulmonary hypertension. They are the endothelin receptor antagonist macitentan, the soluble guanylate cyclase stimulator riociguat, and the prostacyclin IP receptor agonist selexipag. The first two were approved in 2013 and the last one in 2015.

Unit IV is on acute coronary syndromes and other thrombotic disorders, and comprises three chapters (Chapters 8–10). Chapter 8 first gives an overview on acute coronary syndromes (ACS), including definition, classification, epidemiology, and molecular pathophysiology. It then introduces the various classes of drugs, including emerging therapeutic modalities, for both acute and long-term management of ACS. Chapter 9 considers two new US FDA-approved drugs for ACS, and they are the $P2Y_{12}$ receptor inhibitor cangrelor (approved in 2015) and the thrombin receptor antagonist vorapaxar (approved in 2014). The two new selective factor Xa inhibitors edoxaban (approved in 2015) and betrixaban (approved in 2017) for the management of other thromboembolic disorders are covered in Chapter 10.

Unit V, the last unit of the book, is on heart failure, and contains two chapters (Chapters 11 and 12). Chapter 11 introduces the various aspects of heart failure, especially heart failure with reduced ejection fraction, and outlines the diverse classes of drugs for treating heart failure. This is followed by Chapter 12, the last chapter of the book, that surveys ivabradine (an I_f channel inhibitor) and Entresto (a fixed dose combination of sacubitril and valsartan), both approved in 2015. They are also the only two new drugs that have been approved by the US FDA for treating chronic heart failure in more than a decade.

To help the reader understand the various topics and retain new knowledge, each of the above 12 chapters is supplemented at the beginning with chapter highlights of key points, and at the end with a list of self-assessment questions. It is worth noting that peer-reviewed scholarly journals of high quality are instrumental in disseminating the leading-edge research findings so as to advance our scientific knowledge. In this context, the contents of this book are written based primarily on the original scientific findings published in the highly influential peer-reviewed journals. Due to space limitations, only original and/or representative references are cited.

It is hoped that this book by integrating fundamental concepts with forefront discoveries and translating essential bioscience to clinical medicine, will provide the reader a unique approach to understanding the rapidly evolving field of cardiovascular medicine, particularly cardiovascular therapeutics. In view of the rapidly evolving nature of the field (and medicine as a whole), the information contained in this book is subject to change based on new scientific knowledge and clinical investigations. Although the author of the book has checked with sources believed to be reliable and accurate at the time of publication, information included in the book may not be accurate in every respect due to the possibility of human errors and rapid changes in biomedical sciences. As such, the author of the book does not warrant that the information contained in the work is in every respect accurate and complete. The author disclaims all responsibility for any errors or omissions or for the results obtained from the use of the information contained in this book. The reader is advised to seek independent verification for any data, advice, or recommendations contained in the work.

"Cardiovascular Medicine: New Therapeutic Drugs Approved by the US FDA (2013–2017)" would not have been possible without the original essential scientific findings published by numerous scientists in influential scholarly journals of high scientific quality. The author is thankful for the time and effort invested by the editorial personnel at Cell Med Press, AIMSCI Inc., which made the work possible and of high quality.

Y. Robert Li
North Carolina, USA

UNIT I

DYSLIPIDEMIAS

UNIT I

DYSLIPIDEMIAS

CHAPTER 1

Overview of Dyslipidemias and Drug Therapy

CHAPTER HIGHLIGHTS

- Dyslipidemias constitute a chief risk factor of atherosclerotic cardiovascular diseases, a major cause of death globally.
- Common forms of dyslipidemias include hypercholesterolemia, hypertriglyceridemia, and mixed hyperlipidemia.
- The United Stated Food and Drug Administration (US FDA)-approved drugs for dyslipidemias include 9 classes, with statins being the most important class of cholesterol-lowering drugs.
- PCSK9 inhibitors are the newest drug class for reducing cholesterol levels.

KEYWORDS | ApoB-100 antisense; Bile acid sequestrant; Dyslipidemia; Ezetimibe; Fibrate; Hypercholesterolemia; MTP inhibitor; Niacin; Omega-3-fatty acid; PCSK9 inhibitors; Statin

CITATION | *Li YR. Cardiovascular Medicine: New Therapeutic Drugs Approved by the US FDA (2013–2017). Cell Med Press, Raleigh, NC, USA. 2018. http://dx.doi.org/10.20455/ndcvd.2018.01*

ABBREVIATIONS | ANGPTL3, angiopoietin-like 3; ApoA-I, apolipoprotein A-I; ApoC-II, apolipoprotein C-II; CETP, cholesteryl ester transfer protein; HDL, high-density lipoprotein; LCAT, lecithin-cholesterol acyltransferase; LDL, low-density lipoprotein; MTP, microsomal triglyceride transfer protein; NPC1L1, Niemann-Pick C1-Like 1; PCSK9, proprotein convertase subtilisin/kexin type 9; US FDA, the United States Food and Drug Administration; VLDL, very low-density lipoprotein

CHAPTER AT A GLANCE

1. INTRODUCTION

Dyslipidemias constitute a chief cause of atherosclerosis and athero-sclerosis-associated conditions, such as coronary artery disease, ischemic cerebrovascular disease, and peripheral vascular disease. Hence, effective management of dyslipidemias is an essential component of preventive cardiology. This chapter introduces the basic molecular medicine of dyslipidemias focusing on the underlying molecular etiologies. It then provides a brief overview of the mechanistically based drug therapy. This will set a stage for the subsequent coverage of the newly approved drugs for treating the different forms of dyslipidemias.

2. MOLECULAR MEDICINE OF DYSLIPIDEMIAS

2.1. Definitions

Dyslipidemias and lipoprotein disorders (also known as disorders of lipoprotein metabolism) are probably among the most commonly encountered terms in cardiovascular medicine. The term "lipoprotein disorders" emphasizes the molecular etiology and pathophysiology, whereas the term "dyslipidemias" focuses on the plasma lipid profile (primarily cholesterol and triglycerides) of the lipoprotein disorders. The Merriam–Webster medical dictionary definition of dyslipidemia is "a condition marked by abnormal concentrations of lipids or lipoproteins in the blood".

The abnormal concentrations can be either higher or lower than the normal values, with the former known as hyperlipidemias (e.g., hypercholesterolemia, hypertriglyceridemia) and the latter as hypolipidemias (e.g., low levels of high-density lipoprotein cholesterol). Hence, dyslipidemias do not necessarily always involve increased levels of blood lipids. For this reason, when referring to lipid disorders, the term dyslipidemias is preferred over hyperlipidemias to encompass the entire spectrum of the lipid abnormalities.

2.2. Classification Schemes

Dyslipidemias are classified in various ways based on different criteria. The two commonly used criteria are lipid profiles and underlying etiologies.

2.2.1. Classification Based on Lipid Profiles

Based on lipid profiles, dyslipidemias are usually classified into four categories, as listed below.

- Hypercholesterolemia (see Section 2.3.1)

- Hypertriglyceridemia (see Section 2.3.2)
- Mixed hyperlipidemia (see Section 2.3.3)
- Hypoalphalipoproteinemia (see Section 2.3.4)

2.2.2. Classification Based on Underlying Etiologies

Dyslipidemias may stem from lipoprotein disorders caused by genetic alterations in the genes encoding the various components of the lipoproteins, the receptors of the lipoproteins, or the enzymes involved in the metabolism of lipoproteins [1–3]. As described below, a particular type of dyslipidemia may result from more than one lipoprotein disorders. Dyslipidemias resulting from genetic lipoprotein disorders are frequently called primary dyslipidemias. Most cases of primary dyslipidemias do not result from a single gene defect but instead stem from the cumulative burden of multiple genes (polygenic) that predisposes the individuals to milder forms of dyslipidemias, particularly in the presence of unhealthy life-style, including excessive dietary intake of saturated fats and lack of physical activity.

On the other hand, dyslipidemias may also result from a variety of other diseases and conditions, including obesity, diabetes mellitus (diabetes for short), lipodystrophy, thyroid diseases, kidney disorders, hepatic disorders, lysosomal storage diseases, Cushing's syndrome, alcohol intake, and use of estrogens and many other medications (e.g., thiazide diuretics, β-adrenergic receptor blockers, anti-human immunodeficiency virus protease inhibitors, and antischizophrenic drugs). Dyslipidemias resulting from the above diseases and conditions are known as secondary dyslipidemias.

2.3. Major Types of Primary Dyslipidemias and Their Underlying Genetic Lipoprotein Disorders

This section describes the four major types of primary dyslipidemias and their underlying genetic lipoprotein disorders, which provide a foundation for understanding drug therapy of dyslipidemias.

2.3.1. Hypercholesterolemia

Primary hypercholesterolemia is characterized by increased levels of total plasma cholesterol and low-density lipoprotein (LDL) cholesterol with normal plasma concentrations of triglycerides. The causes of primary hypercholesterolemia include familial hypercholesterolemia, familial defective apolipoprotein B-100 (ApoB-100), autosomal dominant hypercholesterolemia, and more commonly, polygenic hypercholesterolemia [4, 5] (**Table 1.1**).

2.3.2. Hypertriglyceridemia

Primary hypertriglyceridemia is characterized by high fasting plasma levels of triglycerides (200–500 mg/dl or higher) and frequently normal plasma levels of LDL cholesterol. The major causes of primary hypertriglyceridemia include familial hypertriglyceridemia, lipoprotein lipase deficiency, and apolipoprotein C-II (ApoC-II) deficiency [6] (**Table 1.2**).

TABLE 1.1. Major LDL disorders leading to increased LDL cholesterol

Name of disorder	Genetic etiology	Prevalence
Familial hypercholesterolemia	LDL receptor gene mutations, causing decreased expression of LDL receptors, leading to reduced uptake of LDL by hepatocytes	1/500 (heterozygous); 1/1,000,000 (homozygous)
Familial defective ApoB-100	Mutations of the ApoB-encoding gene, causing disruption of LDL receptor-binding domain of ApoB-100 and the consequent decreased hepatic uptake of LDL	<1/1000 (in individuals of German descent)
Autosomal dominant hypercholesterolemia	Gain-of-function mutations in the PCSK9-encoding gene, leading to increased LDL receptor degradation. PCSK9 binds to LDL receptors, causing receptor degradation	<1/1,000,000
Autosomal recessive hypercholesterolemia	Mutations in the LDL receptor adaptor protein (LDLRAP)-encoding gene. LDLRAP is a protein involved in LDL receptor-mediated endocytosis of LDL	<1/1,000,000
Sitosterolemia (also known as phytosterolemia)	Mutations in either ABCG5- or ABCG8-encoding gene, leading to decreased pumping of cholesterol from enterocytes into the gut lumen and from the hepatocytes into the bile. ABCG5 and ABCG8 are two ATP-binding cassette (ABC) proteins that are expressed in enterocytes and hepatocytes. Heterodimerization of the 2 proteins forms a functional complex that pumps both plant steroids and animal steroids (mainly cholesterol) into the gut lumen and into the bile	<1/1,000,000
Familial lipoprotein(a) hyperlipoproteinemia[1]	Variation in the Apo(a)-encoding gene	Up to 30%[2]

Note: [1]Lipoprotein(a) is considered as an LDL-like lipoprotein; [2]based on *Arterioscler Thromb Vasc Biol* 2016; 36(11):2239–45.

2.3.3. Mixed Hyperlipidemia

Individuals with primary mixed hyperlipidemia exhibit complex lipid profiles, which are frequently characterized by increased plasma levels of total cholesterol, LDL cholesterol, and triglycerides. The plasma level of high-density lipoprotein (HDL) cholesterol is often reduced. Mixed hyperlipidemia mainly results from familial combined hyperlipidemia (one of the most common genetic hyperlipidemias in the general population with an estimated prevalence of 0.5%–2.0%) and dysbetalipoproteinemia [7] (**Table 1.2**).

2.3.4. Hypoalphalipoproteinemia

The low plasma level of HDL cholesterol is referred to as hypoalphalipoproteinemia because HDL is the "alpha lipoprotein". Decreased HDL cholesterol or cholesterol efflux capacity is an independent risk factor of atherosclerotic cardiovascular diseases [8–

10]. The causes of decreased HDL cholesterol include apolipoprotein A-I (ApoA-I) deficiency, Tangier disease, familial HDL deficiency, and lecithin-cholesterol acyltransferase (LCAT) deficiency, among others (**Table 1.3**).

TABLE 1.2. Major triglyceride-rich lipoprotein disorders leading to hypertriglyceridemia

Name of disorder	Genetic etiology	Prevalence
Familial hypertriglyceridemia (mainly increased VLDL levels)	Polygenic (the disorder results from the cumulative burden of multiple genes)	1/500
Familial combined hyperlipidemia (elevated levels of both VLDL triglycerides and LDL cholesterol)	Polygenic (see above for definition), and one of the most common genetic hyperlipidemias in the general population, being the most frequent in patients affected by coronary heart disease (10%)	0.5–2%
Lipoprotein lipase deficiency (mainly chylomicronemia, also elevated plasma levels of VLDL)	Mutations in the lipoprotein lipase-encoding gene, leading to lipoprotein lipase deficiency and thereby decreased catabolism of VLDL and chylomicrons	1/1,000,000
Familial ApoC-II deficiency (mainly chylomicronemia, also elevated plasma levels of VLDL)	Mutations in the ApoC-II-encoding gene, leading to ApoC-II deficiency. ApoC-II is a co-factor of lipoprotein lipase, and deficiency of ApoC-II disables lipoprotein lipase	<1/1,000,000
ApoA-V deficiency (chylomicronemia)	Mutations in the ApoA-V-encoding gene, leading to ApoA-V deficiency. ApoA-V is present in chylomicrons, VLDL, and HDL, and is involved in triglyceride metabolism. Deficiency of ApoA-V results in elevated levels of triglyceride-rich lipoproteins	<1/1,000,000
Familial hepatic lipase deficiency	Mutations in the hepatic lipase-encoding gene, leading to hepatic lipase deficiency. Hepatic lipase is involved in the conversion of IDL to LDL, and deficiency of this enzyme results in increased levels of IDL particles, also called VLDL remnants	<1/1,000,000
Familial dysbetalipoproteinemia	Genetic variations in the ApoE-encoding gene, leading to ApoE dysfunction. ApoE is present on the surface of chylomicron remnants and essential for the receptor-mediated endocytosis of the particles (via hepatic receptors). Several types of mutations of the ApoE gene can cause a deficiency in the clearance of these remnant particles	1/10,000

Note: Those with prevalence <1/1,000,000 are considered rare diseases, and the exact number of the prevalence is often unknown. IDL, intermediate-density lipoprotein; VLDL, very low-density lipoprotein.

TABLE 1.3. Major HDL disorders leading to decreased HDL cholesterol

Name of disorder	Genetic etiology	Prevalence
ApoA-I deficiency	Deletion of the ApoA-I-encoding gene, leading to ApoA-I deficiency. ApoA-I is a major apolipoprotein of HDL and required for LCAT activity	Rare (only a few dozens of cases have been described)
ABCA1 deficiency, also known as Tangier disease	Mutations in the ABCA1-encoding gene, leading to ABCA1 deficiency ABCA1 is a cellular transporting protein that facilitates efflux of unesterified cholesterol and phospholipids from peripheral cells to ApoA-I. Hence, ABCA1 deficiency affects HDL maturation	Rare (about 50 cases have been described)
Familial HDL deficiency	Mutations in the ABCA1- or ApoA-I-encoding gene, leading to decreased formation of ABCA1 or ApoA-I	Rare (unknown)
LCAT deficiency (There are two forms of LCAT deficiency: complete deficiency, also called classic LCAT deficiency, and partial deficiency, also known as fish-eye disease.)	Mutations in the LCAT-encoding gene, leading to LCAT deficiency LCAT is activated by ApoA-I and catalyzes the esterification of cholesterol to form cholesteryl esters. LCAT deficiency results in increased proportion of free cholesterol in circulating lipoproteins and impairs the functional maturation of HDL, leading to the rapid catabolism of circulating ApoA-I	Rare (about 100 cases have been described)

Note: The number of cases under Prevalence refers to the number of cases that have been described in the scientific literature or in the world.

3. OVERVIEW OF THE MECHANISTICALLY BASED DRUG THERAPY

The in-depth understanding of lipoprotein metabolism and lipoprotein disorders at the molecular and genetic levels over the past decades has dramatically advanced the development of mechanistically based pharmacological modalities to treat dyslipidemias and/or to reduce the risk of atherosclerotic cardiovascular diseases [5, 11–15]. Currently, the United States Food and Drug Administration (US FDA)-approved drugs for dyslipidemias may be classified into 9 classes. This section briefly introduces these drugs regarding their major mechanisms of action and clinical indications. The name in the parentheses after the drug name is the trade name (or proprietary name), and the date denotes the initial approval date by the US FDA.

3.1. Statins

- Lovastatin (Mevacor) (August 1987); Lovastatin extended-release (Altocor) (June 2002)
- Pravastatin (Pravachol) (October 1991)

- Simvastatin (Zocor) (December 1991)
- Fluvastatin (Lescol) (December1993)
- Atorvastatin (Lipitor) (December 1996)
- Rosuvastatin (Crestor) (August 2003)
- Pitavastatin (Livalo) (August 2009)

Statins are the commonly used names for a class of drugs known as 3-hydroxy-3-methylglutaryl-coenzyme A (HMG-CoA) reductase inhibitors. These drugs inhibit the de novo cholesterol synthesis in the liver, leading to the upregulation of hepatocyte LDL receptors and the consequent augmented clearance of LDL particles from the plasma (**Figure 1.1**). As listed above in chronological order of approval date, there are currently 7 statins approved by the US FDA (structures shown in **Figure 1.2**). Among the 7 statins, pitavastatin is the newest member approved by the US FDA in 2009. It is also the most potent statin drug, followed by rosuvastatin and atorvastatin. The clinical efficacy of statins in the management of cardiovascular disorders stems from both the lipid-lowering activity and the other novel effects (e.g., anti-inflammation, anti-oxidative stress, anti-tissue remodeling, inhibition of platelet activation and aggregation, and stabilization of atherosclerotic plaque) of this drug class. Presently, statins are considered as the most important and effective drugs with an established safety profile in treating hypercholesterolemia to prevent atherosclerotic cardiovascular diseases [16–19].

3.2. Cholesterol Absorption Inhibitors

- Ezetimibe (Zetia) (October 2002)

These drugs block the absorption of cholesterol from the intestine. Currently, ezetimibe is the only member in this class that has been approved by the US FDA. The molecular target of ezetimibe has been shown to be the sterol transporter, namely, Niemann-Pick C1-Like 1 (NPC1L1), located on the brush border of small intestinal epithelial cells. This transporter is involved in the intestinal uptake of cholesterol and phytosterols. NPC1L1 is also present in the liver. Naturally occurring mutations that disrupt NPC1L1 function were found to be associated with reduced plasma LDL cholesterol levels and a decreased risk of coronary heart disease [20].

Inhibition of NPC1L1 by ezetimibe leads to a decrease in the delivery of intestinal cholesterol to the liver. This causes a reduction of hepatic cholesterol stores, which results in the upregulation of hepatocyte LDL receptors and the consequent augmented clearance of LDL particles from the plasma. Because statins and ezetimibe act via different mechanisms to lower cholesterol, combination of a statin and ezetimibe represents an effective approach to reducing LDL cholesterol, retarding atherosclerotic plaque progression, and improving cardiovascular outcomes [21–23]. In this context, two fixed-dose combinations of ezetimibe and a statin have been approved by the US FDA. They are listed below.

- Ezetimibe/simvastatin (Vytorin) (July 2004)
- Ezetimibe/atorvastatin (Liptruzet) (May 2013)

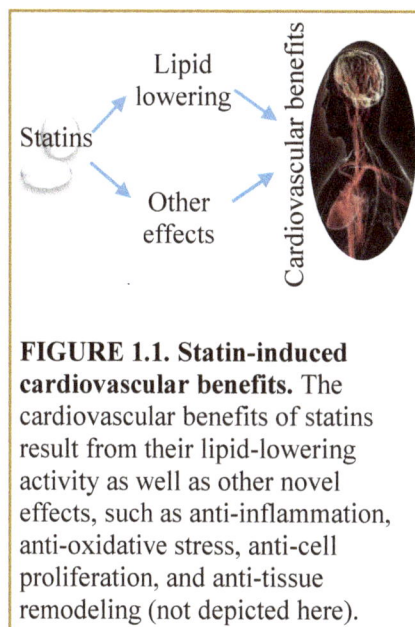

FIGURE 1.1. Statin-induced cardiovascular benefits. The cardiovascular benefits of statins result from their lipid-lowering activity as well as other novel effects, such as anti-inflammation, anti-oxidative stress, anti-cell proliferation, and anti-tissue remodeling (not depicted here).

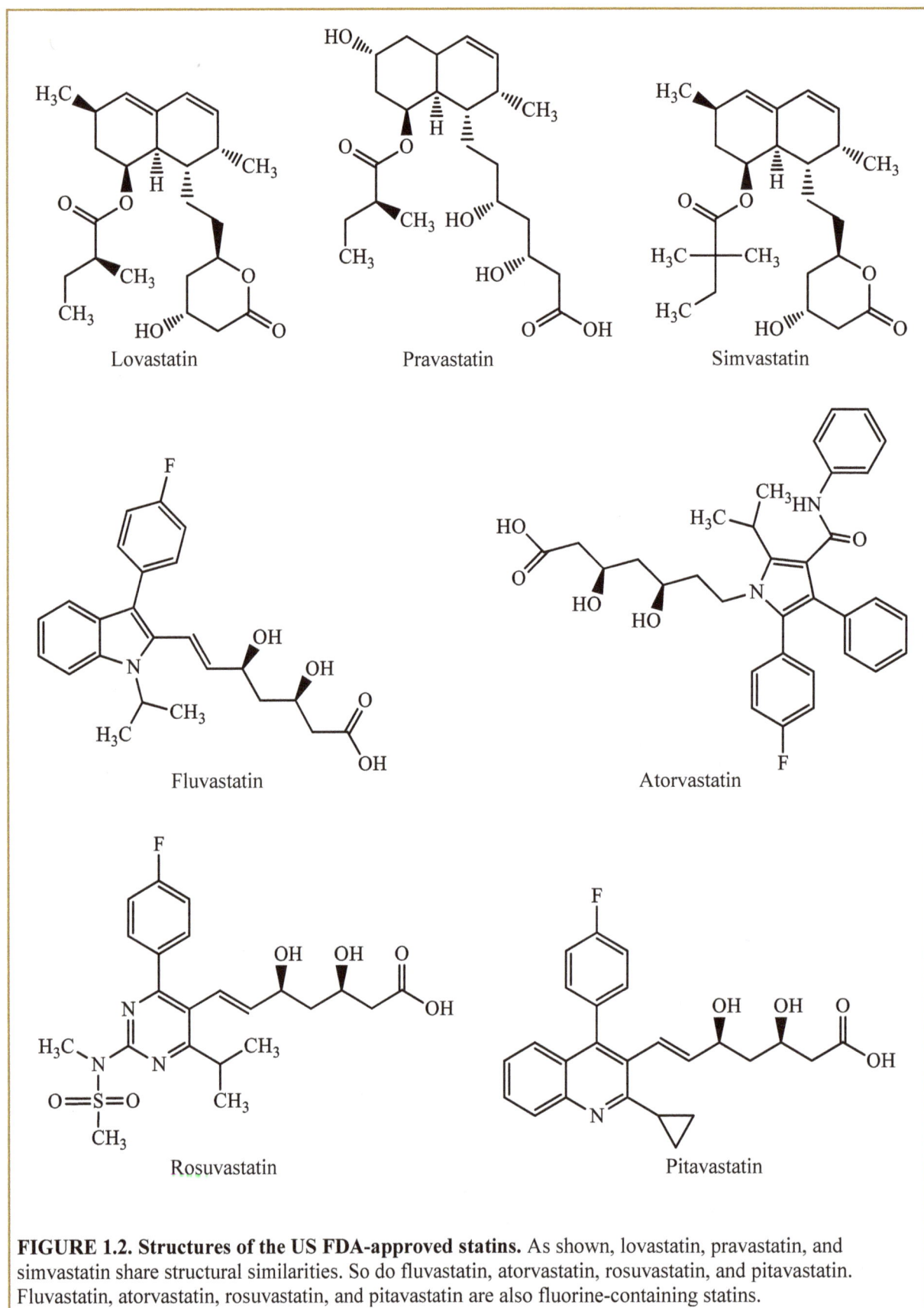

FIGURE 1.2. Structures of the US FDA-approved statins. As shown, lovastatin, pravastatin, and simvastatin share structural similarities. So do fluvastatin, atorvastatin, rosuvastatin, and pitavastatin. Fluvastatin, atorvastatin, rosuvastatin, and pitavastatin are also fluorine-containing statins.

As ezetimibe inhibits NPC1L1-mediated uptake of phytosterols from gut lumen into enterocytes, this drug is indicated as adjunctive therapy to diet for the reduction of elevated sitosterol and campesterol levels in patients with homozygous familial sitosterolemia.

3.3. Bile Acid Sequestrants

- Cholestyramine (Questran) (Prior to January 1, 1982)
- Colestipol (Colestid) (Prior to January 1, 1982)
- Colesevelam (Welchol) (May 2000)

These drugs block the enterohepatic circulation of bile acids, thereby causing increased synthesis of bile acids from cholesterol, and the decreased cholesterol levels in hepatocytes. Decreased cholesterol in hepatocytes results in upregulation of hepatocyte LDL receptors and the consequent augmented clearance of LDL particles from the plasma (**Figure 1.3**). As listed above, this drug class has three members approved by the US FDA. Bile acid sequestrants are among the safest lipid-lowering drugs due to their inability to enter the systemic circulation. A recent systematic review and meta-analysis of randomized controlled trials suggested that the cholesterol lowering effect of bile acid sequestrants may translate into a clinically relevant reduction in coronary artery disease [24]. This is in line with a recent meta-regression analysis showing that use of statin and non-statin therapies that act via upregulation of LDL receptor expression to reduce LDL cholesterol was associated with similar relative risks of major vascular events per change in LDL cholesterol, and that lower achieved LDL cholesterol levels were associated with lower rates of major coronary events [25].

3.4. Fibrate Drugs

- Gemfibrozil (Lopid) (Prior to January 1, 1982)
- Fenofibrate (Tricor, Antara, Lofibra) (December 1993)
- Fenofibric acid, delayed-release (Trilipix) (December 2008)

As illustrated in **Figure 1.4**, fibrate drugs act to enhance the activity of lipoprotein lipase, thereby promoting the catabolism of triglyceride-enriched lipoproteins. Listed above are the three members of this drug class currently approved by the US FDA. Fibrate drugs are effective and commonly prescribed for treating patients with hypertriglyceridemia [26]. They also increase HDL cholesterol. Despite the concerns on the efficacy of fibrate drugs in primary prevention of cardiovascular morbidity and mortality [27–29], multiple recent systemic reviews and meta-analyses have demonstrated that fibrates can reduce the risk of major cardiovascular events predominantly by prevention of coronary events, and might have a significant role in the management of individuals at high risk of cardiovascular events and those with combined dyslipidemia [30, 31].

3.5. Niacin

- Niacin extended-release (Niaspan) (October 1999)

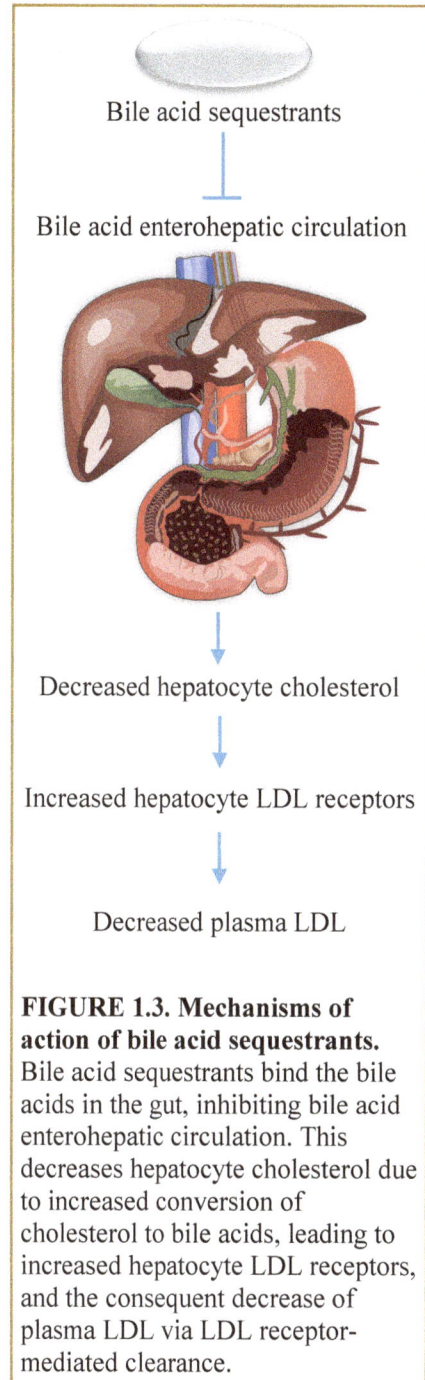

Bile acid sequestrants

Bile acid enterohepatic circulation

Decreased hepatocyte cholesterol

Increased hepatocyte LDL receptors

Decreased plasma LDL

FIGURE 1.3. Mechanisms of action of bile acid sequestrants. Bile acid sequestrants bind the bile acids in the gut, inhibiting bile acid enterohepatic circulation. This decreases hepatocyte cholesterol due to increased conversion of cholesterol to bile acids, leading to increased hepatocyte LDL receptors, and the consequent decrease of plasma LDL via LDL receptor-mediated clearance.

Niaspan acts via different mechanisms to decease triglyceride synthesis and increase HDL level. The mechanism by which Niaspan alters lipid profiles has not been well defined. It may involve several actions including partial inhibition of release of free fatty acids from adipose tissue, and increased lipoprotein lipase activity, which may increase the rate of chylomicron triglyceride removal from the plasma. Niaspan increases HDL cholesterol likely by elevating the level of ApoA-I, a major component of the HDL particles. Niaspan is probably the most effective drug for raising HDL cholesterol [32]. Adding Niaspan to statin therapy was shown to cause a significant regression of carotid intima-media thickness in patients with coronary heart disease or a coronary heart disease risk equivalent [33]. However, among patients with atherosclerotic cardiovascular disease and LDL cholesterol levels of less than 70 mg/dl (due to intensive statin therapy), there was no incremental clinical benefit from the addition of Niaspan to statin therapy during a 3-year follow-up period, despite significant improvements in HDL cholesterol and triglyceride levels [34]. A randomized controlled trial (HPS2-THRIVE) involving 25,673 adults with atherosclerotic vascular disease demonstrated that the addition of Niaspan-laropiprant to statin-based LDL cholesterol-lowering therapy did not significantly reduce the risk of major vascular events but did increase the risk of serious adverse events [35]. A systemic review and meta-analysis of 23 randomized controlled trials published between 1968 and 2015 concluded that moderate- to high-quality evidence suggests that niacin does not reduce mortality, cardiovascular mortality, non-cardiovascular mortality, the number of fatal or non-fatal myocardial infarctions, nor the number of fatal or non-fatal strokes but is associated with side effects, and that benefits from niacin therapy in the prevention of cardiovascular disease events are unlikely [36].

3.6. Omega-3 Fatty Acids

- Omega-3-acid ethyl esters (Lovaza) (November 2004)
- Icosapent ethyl (Vascepa) (July 2012)
- Omega-3-carboxylic acids (Epanova) (May 2014)

The US FDA has approved three pharmaceutical preparations of omega-3 fatty acids with the newest one, namely, Epanova, approved in 2014. These drugs decrease the synthesis of triglycerides via acting on various pathways leading to decreased synthesis and increased hydrolysis of triglycerides, and are indicated to treat patients with severe hypertriglyceridemia. Omega-3 fatty acids may also provide benefits in disease conditions, including heart failure [37, 38], left ventricular remodeling after acute myocardial infarction [39], diabetic retinopathy [40], and asthma [41].

3.7. ApoB-100 Antisense Drugs

- Mipomersen (Kynamro) (January 2013)

These drugs are oligonucleotides that target the ApoB-100 mRNA, leading to its degradation and thereby the consequent reduction of

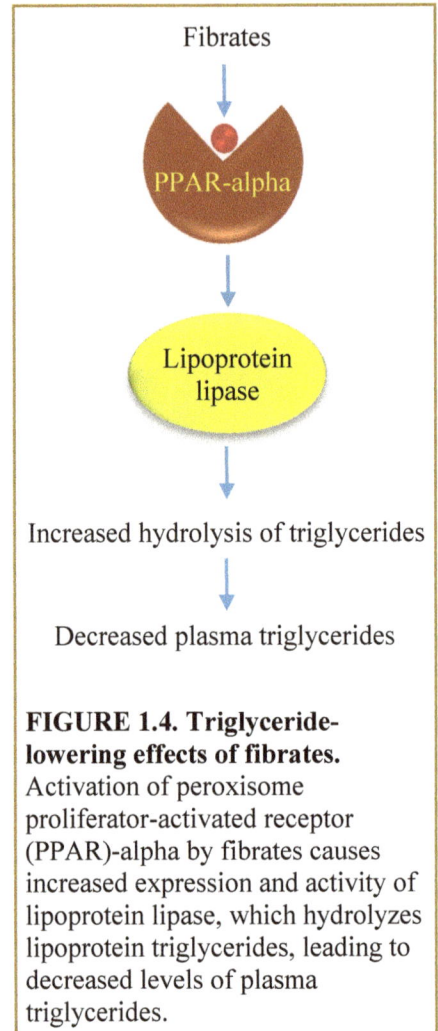

FIGURE 1.4. Triglyceride-lowering effects of fibrates. Activation of peroxisome proliferator-activated receptor (PPAR)-alpha by fibrates causes increased expression and activity of lipoprotein lipase, which hydrolyzes lipoprotein triglycerides, leading to decreased levels of plasma triglycerides.

ApoB-100-containig lipoproteins [42, 43]. Currently, mipomersen is the only class member approved by the US FDA. This drug is indicated for cholesterol-lowering in patients with homozygous familial hypercholesterolemia.

3.8. MTP Inhibitors

- Lomitapide (Juxtapid) (December 2012)

These drugs inhibit microsomal triglyceride transfer protein (MTP) (**Figure 1.5**), an enzyme involved in the assembly of VLDL in the liver [44]. Currently, lomitapide is the only member approved by the US FDA and indicated for cholesterol-lowering in patients with homozygous familial hypercholesterolemia [45].

3.9. PCSK9 Inhibitors

- Alirocumab (Praluent) (July 2015)
- Evolocumab (Repatha) (August 2015)

These drugs inhibit proprotein convertase subtilisin/kexin type 9 (PCSK9), a negative regulator of LDL receptors [46]. Inhibition of PCSK9 in hepatocytes results in increases in LDL receptors [47–49], thereby leading to augmented clearance of LDL particles from the plasma. Listed above are the only two drug class members approved by the US FDA. They are monoclonal antibodies against PCSK9 in the circulation, and indicated for cholesterol-lowering in patients with heterozygous familial hypercholesterolemia or clinical atherosclerotic cardiovascular disease, who require additional lowering of LDL-C. Evolocumab is also indicated for cholesterol-lowering in patients with homozygous familial hypercholesterolemia.

4. EMERGING THERAPEUTIC MODALITIES

As our understanding of the molecular etiology and pathophysiology of lipoprotein disorders increases, more effective drugs will continue to emerge. In this context, emerging pharmacological modalities include (1) agents that inhibit cholesteryl ester transfer protein (CETP) to augment HDL cholesterol [50–53]; (2) antisense inhibitors of apolipoprotein C-III to treat hypertriglyceridemia [54]; (3) angiopoietin-like 3 (ANGPTL3) inhibitors to lower both triglycerides and cholesterol [55]; and (4) antisense inhibitors of lipoprotein(a) [56], a causal factor of coronary artery disease [57].

5. SELF-ASSESSMENT QUESTIONS

5.1. Heterozygous familial hypercholesterolemia is a common form of dyslipidemia, affecting 0.2% of the general population. It is a major risk factor for atherosclerotic cardiovascular diseases. The genetic etiology of this dyslipidemia is believed to be mutations in a gene encoding which of the following protein?

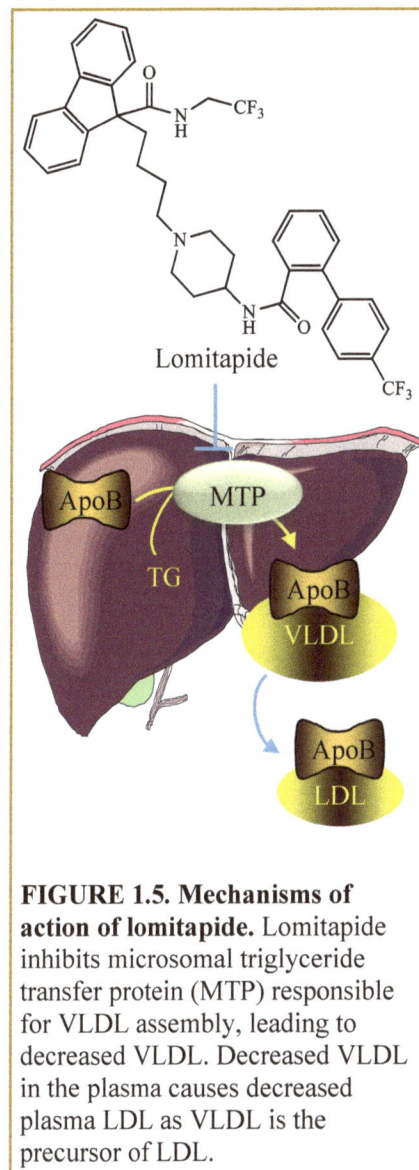

FIGURE 1.5. Mechanisms of action of lomitapide. Lomitapide inhibits microsomal triglyceride transfer protein (MTP) responsible for VLDL assembly, leading to decreased VLDL. Decreased VLDL in the plasma causes decreased plasma LDL as VLDL is the precursor of LDL.

A. Apolipoprotein B-100
B. Apolipoprotein C-II
C. 3-Hydroxy-3-methylglutaryl-coenzyme A reductase
D. Low-density lipoprotein receptor
E. Proprotein convertase subtilisin/kexin type 9

5.2. Which of the following is the closest estimation of the prevalence of homozygous familiar hypercholesterolemia?

A. One in 100
B. One in 1,000
C. One in 10,000
D. One in 100,000
E. One in 1,000,000

5.3. Statins are now recognized as the most important medications for treating hypercholesterolemia to reduce cardiovascular mortality and morbidity. Which of the following is the newest member of this drug class?

A. Atorvastatin
B. Lovastatin
C. Pitavastatin
D. Rosuvastatin
E. Simvastatin

5.4. Niemann-Pick C1-Like 1 (NPC1L1) is located on the brush border of small intestinal epithelial cells. Inhibition of this protein transporter most likely leads to which of the following?

A. Deceased absorption of sitosterol
B. Decreased absorption of vitamin D
C. Decreased plasma level of high-density lipoprotein cholesterol
D. Increased absorption of calcium
E. Increased plasma level of triglycerides

5.5. The microsomal triglyceride transfer protein (MTP) is an enzyme involved in the assembly of very low-density lipoprotein in the liver. This enzyme serves as the primary molecular target for which of the following drugs?

A. Alirocumab
B. Fenofibrate
C. Lomitapide
D. Pitavastatin
E. Vascepa

ANSWERS AND EXPLANATIONS

5.1. The correct answer is D. Mutations in the low-density lipoprotein (LDL) receptor gene cause decreased expression of LDL receptors in hepatocytes, leading to reduced uptake of the plasma LDL particles by the liver cells and consequent elevation of the plasma LDL cholesterol. Mutations of the apolipoprotein (Apo) B-100-encoding gene cause familial defective ApoB-100. Mutations in ApoC-II-encoding gene cause ApoC-II deficiency, resulting in hypertriglyceridemia. 3-Hydroxy-3-methylglutaryl-coenzyme A reductase is the target of statin drugs.

5.2. The correct answer is E. Homozygous familial hypercholesterolemia is a rare genetic disorder affecting one in a million in the general population (approximately a total of 300 individuals in the United States).

5.3. The correct answer is C. Pitavastatin is the newest member of the statin drug class that currently consists of 7 members, and it was initially approved by the US FDA in August 2009.

5.4. The correct answer is A. Niemann-Pick C1-Like 1 (NPC1L1) protein is a cholesterol transporting protein. It also mediates the uptake of phytosterols from the gut lumen into enterocytes. Inhibition of this protein by ezetimibe is indicated as adjunctive therapy to diet for the reduction of elevated sitosterol and campesterol levels in patients with homozygous familial sitosterolemia.

5.5. The correct answer is C. Lomitapide is the only MTP inhibitor approved by the US FDA for cholesterol-lowering in patients with homozygous familial hypercholesterolemia. Alirocumab is a monoclonal antibody-based inhibitor of proprotein convertase subtilisin/kexin type 9 (PCSK9). Fenofibrate activates peroxisome proliferator-activated receptor (PPAR)-alpha, resulting in increased expression and activity of lipoprotein lipase. Pitavastatin is an inhibitor of 3-hydroxy-3-methylglutaryl-coenzyme A reductase. Vascepa is an n-3 fatty acid-based pharmaceutical preparation approved by the US FDA for treating severe hypertriglyceridemia. The molecular target of Vascepa remains to be defined.

REFERENCES

1. Mahley RW, Weisgraber KH, Innerarity TL, Rall SC, Jr. Genetic defects in lipoprotein metabolism. Elevation of atherogenic lipoproteins caused by impaired catabolism. *JAMA* 1991; 265(1):78–83.
2. Hegele RA, Ginsberg HN, Chapman MJ, Nordestgaard BG, Kuivenhoven JA, Averna M, Boren J, Bruckert E, Catapano AL, Descamps OS, Hovingh GK, Humphries SE, et al. The polygenic nature of hypertriglyceridaemia: implications for definition, diagnosis, and management. *Lancet Diabetes Endocrinol* 2014; 2(8):655–66.
3. Rader DJ. New Therapeutic approaches to the treatment of dyslipidemia. *Cell Metab* 2016; 23(3):405–12.
4. Talmud PJ, Shah S, Whittall R, Futema M, Howard P, Cooper JA, Harrison SC, Li K, Drenos F, Karpe F, Neil HA, Descamps OS, et al. Use of low-density lipoprotein cholesterol gene score to distinguish patients with polygenic and monogenic familial hypercholesterolaemia: a case-control study. *Lancet* 2013; 381(9874):1293–301.
5. Ridker PM. LDL cholesterol: controversies and future therapeutic directions. *Lancet* 2014; 384(9943):607–17.
6. Nordestgaard BG. Triglyceride-rich lipoproteins and atherosclerotic cardiovascular disease: new insights from epidemiology, genetics, and biology. *Circ Res* 2016; 118(4):547–63.
7. Ellis KL, Hooper AJ, Burnett JR, Watts GF.

Progress in the care of common inherited atherogenic disorders of apolipoprotein B metabolism. *Nat Rev Endocrinol* 2016; 12(8):467–84.

8. Feig JE, Hewing B, Smith JD, Hazen SL, Fisher EA. High-density lipoprotein and atherosclerosis regression: evidence from preclinical and clinical studies. *Circ Res* 2014; 114(1):205–13.

9. Rohatgi A, Khera A, Berry JD, Givens EG, Ayers CR, Wedin KE, Neeland IJ, Yuhanna IS, Rader DR, de Lemos JA, Shaul PW. HDL cholesterol efflux capacity and incident cardiovascular events. *N Engl J Med* 2014; 371(25):2383–93.

10. Saleheen D, Scott R, Javad S, Zhao W, Rodrigues A, Picataggi A, Lukmanova D, Mucksavage ML, Luben R, Billheimer J, Kastelein JJ, Boekholdt SM, et al. Association of HDL cholesterol efflux capacity with incident coronary heart disease events: a prospective case-control study. *Lancet Diabetes Endocrinol* 2015; 3(7):507–13.

11. Rader DJ, Hovingh GK. HDL and cardiovascular disease. *Lancet* 2014; 384(9943):618–25.

12. Nordestgaard BG, Varbo A. Triglycerides and cardiovascular disease. *Lancet* 2014; 384(9943):626–35.

13. Rodriguez F, Harrington RA. Cholesterol, cardiovascular risk, statins, PCSK9 inhibitors, and the future of LDL-C lowering. *JAMA* 2016; 316(19):1967–8.

14. Writing C, Lloyd-Jones DM, Morris PB, Ballantyne CM, Birtcher KK, Daly DD, Jr., DePalma SM, Minissian MB, Orringer CE, Smith SC, Jr. 2016 ACC expert consensus decision pathway on the role of non-statin therapies for LDL-cholesterol lowering in the management of atherosclerotic cardiovascular disease risk: a report of the American College of Cardiology Task Force on Clinical Expert Consensus Documents. *J Am Coll Cardiol* 2016; 68(1):92–125.

15. Narasimhan SD. Beyond statins: new therapeutic frontiers for cardiovascular disease. *Cell* 2017; 169(6):971–3.

16. Yusuf S, Bosch J, Dagenais G, Zhu J, Xavier D, Liu L, Pais P, Lopez-Jaramillo P, Leiter LA, Dans A, Avezum A, Piegas LS, et al. Cholesterol lowering in intermediate-risk persons without cardiovascular disease. *N Engl J Med* 2016; 374(21):2021–31.

17. Chou R, Dana T, Blazina I, Daeges M, Jeanne

TL. Statins for prevention of cardiovascular disease in adults: evidence report and systematic review for the US Preventive Services Task Force. *JAMA* 2016; 316(19):2008–24.

18. Gupta A, Thompson D, Whitehouse A, Collier T, Dahlof B, Poulter N, Collins R, Sever P, ASCOT Investigators. Adverse events associated with unblinded, but not with blinded, statin therapy in the Anglo-Scandinavian Cardiac Outcomes Trial-Lipid-Lowering Arm (ASCOT-LLA): a randomised double-blind placebo-controlled trial and its non-randomised non-blind extension phase. *Lancet* 2017; 389(10088):2473–81.

19. Heller DJ, Coxson PG, Penko J, Pletcher MJ, Goldman L, Odden MC, Kazi DS, Bibbins-Domingo K. Evaluating the impact and cost-effectiveness of statin use guidelines for primary prevention of coronary heart disease and stroke. *Circulation* 2017; 136(12):1087–98.

20. Myocardial Infarction Genetics Consortium I, Stitziel NO, Won HH, Morrison AC, Peloso GM, Do R, Lange LA, Fontanillas P, Gupta N, Duga S, Goel A, Farrall M, et al. Inactivating mutations in NPC1L1 and protection from coronary heart disease. *N Engl J Med* 2014; 371(22):2072–82.

21. Cannon CP, Blazing MA, Giugliano RP, McCagg A, White JA, Theroux P, Darius H, Lewis BS, Ophuis TO, Jukema JW, De Ferrari GM, Ruzyllo W, et al. Ezetimibe added to statin therapy after acute coronary syndromes. *N Engl J Med* 2015; 372(25):2387–97.

22. Tsujita K, Sugiyama S, Sumida H, Shimomura H, Yamashita T, Yamanaga K, Komura N, Sakamoto K, Oka H, Nakao K, Nakamura S, Ishihara M, et al. Impact of dual lipid-lowering strategy with ezetimibe and atorvastatin on coronary plaque regression in patients with percutaneous coronary intervention: the multicenter randomized controlled PRECISE-IVUS trial. *J Am Coll Cardiol* 2015; 66(5):495–507.

23. Baigent C, Landray MJ, Reith C, Emberson J, Wheeler DC, Tomson C, Wanner C, Krane V, Cass A, Craig J, Neal B, Jiang L, et al. The effects of lowering LDL cholesterol with simvastatin plus ezetimibe in patients with chronic kidney disease (Study of Heart and Renal Protection): a randomised placebo-controlled trial. *Lancet* 2011; 377(9784):2181–92.

24. Ross S, D'Mello M, Anand SS, Eikelboom J,

Consortium CAD, Stewart AF, Samani NJ, Roberts R, Pare G. Effect of bile acid sequestrants on the risk of cardiovascular events: a Mendelian randomization analysis. *Circ Cardiovasc Genet* 2015; 8(4):618–27.

25. Silverman MG, Ference BA, Im K, Wiviott SD, Giugliano RP, Grundy SM, Braunwald E, Sabatine MS. Association between lowering LDL-C and cardiovascular risk reduction among different therapeutic interventions: a systematic review and meta-analysis. *JAMA* 2016; 316(12):1289–97.

26. Jackevicius CA, Tu JV, Ross JS, Ko DT, Carreon D, Krumholz HM. Use of fibrates in the United States and Canada. *JAMA* 2011; 305(12):1217–24.

27. Group AS, Ginsberg HN, Elam MB, Lovato LC, Crouse JR, 3rd, Leiter LA, Linz P, Friedewald WT, Buse JB, Gerstein HC, Probstfield J, Grimm RH, et al. Effects of combination lipid therapy in type 2 diabetes mellitus. *N Engl J Med* 2010; 362(17):1563–74.

28. Goldfine AB, Kaul S, Hiatt WR. Fibrates in the treatment of dyslipidemias: time for a reassessment. *N Engl J Med* 2011; 365(6):481–4.

29. Jakob T, Nordmann AJ, Schandelmaier S, Ferreira-Gonzalez I, Briel M. Fibrates for primary prevention of cardiovascular disease events. *Cochrane Database Syst Rev* 2016; 11:CD009753.

30. Jun M, Foote C, Lv J, Neal B, Patel A, Nicholls SJ, Grobbee DE, Cass A, Chalmers J, Perkovic V. Effects of fibrates on cardiovascular outcomes: a systematic review and meta-analysis. *Lancet* 2010; 375(9729):1875–84.

31. Jun M, Zhu B, Tonelli M, Jardine MJ, Patel A, Neal B, Liyanage T, Keech A, Cass A, Perkovic V. Effects of fibrates in kidney disease: a systematic review and meta-analysis. *J Am Coll Cardiol* 2012; 60(20):2061–71.

32. Ashen MD, Blumenthal RS. Clinical practice. Low HDL cholesterol levels. *N Engl J Med* 2005; 353(12):1252–60.

33. Taylor AJ, Villines TC, Stanek EJ, Devine PJ, Griffen L, Miller M, Weissman NJ, Turco M. Extended-release niacin or ezetimibe and carotid intima-media thickness. *N Engl J Med* 2009; 361(22):2113–22.

34. AIM-HIGH Investigators, Boden WE, Probstfield JL, Anderson T, Chaitman BR, Desvignes-Nickens P, Koprowicz K, McBride R, Teo K, Weintraub W. Niacin in patients with low HDL cholesterol levels receiving intensive statin therapy. *N Engl J Med* 2011; 365(24):2255–67.

35. Group HTC, Landray MJ, Haynes R, Hopewell JC, Parish S, Aung T, Tomson J, Wallendszus K, Craig M, Jiang L, Collins R, Armitage J. Effects of extended-release niacin with laropiprant in high-risk patients. *N Engl J Med* 2014; 371(3):203–12.

36. Schandelmaier S, Briel M, Saccilotto R, Olu KK, Arpagaus A, Hemkens LG, Nordmann AJ. Niacin for primary and secondary prevention of cardiovascular events. *Cochrane Database Syst Rev* 2017; 6:CD009744.

37. Tavazzi L, Maggioni AP, Marchioli R, Barlera S, Franzosi MG, Latini R, Lucci D, Nicolosi GL, Porcu M, Tognoni G, GISSI-HF Investigators. Effect of n-3 polyunsaturated fatty acids in patients with chronic heart failure (the GISSI-HF trial): a randomised, double-blind, placebo-controlled trial. *Lancet* 2008; 372(9645):1223–30.

38. Nodari S, Triggiani M, Campia U, Manerba A, Milesi G, Cesana BM, Gheorghiade M, Dei Cas L. Effects of n-3 polyunsaturated fatty acids on left ventricular function and functional capacity in patients with dilated cardiomyopathy. *J Am Coll Cardiol* 2011; 57(7):870–9.

39. Heydari B, Abdullah S, Pottala JV, Shah R, Abbasi S, Mandry D, Francis SA, Lumish H, Ghoshhajra BB, Hoffmann U, Appelbaum E, Feng JH, et al. Effect of Omega-3 acid ethyl esters on left ventricular remodeling after acute myocardial infarction: the OMEGA-REMODEL randomized clinical trial. *Circulation* 2016; 134(5):378–91.

40. Sala-Vila A, Diaz-Lopez A, Valls-Pedret C, Cofan M, Garcia-Layana A, Lamuela-Raventos RM, Castaner O, Zanon-Moreno V, Martinez-Gonzalez MA, Toledo E, Basora J, Salas-Salvado J, et al. Dietary marine omega-3 fatty acids and incident sight-threatening retinopathy in middle-aged and older individuals with type 2 diabetes: prospective investigation from the PREDIMED trial. *JAMA Ophthalmol* 2016; 134(10):1142–9.

41. Bisgaard H, Stokholm J, Chawes BL, Vissing NH, Bjarnadottir E, Schoos AM, Wolsk HM, Pedersen TM, Vinding RK, Thorsteinsdottir S, Folsgaard NV, Fink NR, et al. Fish oil-derived fatty acids in pregnancy and wheeze and asthma in offspring. *N Engl J Med* 2016; 375(26):2530–9.

42. Neely RD, Bassendine MF. Antisense

technology to lower LDL cholesterol. *Lancet* 2010; 375(9719):959–61.

43. Reyes-Soffer G, Moon B, Hernandez-Ono A, Dionizovik-Dimanovski M, Jimenez J, Obunike J, Thomas T, Ngai C, Fontanez N, Donovan DS, Karmally W, Holleran S, et al. Complex effects of inhibiting hepatic apolipoprotein B100 synthesis in humans. *Sci Transl Med* 2016; 8(323):323ra12.

44. Hooper AJ, Burnett JR, Watts GF. Contemporary aspects of the biology and therapeutic regulation of the microsomal triglyceride transfer protein. *Circ Res* 2015; 116(1):193–205.

45. Cuchel M, Meagher EA, du Toit Theron H, Blom DJ, Marais AD, Hegele RA, Averna MR, Sirtori CR, Shah PK, Gaudet D, Stefanutti C, Vigna GB, et al. Efficacy and safety of a microsomal triglyceride transfer protein inhibitor in patients with homozygous familial hypercholesterolaemia: a single-arm, open-label, phase 3 study. *Lancet* 2013; 381(9860):40–6.

46. Attie AD, Seidah NG. Dual regulation of the LDL receptor: some clarity and new questions. *Cell Metab* 2005; 1(5):290–2.

47. Stein EA, Mellis S, Yancopoulos GD, Stahl N, Logan D, Smith WB, Lisbon E, Gutierrez M, Webb C, Wu R, Du Y, Kranz T, et al. Effect of a monoclonal antibody to PCSK9 on LDL cholesterol. *N Engl J Med* 2012; 366(12):1108–18.

48. Fitzgerald K, Frank-Kamenetsky M, Shulga-Morskaya S, Liebow A, Bettencourt BR, Sutherland JE, Hutabarat RM, Clausen VA, Karsten V, Cehelsky J, Nochur SV, Kotelianski V, et al. Effect of an RNA interference drug on the synthesis of proprotein convertase subtilisin/kexin type 9 (PCSK9) and the concentration of serum LDL cholesterol in healthy volunteers: a randomised, single-blind, placebo-controlled, phase 1 trial. *Lancet* 2014; 383(9911):60–8.

49. Raal FJ, Giugliano RP, Sabatine MS, Koren MJ, Langslet G, Bays H, Blom D, Eriksson M, Dent R, Wasserman SM, Huang F, Xue A, et al. Reduction in lipoprotein(a) with PCSK9 monoclonal antibody evolocumab (AMG 145): a pooled analysis of more than 1,300 patients in 4 phase II trials. *J Am Coll Cardiol* 2014; 63(13):1278–88.

50. Schwartz GG, Olsson AG, Abt M, Ballantyne CM, Barter PJ, Brumm J, Chaitman BR, Holme IM, Kallend D, Leiter LA, Leitersdorf E, McMurray JJ, et al. Effects of dalcetrapib in patients with a recent acute coronary syndrome. *N Engl J Med* 2012; 367(22):2089–99.

51. van Capelleveen JC, Brewer HB, Kastelein JJ, Hovingh GK. Novel therapies focused on the high-density lipoprotein particle. *Circ Res* 2014; 114(1):193–204.

52. Lincoff AM, Nicholls SJ, Riesmeyer JS, Barter PJ, Brewer HB, Fox KAA, Gibson CM, Granger C, Menon V, Montalescot G, Rader D, Tall AR, et al. Evacetrapib and cardiovascular outcomes in high-risk vascular disease. *N Engl J Med* 2017; 376(20):1933–42.

53. Ballantyne CM, Shah S, Sapre A, Ashraf TB, Tobias SC, Sahin T, Ye P, Dong Y, Sheu WH, Kang DH, Ferreira Rossi PR, Moiseeva Y, et al. A multiregional, randomized evaluation of the lipid-modifying efficacy and tolerability of anacetrapib added to ongoing statin therapy in patients with hypercholesterolemia or low high-density lipoprotein cholesterol. *Am J Cardiol* 2017; 120(4):569–76.

54. Gaudet D, Alexander VJ, Baker BF, Brisson D, Tremblay K, Singleton W, Geary RS, Hughes SG, Viney NJ, Graham MJ, Crooke RM, Witztum JL, et al. Antisense inhibition of apolipoprotein C-III in patients with hypertriglyceridemia. *N Engl J Med* 2015; 373(5):438–47.

55. Dewey FE, Gusarova V, Dunbar RL, O'Dushlaine C, Schurmann C, Gottesman O, McCarthy S, Van Hout CV, Bruse S, Dansky HM, Leader JB, Murray MF, et al. Genetic and pharmacologic inactivation of ANGPTL3 and cardiovascular disease. *N Engl J Med* 2017; 377(3):211–21.

56. Viney NJ, van Capelleveen JC, Geary RS, Xia S, Tami JA, Yu RZ, Marcovina SM, Hughes SG, Graham MJ, Crooke RM, Crooke ST, Witztum JL, et al. Antisense oligonucleotides targeting apolipoprotein(a) in people with raised lipoprotein(a): two randomised, double-blind, placebo-controlled, dose-ranging trials. *Lancet* 2016; 388(10057):2239–53.

57. Saleheen D, Haycock PC, Zhao W, Rasheed A, Taleb A, Imran A, Abbas S, Majeed F, Akhtar S, Qamar N, Zaman KS, Yaqoob Z, et al. Apolipoprotein(a) isoform size, lipoprotein(a) concentration, and coronary artery disease: a mendelian randomisation analysis. *Lancet Diabetes Endocrinol* 2017; 5(7):524–33.

CHAPTER 2

New Drugs for Hypercholesterolemia

CHAPTER HIGHLIGHTS

- Elevation of blood cholesterol, especially low-density lipoprotein (LDL) cholesterol is a major risk factor of atherosclerotic cardiovascular diseases (ASCVDs).
- Treatment of hypercholesterolemia is an effective approach to preventing ASCVDs.
- Commonly used cholesterol-lowering drugs include statins, cholesterol absorption inhibitors, and bile acid sequestrants, among others.
- The United States Food and Drug Administration has recently approved three novel drugs and one fixed-dose combination drug for treating hypercholesterolemia.
- These new drugs include mipomersen (an apolipoprotein B-100 antisense), Liptruzet (a fixed-dose combination of ezetimibe and atorvastatin), and two PCSK9 inhibitors alirocumab and evolocumab.

KEYWORDS | Alirocumab; Atorvastatin; Evolocumab; Ezetimibe; Hypercholesterolemia; Liptruzet; Mipomersen; Vytorin

CITATION | *Li YR. Cardiovascular Medicine: New Therapeutic Drugs Approved by the US FDA (2013–2017). Cell Med Press, Raleigh, NC, USA. 2018. http://dx.doi.org/10.20455/ndcvd.2018.02*

ABBREVIATIONS | ALT, alanine transaminase; ApoA-I, apolipoprotein A-I; ApoB-100, apolipoprotein B-100; AST, aspartate transaminase; CYP, cytochrome P450; HDL, high-density lipoprotein; HMG-CoA, 3-hydroxy-3-methylglutaryl-coenzyme A; HeFH, heterozygous familial hypercholesterolemia; HoFH, homozygous familial hypercholesterolemia; LDL, low-density lipoprotein; LDLR, low-density lipoprotein receptor; MTP, microsomal triglyceride transfer protein; PCSK9, proprotein convertase subtilisin/kexin type 9; RNAi, RNA interference; US FDA, the United States Food and Drug Administration; VLDL, very low-density lipoprotein

CHAPTER AT A GLANCE

1. INTRODUCTION

Although dyslipidemias can be manifested as any changes in the plasma lipid profiles, elevation of total cholesterol and low-density lipoprotein (LDL) cholesterol has received the most attention. This is due primarily to two reasons: (1) both total and LDL cholesterol can be effectively modified by lifestyle changes and drug therapies; and (2) reducing total and LDL cholesterol, especially LDL cholesterol, prevents cardiovascular diseases and decreases cardiovascular mortality. Data suggest that for every 30 mg/dl change in LDL cholesterol, the relative risk for coronary heart disease is changed in proportion by 30% [1]. Plasma levels of total cholesterol and LDL cholesterol, particularly LDL cholesterol, continue to constitute the primary targets of medical therapy to reduce the atherosclerotic cardiovascular risk. Indeed, LDL cholesterol reduction is one of the most important criteria used in the development of new lipid-lowering drugs.

As introduced in Chapter 1, several classes of drugs have been developed and approved by the United States Food and Drug Administration (US FDA) over the past decades for the treatment of hypercholesterolemia. Major cholesterol-lowering drugs include: (1) the widely used statins, also known as 3-hydroxy-3-methylglutaryl-coenzyme A (HMG-CoA) reductase inhibitors (atorvastatin, fluvastatin, lovastatin, pitavastatin, pravastatin, rosuvastatin, simvastatin); (2) the cholesterol absorption inhibitor ezetimibe; (3) the bile acid sequestrants (cholestyramine, colesevelam, colestipol); and (4) the microsomal triglyceride transfer protein (MTP) inhibitor lomitapide, among others.

This chapter covers the new drugs for treating hypercholesterolemia approved by the US FDA over the past five years (2013–2017). These include: (1) an apolipoprotein (Apo) B-100 antisense drug mipomersen (approved in January 2013); (2) a fixed-dose combination of ezetimibe and atorvastatin (approved in May 2013), and (3) two proprotein convertase subtilisin/kexin type 9 (PCSK9) inhibitors—alirocumab (approved in July 2015) and evolocumab (approved in August 2015).

2. THE APOB-100 ANTISENSE DRUG: MIPOMERSEN (KYNAMRO)

2.1. Overview

The Approval of mipomersen (Genzyme Corporation, Cambridge, MA, USA) for treating homozygous familial hypercholesterolemia (HoFH) by the US FDA was primarily based on a randomized controlled trial in 51 patients aged 12 years and older with HoFH, which was reported in Lancet in 2010 [2]. Of the 51 patients, 45 completed the 26-week treatment period (28 mipomersen, 17 placebo). Mean concentrations of LDL cholesterol at baseline were 441 mg/dl in the mipomersen group and 402 mg/dl in the placebo group. The mean percentage change in LDL cholesterol concentration was significantly greater with mipomersen (−24.7%) than with placebo (−3.3%) [2]. More recently, multiple clinical trials have also demonstrated an efficacy for mipomersen in non-homozygous familial hypercholesterolemic patients with high LDL cholesterol refractory to conventional lipid-lowering therapy. These include patients with heterozygous familial hypercholesterolemia and severe hypercholesterolemia at high cardiovascular risk [3, 4].

2.2. Chemistry and Pharmacokinetics

Mipomersen is a synthetic phosphorothioate oligonucleotide drug (20 nucleotides in length). It is a specific antisense inhibitor of ApoB-100 synthesis (**Figure 2.1**). Following subcutaneous injection, the peak plasma concentrations of mipomersen are typically reached in 3 to 4 h, and the bioavailability ranges from 54% to 78%. Mipomersen is highly bound to human plasma proteins (≥90%). It is not a substrate for cytochrome P450 (CYP) enzyme-mediated metabolism, and is metabolized in tissues by endonucleases to form shorter oligonucleotides that are further metabolized by exonucleases. The elimination of mipomersen involves both metabolism in tissues and excretion primarily in the urine. Following subcutaneous administration, the elimination half-life of mipomersen is approximately 1–2 months.

2.3. Molecular Mechanisms and Pharmacological Effects

Mipomersen is an antisense oligonucleotide targeted to human mRNA for ApoB-100, the principal apolipoprotein of LDL and its metabolic precursor, very low-density lipoprotein (VLDL). Mipomersen is complementary to the coding region of the mRNA for ApoB-100, and binds by Watson and Crick base pairing. The hybridization of mipomersen to the cognate mRNA results in RNase H-mediated degradation of the cognate mRNA, thus inhibiting the translation of ApoB-100 mRNA to ApoB-100 protein (**Figure 2.1**).

In cultured hepatocytes, mipomersen selectively reduces ApoB-100 mRNA, protein, and secreted protein in a concentration- and time-dependent manner. ApoB-100 is also a major component of other lipoproteins, including VLDL, intermediate-density lipoprotein (IDL), and lipoprotein(a) [Lp(a)]. In this context, mipomersen reduces Lp(a) levels in both experimental animals and humans [5, 6].

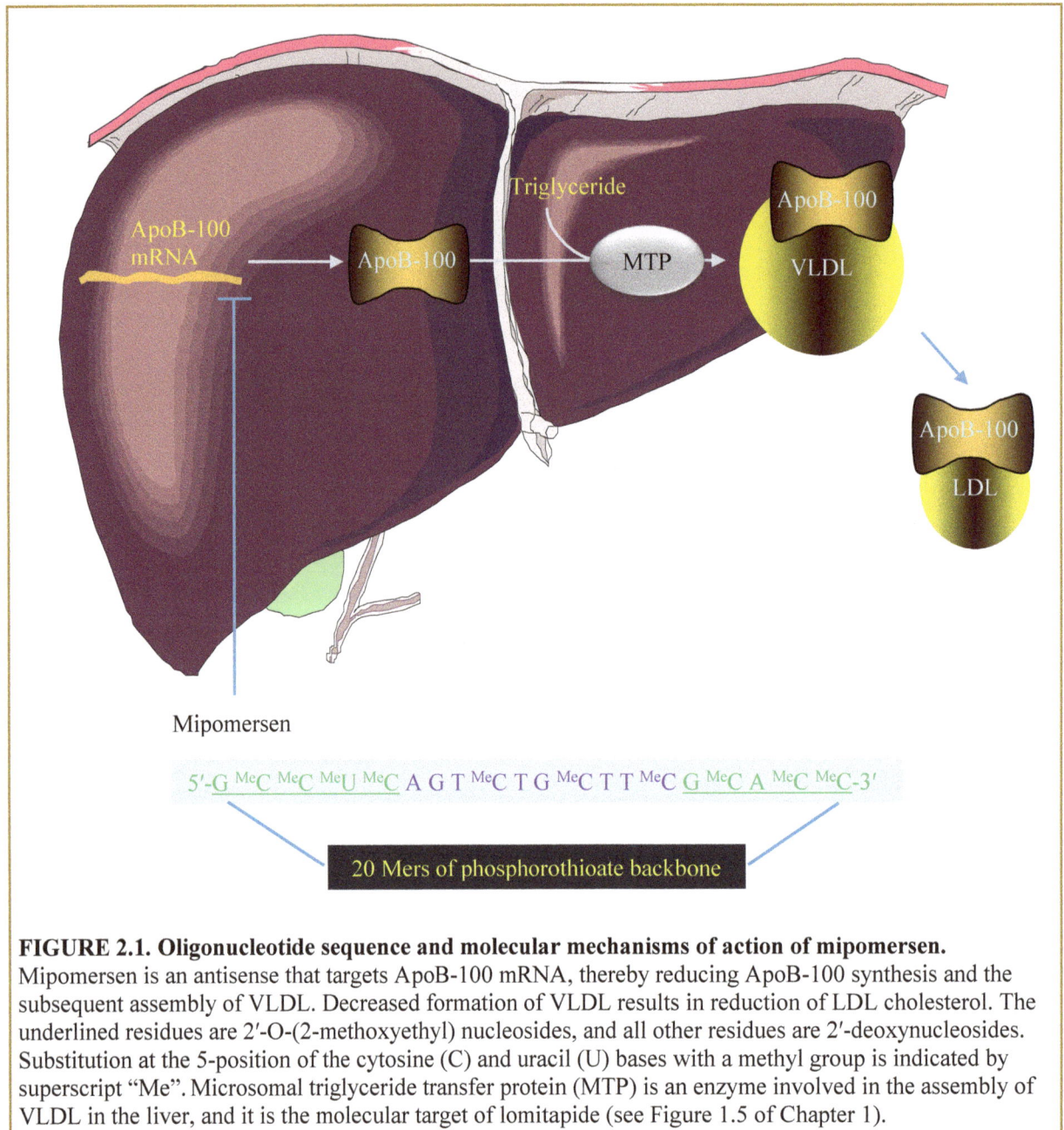

FIGURE 2.1. Oligonucleotide sequence and molecular mechanisms of action of mipomersen.
Mipomersen is an antisense that targets ApoB-100 mRNA, thereby reducing ApoB-100 synthesis and the subsequent assembly of VLDL. Decreased formation of VLDL results in reduction of LDL cholesterol. The underlined residues are 2′-O-(2-methoxyethyl) nucleosides, and all other residues are 2′-deoxynucleosides. Substitution at the 5-position of the cytosine (C) and uracil (U) bases with a methyl group is indicated by superscript "Me". Microsomal triglyceride transfer protein (MTP) is an enzyme involved in the assembly of VLDL in the liver, and it is the molecular target of lomitapide (see Figure 1.5 of Chapter 1).

The major effects of mipomersen on lipid profiles in patients with HoFH are given in **Table 2.1**.

2.4. Clinical Uses

2.4.1. Clinical Indications

Mipomersen is indicated as an adjunct to lipid-lowering medications and diet to reduce LDL cholesterol, ApoB-100, total cholesterol, and non-high-density lipoprotein (HDL) cholesterol in HoFH patients.

TABLE 2.1. Effects of mipomersen on lipid profiles in patients with HoFH

Lipid	Change (% compared with placebo)
ApoB-100	−24
LDL cholesterol	−21
Lipoprotein(a)	−23
Non-HDL cholesterol	−22
Total cholesterol	−19
Triglycerides	−18
VLDL cholesterol	−20
HDL cholesterol	+11

Note: The data are based on *Lancet* 2010; 375:998–1006 and the US FDA drug label information for mipomersen. The minus sign indicates reduction, and the plus sign indicates elevation.

2.4.2. Limitations of Use

- The safety and effectiveness of mipomersen have not been well-established in patients with hypercholesterolemia who do not have HoFH. A planned interim analysis of an ongoing, open-label extension trial in 141 patients with familial hypercholesterolemia receiving a subcutaneous injection of 200 mg mipomersen weekly plus maximally tolerated lipid-lowering therapy for up to 104 weeks, suggested that long-term treatment with mipomersen for up to 104 weeks provided sustained reductions in all atherosclerotic lipoproteins measured and a safety profile consistent with prior controlled trials in these high-risk patient populations.
- The effect of mipomersen on cardiovascular morbidity and mortality has not been determined.
- The safety and effectiveness of mipomersen as an adjunct to LDL apheresis have not been established. Accordingly, the use of mipomersen as an adjunct to LDL apheresis is not recommended.

2.5. Therapeutic Dosages

The dosage forms and strengths of mipomersen are listed below.

- Subcutaneous injection: single-use vial containing 1 ml of a 200 mg/ml solution; single-use pre-filled syringe containing 1 ml of a 200 mg/ml solution

The drug is given at 200 mg once weekly as a subcutaneous injection. The injection sites may include abdomen, thigh region, or outer area of the upper arm. Before treatment, alanine transaminase (ALT), aspartate transaminase (AST), alkaline phosphatase, and total bilirubin should be measured because the drug may cause liver injury (also see Section 2.6.1).

> **LDL apheresis**
> LDL apheresis is a type of "extracorporeal" (blood taken outside the body) procedure to remove LDL cholesterol from the blood. During LDL apheresis, the plasma portion of the blood, which contains LDL particles, is separated and run through a machine that removes the LDL particles. LDL apheresis is indicated in patients, such as those with homozygous familial hypercholesterolemia, who, despite the maximum amount of drug treatment and a cholesterol-lowering diet, still have higher LDL cholesterol levels.

2.6. Adverse Effects and Drug Interactions

2.6.1. Adverse Effects

The most commonly reported adverse reactions are injection site reactions, flu-like symptoms, nausea, headache, and elevations in serum transaminases, specifically ALT. Mipomersen may also increase the risk of hepatic steatosis, a risk factor for progressive liver disease, including steatohepatitis and cirrhosis. Risk of hepatotoxicity is a US FDA black box warning for mipomersen.

2.6.2. Drug Interactions

No significant drug interactions have been reported with mipomersen. For example, no clinically significant interactions have been documented between mipomersen and drugs, such as warfarin, simvastatin, and ezetimibe. This is likely due to its unique pharmacokinetic characteristics including its inability to affect CYP enzymes as well as the novel mechanism of its metabolism, which is not shared by most other drugs.

2.6.3. Contraindications and FDA Pregnancy Category

- Moderate or severe hepatic impairment, or active liver disease, including unexplained persistent elevations of serum transaminases
- Known sensitivity to product components
- FDA pregnancy category: B

2.7. Comparison with Existing Members and New Development since the US FDA Approval

Mipomersen is the first-in-class drug and, currently, the only member of the drug class approved by the US FDA. In addition to its efficacy in HoFH, the LDL cholesterol-lowering effects of mipomersen have recently also been reported in different patient populations, including pediatric patients and patients with heterozygous familial hypercholesterolemia [7–9]. Long-term treatment with mipomersen may reduce the risk of cardiovascular events in patients with familial hypercholesterolemia [8]. In addition to LDL cholesterol lowering, mipomersen can effectively reduce Lp(a) levels [4, 10] as well as the number of small LDL particles [10]. Lp(a) is an independent risk factor for atherosclerotic cardiovascular diseases [11].

Although multiple clinical studies have demonstrated that mipomersen therapy is associated with liver injury [3, 12, 13] (a black box warning, see Section 2.6.1.), the exact mechanism underlying its hepatotoxicity remains unknown. In this context, recent advances in the stereochemistry of phosphorothioate oligonucleotide therapeutics [14], along with the enhanced understanding of the intracellular trafficking of antisense oligonucleotide drugs [15], may help delineate the mechanisms of toxicity. Such advances would provide opportunities for improving the therapeutic index of mipomersen and related therapeutic modalities that involve the use of antisense techniques to alter specific molecular targets.

Black box warning
A boxed warning, commonly known as a "black box warning", is the most serious type of warning mandated by the US FDA for certain prescription drugs. It is so called because the US FDA specifies that it is formatted with a box or border around the text. The black box warning is prominently featured in the drug labelling to warn prescribers about a significant risk of serious or even life-threatening adverse reactions.

FDA pregnancy categories
Category A: Adequate and well-controlled studies have failed to demonstrate a risk to the fetus in the first trimester of pregnancy (and there is no evidence of risk in later trimesters).
Category B: Animal studies have failed to demonstrate a risk to the fetus and there are no adequate and well-controlled studies in pregnant women.
Category C: Animal studies have shown an adverse effect on the fetus and there are no adequate and well-controlled studies in humans, but potential benefits may warrant use of the drug in pregnant women despite potential risks.
Category D: There is positive evidence of human fetal risk based on adverse reaction data from investigational or marketing experience or studies in humans, but potential benefits may warrant use of the drug in pregnant women despite potential risks.
Category X: Studies in animals or humans have demonstrated fetal abnormalities and/or there is positive evidence of human fetal risk based on adverse reaction data from investigational or marketing experience, and the risks involved in use of the drug in pregnant women clearly outweigh potential benefits.

3. FIXED-DOSE COMBINATION OF EZETIMIBE AND ATORVASTATIN (LIPTRUZET)

3.1. Overview

The first fixed-dose combination of ezetimibe and a statin (simvastatin), with the trade name of Vytorin (Merck & Co., Inc., New Jersey, USA), was approved by the US FDA in 2004. Liptruzet (Merck & Co., Inc.) is the second one of this type of fixed-dose combination of ezetimibe and a statin. The US FDA approval of Liptruzet in May 2013 was based on randomized controlled clinical trials demonstrating the efficacy of Liptruzet in patients with hypercholesterolemia, including HoFH [16, 17].

3.2. Chemistry and Pharmacokinetics

Liptruzet contains ezetimibe (a selective inhibitor of the absorption of intestinal cholesterol and related phytosterols), and atorvastatin (an HMG-CoA reductase inhibitor). The chemical structures of the above two active ingredients are shown in **Figure 2.2**.

Liptruzet has been shown to be bioequivalent and clinically equivalent in LDL cholesterol reduction to co-administration of the corresponding doses of ezetimibe and atorvastatin. The pharmacokinetic properties of Liptruzet reflect those of the individual drug component, which are summarized in **Table 2.2**. The reader is advised to refer to Ref. [18] for details on clinical pharmacokinetics of ezetimibe and atorvastatin.

3.3. Molecular Mechanisms and Pharmacological Effects

3.3.1. Molecular Mechanisms

Total body cholesterol, including LDL cholesterol is derived from intestinal absorption and endogenous synthesis. Liptruzet contains ezetimibe and atorvastatin, two lipid-lowering drugs with complementary mechanisms of action (**Figure 2.2**). In this context, ezetimibe reduces blood cholesterol by inhibiting the absorption of cholesterol by the small intestine. The molecular target of ezetimibe is a sterol transporter, known as Niemann-Pick C1-Like 1 (NPC1L1), which is involved in the intestinal uptake of cholesterol and phytosterols [19–21]. On the other hand, atorvastatin reduces LDL cholesterol by inhibiting the HMG-CoA reductase and cholesterol synthesis in the liver. This increases the number of hepatic LDL receptors on the cell surface, leading to enhanced uptake and catabolism of plasma LDL particles.

3.3.2. Pharmacological Effects

Liptruzet is significantly more effective than doubling the dose of atorvastatin in further reducing the levels of total cholesterol, LDL cholesterol, triglycerides, and non-HDL cholesterol. In patients with HoFH, increasing the dose of atorvastatin from 40 to 80 mg reduced LDL cholesterol by only 2% from baseline on atorvastatin 40 mg. In

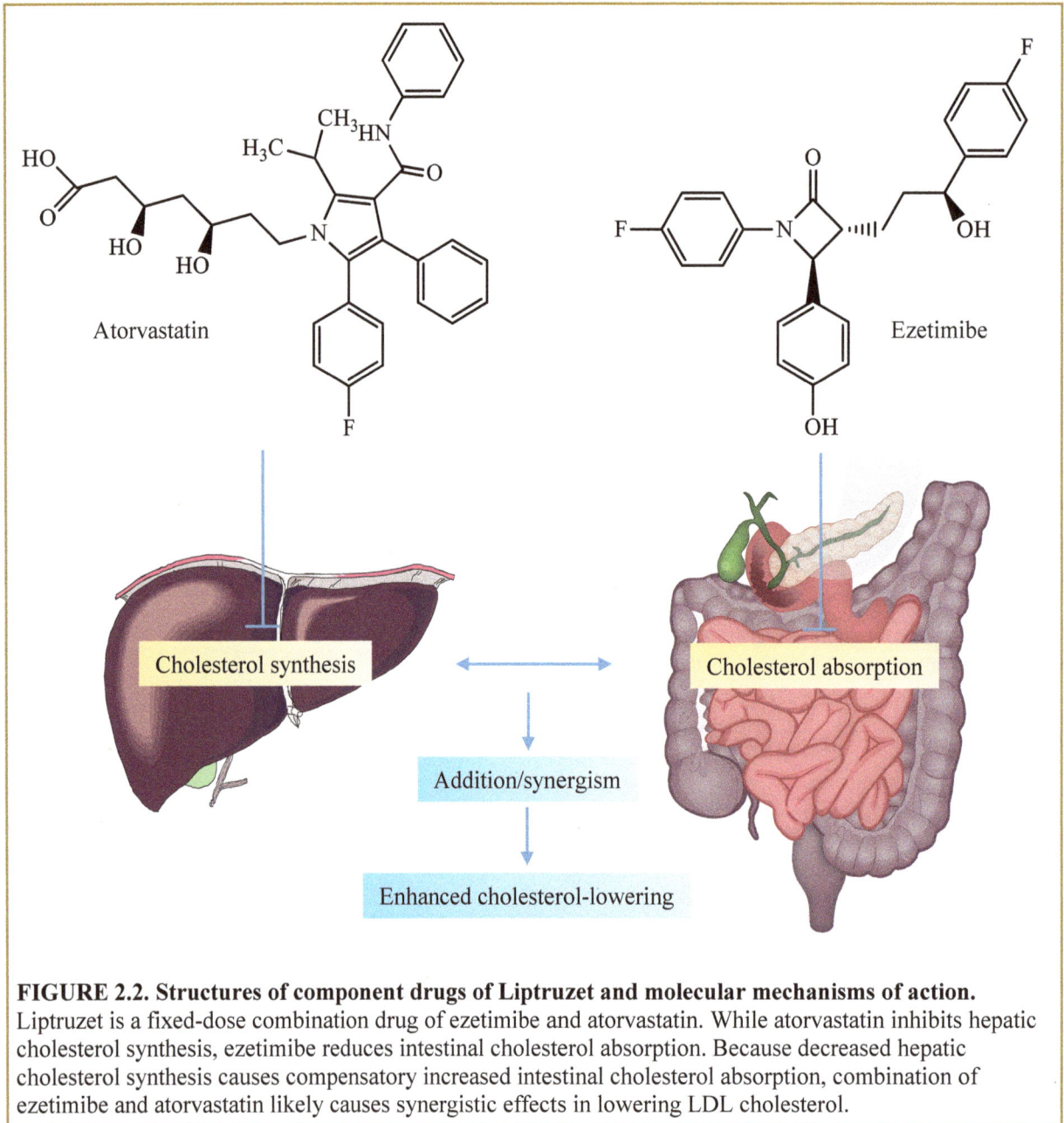

FIGURE 2.2. Structures of component drugs of Liptruzet and molecular mechanisms of action.
Liptruzet is a fixed-dose combination drug of ezetimibe and atorvastatin. While atorvastatin inhibits hepatic cholesterol synthesis, ezetimibe reduces intestinal cholesterol absorption. Because decreased hepatic cholesterol synthesis causes compensatory increased intestinal cholesterol absorption, combination of ezetimibe and atorvastatin likely causes synergistic effects in lowering LDL cholesterol.

contrast, co-administered ezetimibe and atorvastatin equivalent to Liptruzet (10/40 and 10/80 mg) produced a reduction of LDL cholesterol of 19% from baseline on atorvastatin 40 mg. In those patients co-administered ezetimibe and atorvastatin equivalent to Liptruzet (10/80 mg), a reduction of LDL cholesterol of 25% from baseline on atorvastatin 40 mg was produced. Hence, adding ezetimibe to atorvastatin is much more effective than doubling the statin dose in LDL cholesterol reduction in HoFH patients.

In addition to LDL cholesterol reduction, Liptruzet treatment also decreases the levels of total cholesterol, ApoB-100, triglycerides, and non-HDL cholesterol, and increases HDL cholesterol. Elevation of

TABLE 2.2. Major pharmacokinetic properties of ezetimibe and atorvastatin

Property	Ezetimibe	Atorvastatin
Bioavailability	Not available	14%
t_{max}	4–12 h	1–2 h
Plasma protein binding	>90%	≥98%
Vd	Not available	5.4 L/kg bw
Metabolism	Glucuronide conjugation in the small intestine and liver	Hepatic CYP3A4-mediated oxidation
Excretion	Feces (major), urine (minor)	Bile
$t_{1/2}$	22 h	14 h

Note: bw, body weight; $t_{1/2}$, elimination half-life; t_{max}, the time when the maximum plasma concentration is reached; Vd, volume of distribution. Ezetimibe-glucuronide is pharmacologically active.

HDL cholesterol is most likely attributed to atorvastatin. How statin drugs elevate HDL cholesterol remains to be fully elucidated. It has been reported that statins increase ApoA-I mRNA levels in cultured hepatocytes, which might contribute, at least partly, to the increase in HDL cholesterol [22]. In this context, ApoA-I is a major component of HDL particles. Regardless of the mechanisms involved, elevation of HDL cholesterol by statins is likely a contributor to the efficacy of statin therapy in reducing atherosclerotic cardiovascular events.

3.4. Clinical Uses

3.4.1. Clinical Indications

Liptruzet is indicated as adjunctive therapy to diet to:

- Reduce elevated total cholesterol, LDL cholesterol, ApoB-100, triglycerides, and non-HDL cholesterol, and to increase HDL-cholesterol in patients with primary (heterozygous familial and non-familial) hyperlipidemia or mixed hyperlipidemia.
- Reduce elevated total cholesterol and LDL cholesterol in patients with HoFH, as an adjunct to other lipid-lowering treatments.

3.4.2. Limitations of Use

In the recently published IMPROVE-IT trial involving a total of 18,144 patients with a median follow-up of 6 years, Vytorin (ezetimibe/simvastatin) has been demonstrated to incrementally improve cardiovascular outcomes after acute coronary syndromes compared with simvastatin monotherapy [23]. However, up to date, whether Liptruzet causes a similar incremental benefit on cardiovascular morbidity and mortality above that demonstrated for atorvastatin has not been established.

3.5. Therapeutic Dosages

The dosage forms and strengths of Liptruzet are listed below.

- Oral: tablets of 10/10, 10/20, 10/40, and 10/80 (ezetimibe/atorvastatin, mg)

The dosage range of Liptruzet is from 10/10 mg/day to 10/80 mg/day. It is recommended that the starting dosage be 10/10 mg/day or 10/20 mg/day for average patients. For those requiring a greater than 55% reduction in LDL cholesterol, the recommended starting dose is 10/40 mg/day.

3.6. Adverse Effects and Drug Interactions

3.6.1. Adverse Effects

Liptruzet is generally well-tolerated. It may cause muscular skeletal pain, increased liver enzymes, and abdominal pain in some patients. Clinical trial data indicated that the most common adverse effects in patients treated with Liptruzet that led to treatment discontinuation and occurred at a rate greater than placebo were: myalgia (0.8%), abdominal pain (0.8%), and increased hepatic enzymes (0.8%). Rare cases of rhabdomyolysis with acute renal failure secondary to myoglobinuria have been reported with atorvastatin and other statin drugs.

3.6.2. Drug Interactions

The risk of myopathy during treatment with statins, including atorvastatin in Liptruzet is increased with concurrent administration of fibrate drugs, lipid-modifying doses of niacin, cyclosporine, or strong CYP3A4 inhibitors (e.g., clarithromycin, human immunodeficiency virus protease inhibitors, and itraconazole). Bile acid sequestrants, such as cholestyramine can bind and significantly inhibit the absorption of ezetimibe. As such, dosing of Liptruzet should occur either ≥2 hours before or ≥4 hours after administration of a bile acid sequestrant.

3.6.3. Contraindications and FDA Pregnancy Category

- Active liver disease or unexplained persistent elevations of hepatic transaminase levels
- Hypersensitivity to any component of Liptruzet
- Women who are pregnant or may become pregnant
- Nursing mothers
- FDA pregnancy category: X

3.7. Comparison with Existing Members and New Development since the US FDA Approval

Direct comparison of the clinical efficacy between Liptruzet and Vytorin is currently lacking. As noted earlier, an incremental benefit of adding ezetimibe to simvastatin on cardiovascular outcomes has been demonstrated by the IMPROVE-IT trial [23–26]. Such a benefit remains to be established for Liptruzet. Although studies on cardiovascular outcomes are lacking, two recent trials (OCTIVUS and PRECISE-IVUS) reported that compared with atorvastatin monotherapy, the combination of atorvastatin plus ezetimibe showed greater coronary plaque regression in patients with acute coronary syndromes [27, 28].

4. PCSK9 INHIBITORS: ALIROCUMAB (PRALUENT) AND EVOLOCUMAB (REPATHA)

4.1. Overview

PCSK9 is secreted into the plasma primarily by the liver. It binds to the LDL receptor on hepatocytes, preventing the recycling and enhancing the degradation of LDL receptor in endosomes/lysosomes. This results in reduced clearance of plasma LDL cholesterol. Rare gain-of-function PCSK9 variants lead to higher levels of LDL cholesterol and increased risk of cardiovascular diseases; and conversely, loss-of-function PCSK9 variants are associated with reductions in both LDL cholesterol and risk of cardiovascular diseases [29, 30]. Moreover, the level of circulating PCSK9 predicts future risk of cardiovascular events independently of established risk factors [31].

Because of the critical role of PCSK9 in inducing LDL receptor degradation, several anti-PCSK9 therapeutic strategies have recently been developed and tested in clinical trials, among which, monoclonal antibodies are the most advanced PCSK9 inhibitors in development [32–34]. In fact, the US FDA approved two monoclonal antibodies against PCSK9, namely, alirocumab and evolocumab in July 2015 and August 2015, respectively. The former was developed by Sanofi Aventis (Bridgewater, NJ, USA), and the latter by Amgen (Thousand Oaks, CA, USA).

Approval of alirocumab by the US FDA was based on its efficacy demonstrated in five randomized controlled trials that enrolled a total of 3,499 patients: 36% were patients with heterozygous familial hypercholesterolemia (HeFH) and 54% were non-FH patients who had clinical atherosclerotic cardiovascular disease. Among the 5 trials, the ODYSSEY LONG TERM study is the largest one involving 2,341 patients at high risk for cardiovascular events [35]. On the other hand, approval of evolocumab by the US FDA was based on the efficacy demonstrated in randomized controlled trials involving primary hyperlipidemia in patients with clinical atherosclerotic cardiovascular disease, HeFH, and HoFH [36–39].

4.2. Chemistry and Pharmacokinetics

Both alirocumab and evolocumab are human monoclonal antibodies that target PCSK9, and are produced by recombinant DNA technology in cultured Chinese hamster ovary cells. The molecular weights of alirocumab and evolocumab are ~146 and ~144 kDa, respectively. The major pharmacokinetic properties of these two drugs are summarized in **Table 2.3**.

TABLE 2.3. Major pharmacokinetic properties of the PCSK9 inhibitors alirocumab and evolocumab

Property	Alirocumab	Evolocumab
Bioavailability	85%	72%
t_{max}	3–7 days	3–4 days
Vd	0.04–0.05 L/kg bw	0.047 L/kg bw
Metabolism	Degradation to small peptides and amino acids	Degradation to small peptides and amino acids
Elimination	Saturable binding to PCSK9 at low drug concentrations and nonsaturable proteolysis at high drug concentrations	Saturable binding to PCSK9 at low drug concentrations and nonsaturable proteolysis at high drug concentrations
$t_{1/2}$	17–20 days	11–17 days

Note: bw, body weight; $t_{1/2}$, elimination half-life; t_{max}, the time when the maximum plasma concentration is reached; Vd, volume of distribution.

4.3. Molecular Mechanisms and Pharmacological Effects

4.3.1. Molecular Mechanisms

PCSK9 binds to the LDL receptors (LDLR) on the surface of hepatocytes to promote LDLR degradation within the liver. LDLR is the primary receptor that clears circulating LDL. Therefore, the decrease in LDLR levels by PCSK9 results in higher blood levels of LDL cholesterol. By inhibiting the binding of PCSK9 to LDLR, alirocumab and evolocumab increase the number of LDLR available to clear plasma LDL, thereby lowering LDL cholesterol levels (**Figure 2.3**).

4.3.2. Pharmacological Effects

Following a single subcutaneous administration, both alirocumab and evolocumab cause suppression of circulating unbound (free) PCSK9 in a dose-dependent manner. The maximum suppression of the free PCSK9 occurs within 4–8 h (for alirocumab) or by 4 h (for evolocumab). Free PCSK9 concentrations in the blood return toward baseline when the concentrations of the drug decrease below the limit of quantification. Both drugs can cause 40–60% reduction in LDL cholesterol in patients on maximally tolerated statin doses. In patients with HoFH on standard therapy, evolocumab causes ~30% reduction in LDL cholesterol. Up to date, the efficacy of alirocumab in HoFH has not been reported.

4.4. Clinical Uses

4.4.1. Alirocumab

Alirocumab is indicated as an adjunct to diet and maximally tolerated statin therapy for the treatment of adult patients with HeFH or clinical

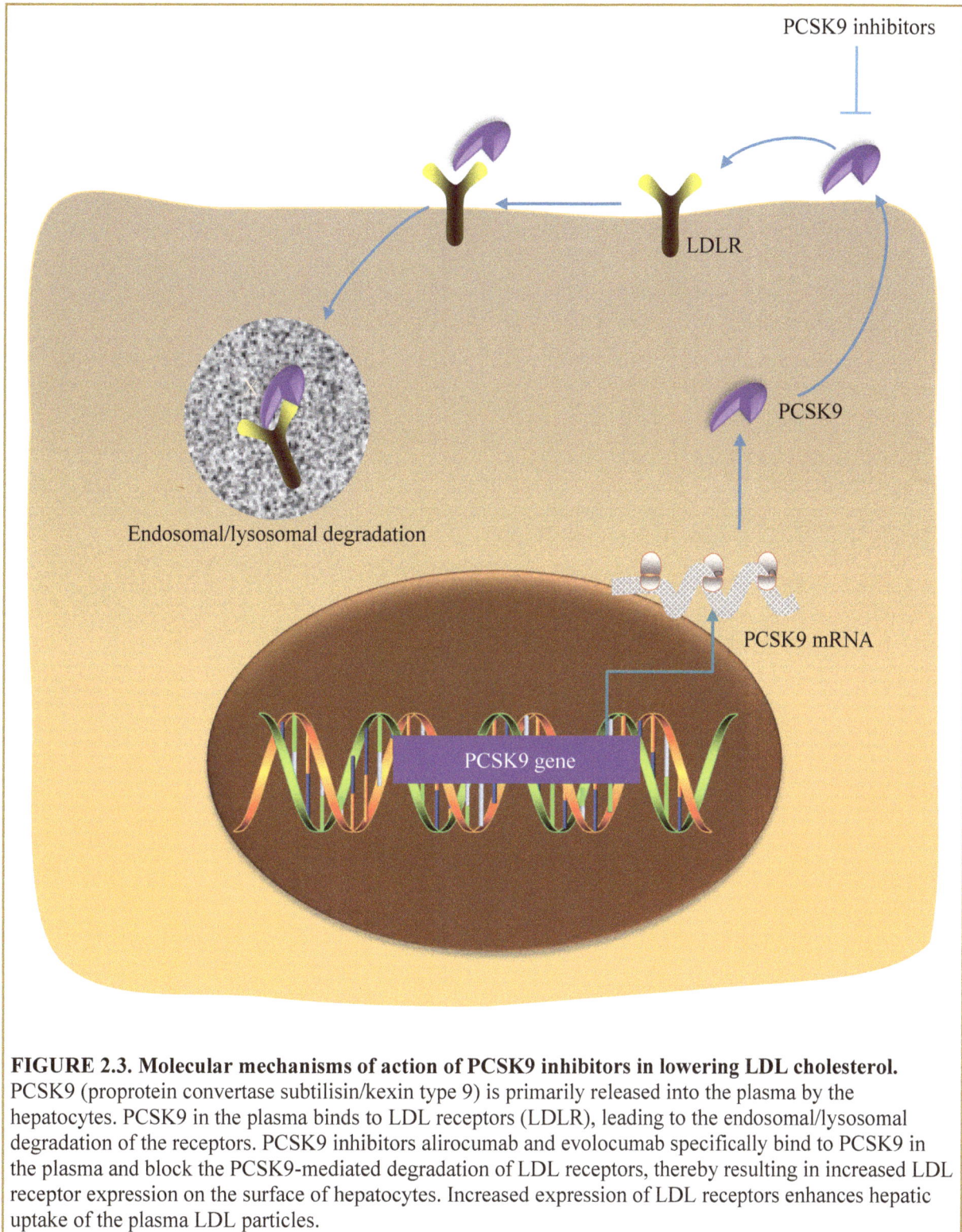

FIGURE 2.3. Molecular mechanisms of action of PCSK9 inhibitors in lowering LDL cholesterol.
PCSK9 (proprotein convertase subtilisin/kexin type 9) is primarily released into the plasma by the
hepatocytes. PCSK9 in the plasma binds to LDL receptors (LDLR), leading to the endosomal/lysosomal
degradation of the receptors. PCSK9 inhibitors alirocumab and evolocumab specifically bind to PCSK9 in
the plasma and block the PCSK9-mediated degradation of LDL receptors, thereby resulting in increased LDL
receptor expression on the surface of hepatocytes. Increased expression of LDL receptors enhances hepatic
uptake of the plasma LDL particles.

atherosclerotic cardiovascular disease, who require additional lowering of LDL cholesterol.

4.4.2. Evolocumab

Evolocumab is indicated as an adjunct to diet and maximally tolerated statin therapy for the treatment of adult patients with HeFH or
clinical atherosclerotic cardiovascular disease, who require additional lowering of LDL cholesterol. Evolocumab is also indicated as
an adjunct to diet and other LDL-lowering therapies (e.g., statins,
ezetimibe, LDL apheresis) for the treatment of patients with HoFH
who require additional lowering of LDL cholesterol.

4.5. Therapeutic Dosages

4.5.1. Alirocumab

The dosage forms and strengths of alirocumab are listed below.

- Subcutaneous injection: 75 mg/ml, 150 mg/ml, in a single-dose
  pre-filled pen or single-dose pre-filled syringe

The recommended starting dose of alirocumab is 75 mg once every 2
weeks administered subcutaneously, which can be increased to the
maximum dosage of 150 mg administered every 2 weeks if the LDL
cholesterol reduction is inadequate. Alternatively, the starting dose
can be 300 mg monthly, and if LDL cholesterol reduction is inadequate, the dosage may be adjusted to 150 mg every 2 weeks.

4.5.2. Evolocumab

The dosage forms and strengths of evolocumab are listed below.

- Subcutaneous injection: 140 mg/ml solution in a single-use pre-
  filled syringe; 140 mg/ml solution in a single-use prefilled
  SureClick® autoinjector; 420 mg/3.5 ml solution in a single-use
  Pushtronex™ system (on-body infusor with prefilled cartridge)

The recommended subcutaneous dosage of evolocumab in patients
with HeFH or patients with primary hyperlipidemia with established
clinical atherosclerotic cardiovascular disease is either 140 mg every
2 weeks or 420 mg once monthly. For HoFH patients, the recommended dose is 420 mg once monthly.

4.6. Adverse Effects and Drug Interactions

4.6.1. Adverse Effects

The adverse effects of alirocumab and evolocumab include allergic
reactions (e.g., pruritus, rash, urticaria), injection site reactions, na-
sopharyngitis, upper respiratory infections, and influenza.

4.6.2. Drug Interactions

Due to the monoclonal antibody nature, drug interactions are generally considered insignificant.

4.6.3. Contraindications and FDA Pregnancy Category

- Contraindications: patients with a history of a serious hypersensitivity reaction
- FDA pregnancy category: not assigned. There are no data available on using alirocumab and evolocumab in pregnant women to inform a drug-associated risk. In animal reproduction studies, these drugs show no effects on pregnancy or neonatal/infant development.

4.7. Comparison with Existing Members and New Development since the US FDA Approval

As noted above, both alirocumab and evolocumab are approved by the US FDA for treating HeFH or clinical atherosclerotic cardiovascular disease. It is of note that evolocumab, but not alirocumab is also indicated for reducing LDL cholesterol in patients with HoFH due to its demonstrated efficacy in this particular patient group [39, 40].

In addition to the LDL cholesterol-lowering efficacy, the benefit in reducing cardiovascular events for both alirocumab and evolocumab has been recently reported in clinical trials [35, 41, 42]. The safety profile of the PCSK9 inhibitors has also been demonstrated in the above trials as well as other clinical studies [43–45]. It is thus safe to state that both alirocumab and evolocumab have become an important part of the medical management of hypercholesterolemia that cannot be adequately controlled with conventional drugs (e.g., statins, ezetimibe, and their combination).

Besides antibody drugs, RNA interference (RNAi) therapeutic modalities are currently under active development for reducing PCSK9 and LDL cholesterol. In this regard, inclisiran, a long-acting RNAi therapeutic agent, is found to markedly reduce PCSK9 and LDL cholesterol for at least 6 months following a single dose in both healthy volunteers [46] and patients at high cardiovascular risk with elevated LDL cholesterol [47]. It is thus likely that the coming years will witness the rapid development of novel drugs targeting PCSK9 to adequately treat hypercholesterolemia and prevent atherosclerotic cardiovascular diseases.

5. SELF-ASSESSMENT QUESTIONS

5.1. Mipomersen is the first-in-class drug that targets specific mRNA. Which of the following is most likely the elimination half-life of this drug?

A. 1–2 minutes
B. 1–2 hours
C. 1–2 days
D. 1–2 weeks
E. 1–2 months

5.2. Following subcutaneous treatment with a newly approved drug that targets apolipoprotein B-100, a patient with homozygous familial hypercholesterolemia shows a reduced plasma level of lipoprotein(a) and elevations in serum transaminases. Which of the following is most likely the drug that the patient receives?

A. Ezetimibe
B. Fenofibrate
C. Mipomersen
D. Niacin
E. Pitavastatin

5.3. A 19-year old man with homozygous familial hypercholesterolemia is being treated with a drug that targets proprotein convertase subtilisin/kexin type 9. Which of the following is most likely the drug that the patient is being treated with?

A. Alirocumab
B. Atorvastatin
C. Evolocumab
D. Ezetimibe
E. Mipomersen

5.4. A 45-year-old man with heterozygous familial hypercholesterolemia has been treated with a maximally tolerated dose of simvastatin for several months, and his blood LDL cholesterol level remains elevated. A decision is made to add a new antibody drug to the treatment regimen to adequately control his hypercholesterolemia. Which of the following is most likely the molecular target of the new lipid-lowering drug?

A. Apolipoprotein B-100 mRNA
B. Cholesteryl ester transfer protein
C. Proprotein convertase subtilisin/kexin type 9
D. Microsomal triglyceride transfer protein
E. Niemann-Pick C1-Like 1

5.5. A 54-year-old female with elevated LDL cholesterol is being treated with a fixed-dose combination drug that reduces both the hepatic cholesterol synthesis and the intestinal absorption of cholesterol. Which of the following is most likely one of the molecular targets of this fixed-dose combination drug?

A. Apolipoprotein C-II
B. Proprotein convertase subtilisin/kexin type 9
C. Microsomal triglyceride transfer protein
D. Niemann-Pick C1-Like 1
E. Peroxisome proliferator-activated receptor alpha

ANSWERS AND EXPLANATIONS

5.1. The correct answer is E. Following subcutaneous administration, the elimination half-life for mipomersen is approximately 1–2 months. The long half-life of this drug enables the once weekly dosing regimen.

5.2. The correct answer is C. Mipomersen is a synthetic phosphorothioate oligonucleotide drug that specifically causes degradation of apolipoprotein B-100 (ApoB-100), leading to the reduction of ApoB-100-containg lipoproteins, including lipoprotein(a). The other drugs listed are given orally.

5.3. The correct answer is C. Among the drugs listed, only alirocumab and evolocumab are proprotein convertase subtilisin/kexin type 9 (PCSK9) inhibitors. While both alirocumab and evolocumab are approved by the US FDA for treating heterozygous familial hypercholesterolemia or clinical atherosclerotic cardiovascular disease, currently, evolocumab, but not alirocumab, is also approved by the US FDA for reducing LDL cholesterol in patients with homozygous familial hypercholesterolemia due to its demonstrated efficacy in this particular patient group.

5.4. The correct answer is C. Currently, only two US FDA-approved lipid-lowering drugs are antibody-based biologic agents, i.e., alirocumab and evolocumab, and both are inhibitors of proprotein convertase subtilisin/kexin type 9. Apolipoprotein B-100 mRNA is the target of mipomersen. Microsomal triglyceride transfer protein and Niemann-Pick C1-Like 1 are the molecular targets of lomitapide and ezetimibe, respectively. Currently, no US FDA-approved lipid-lowering drugs target cholesteryl ester transfer protein, whose inhibition leads to increased HDL cholesterol.

5.5. The correct answer is D. Because the fixed-dose combination drug reduces both cholesterol synthesis and absorption, it is most likely a combination of a statin and ezetimibe. In this context, the US FDA has approved two fixed-dose combination drugs, namely, Vytorin (simvastatin/ezetimibe) and Liptruzet (atorvastatin/ezetimibe). Ezetimibe is a selective inhibitor of Niemann-Pick C1-Like 1, a cholesterol-transporting protein in the enterocytes.

REFERENCES

1. Grundy SM, Cleeman JI, Merz CN, Brewer HB, Jr., Clark LT, Hunninghake DB, Pasternak RC, Smith SC, Jr., Stone NJ, National Heart, Lung, and Blood Institute, American College of Cardiology Foundation. Implications of recent clinical trials for the National Cholesterol Education Program Adult Treatment Panel III guidelines. *Circulation* 2004; 110(2):227–39.

2. Raal FJ, Santos RD, Blom DJ, Marais AD, Charng MJ, Cromwell WC, Lachmann RH, Gaudet D, Tan JL, Chasan-Taber S, Tribble DL, Flaim JD, et al. Mipomersen, an apolipoprotein B synthesis inhibitor, for lowering of LDL cholesterol concentrations in patients with homozygous familial hypercholesterolaemia: a randomised, double-blind, placebo-controlled trial. *Lancet* 2010; 375(9719):998–1006.

3. Stein EA, Dufour R, Gagne C, Gaudet D, East C, Donovan JM, Chin W, Tribble DL, McGowan M. Apolipoprotein B synthesis inhibition with mipomersen in heterozygous familial hypercholesterolemia: results of a randomized, double-blind, placebo-controlled trial to assess efficacy and safety as add-on therapy in patients with coronary artery disease. *Circulation* 2012; 126(19):2283–92.

4. Thomas GS, Cromwell WC, Ali S, Chin W, Flaim JD, Davidson M. Mipomersen, an apolipoprotein B synthesis inhibitor, reduces atherogenic lipoproteins in patients with severe hypercholesterolemia at high cardiovascular risk: a randomized, double-blind, placebo-controlled trial. *J Am Coll Cardiol* 2013; 62(23):2178–84.

5. Merki E, Graham MJ, Mullick AE, Miller ER, Crooke RM, Pitas RE, Witztum JL, Tsimikas S. Antisense oligonucleotide directed to human apolipoprotein B-100 reduces lipoprotein(a) levels and oxidized phospholipids on human apolipoprotein B-100 particles in lipoprotein(a) transgenic mice. *Circulation* 2008; 118(7):743–53.

6. Visser ME, Witztum JL, Stroes ES, Kastelein JJ. Antisense oligonucleotides for the treatment of dyslipidaemia. *Eur Heart J* 2012; 33(12):1451–8.

7. Santos RD, Duell PB, East C, Guyton JR, Moriarty PM, Chin W, Mittleman RS. Long-term efficacy and safety of mipomersen in patients with familial hypercholesterolaemia: 2-year interim results of an open-label extension. *Eur Heart J* 2015; 36(9):566–75.

8. Duell PB, Santos RD, Kirwan BA, Witztum JL, Tsimikas S, Kastelein JJ. Long-term mipomersen treatment is associated with a reduction in cardiovascular events in patients with familial hypercholesterolemia. *J Clin Lipidol* 2016; 10(4):1011–21.

9. Raal FJ, Braamskamp MJ, Selvey SL, Sensinger CH, Kastelein JJ. Pediatric experience with mipomersen as adjunctive therapy for homozygous familial hypercholesterolemia. *J Clin Lipidol* 2016; 10(4):860–9.

10. Santos RD, Raal FJ, Donovan JM, Cromwell WC. Mipomersen preferentially reduces small low-density lipoprotein particle number in patients with hypercholesterolemia. *J Clin Lipidol* 2015; 9(2):201–9.

11. Saleheen D, Haycock PC, Zhao W, Rasheed A, Taleb A, Imran A, Abbas S, Majeed F, Akhtar S, Qamar N, Zaman KS, Yaqoob Z, et al. Apolipoprotein(a) isoform size, lipoprotein(a) concentration, and coronary artery disease: a mendelian randomisation analysis. *Lancet Diabetes Endocrinol* 2017; 5(7):524–33.

12. Akdim F, Stroes ES, Sijbrands EJ, Tribble DL, Trip MD, Jukema JW, Flaim JD, Su J, Yu R, Baker BF, Wedel MK, Kastelein JJ. Efficacy and safety of mipomersen, an antisense inhibitor of apolipoprotein B, in hypercholesterolemic subjects receiving stable statin therapy. *J Am Coll Cardiol* 2010; 55(15):1611–8.

13. Panta R, Dahal K, Kunwar S. Efficacy and safety of mipomersen in treatment of dyslipidemia: a meta-analysis of randomized controlled trials. *J Clin Lipidol* 2015; 9(2):217–25.

14. Iwamoto N, Butler DCD, Svrzikapa N, Mohapatra S, Zlatev I, Sah DWY, Meena, Standley SM, Lu G, Apponi LH, Frank-Kamenetsky M, Zhang JJ, et al. Control of phosphorothioate stereochemistry substantially increases the efficacy of antisense oligonucleotides. *Nat Biotechnol* 2017; 35(9):845–51.

15. Crooke ST, Wang S, Vickers TA, Shen W, Liang XH. Cellular uptake and trafficking of antisense oligonucleotides. *Nat Biotechnol* 2017; 35(3):230–7.

16. Ballantyne CM, Houri J, Notarbartolo A, Melani L, Lipka LJ, Suresh R, Sun S, LeBeaut AP, Sager PT, Veltri EP, Ezetimibe Study Group. Effect of ezetimibe coadministered with atorvastatin in 628 patients with primary hypercholesterolemia: a prospective, randomized, double-blind trial. *Circulation* 2003; 107(19):2409–15.

17. Gagne C, Gaudet D, Bruckert E, Ezetimibe Study Group. Efficacy and safety of ezetimibe coadministered with atorvastatin or simvastatin in patients with homozygous familial hypercholesterolemia. *Circulation* 2002; 105(21):2469–75.

18. Li YR. *Cardiovascular Diseases: From Molecular Pharmacology to Evidence-Based Therapeutics.* John Wiley & Sons, New Jersey, USA. 2015.

19. Altmann SW, Davis HR, Jr., Zhu LJ, Yao X, Hoos LM, Tetzloff G, Iyer SP, Maguire M, Golovko A, Zeng M, Wang L, Murgolo N, et al. Niemann-Pick C1 Like 1 protein is critical for intestinal cholesterol absorption. *Science* 2004; 303(5661):1201–4.

20. Garcia-Calvo M, Lisnock J, Bull HG, Hawes BE, Burnett DA, Braun MP, Crona JH, Davis HR, Jr., Dean DC, Detmers PA, Graziano MP, Hughes M, et al. The target of ezetimibe is Niemann-Pick C1-Like 1 (NPC1L1). *Proc Natl Acad Sci USA* 2005; 102(23):8132–7.

21. Ge L, Wang J, Qi W, Miao HH, Cao J, Qu YX, Li BL, Song BL. The cholesterol absorption inhibitor ezetimibe acts by blocking the sterol-induced internalization of NPC1L1. *Cell Metab* 2008; 7(6):508–19.

22. Martin G, Duez H, Blanquart C, Berezowski V, Poulain P, Fruchart JC, Najib-Fruchart J, Glineur C, Staels B. Statin-induced inhibition of the Rho-signaling pathway activates PPARalpha and induces HDL apoA-I. *J Clin Invest* 2001; 107(11):1423–32.

23. Cannon CP, Blazing MA, Giugliano RP,

McCagg A, White JA, Theroux P, Darius H, Lewis BS, Ophuis TO, Jukema JW, De Ferrari GM, Ruzyllo W, et al. Ezetimibe added to statin therapy after acute coronary syndromes. *N Engl J Med* 2015; 372(25):2387–97.

24. Bohula EA, Giugliano RP, Cannon CP, Zhou J, Murphy SA, White JA, Tershakovec AM, Blazing MA, Braunwald E. Achievement of dual low-density lipoprotein cholesterol and high-sensitivity C-reactive protein targets more frequent with the addition of ezetimibe to simvastatin and associated with better outcomes in IMPROVE-IT. *Circulation* 2015; 132(13):1224–33.

25. Murphy SA, Cannon CP, Blazing MA, Giugliano RP, White JA, Lokhnygina Y, Reist C, Im K, Bohula EA, Isaza D, Lopez-Sendon J, Dellborg M, et al. Reduction in total cardiovascular events with ezetimibe/simvastatin post-acute coronary syndrome: the IMPROVE-IT trial. *J Am Coll Cardiol* 2016; 67(4):353–61.

26. Bohula EA, Morrow DA, Giugliano RP, Blazing MA, He P, Park JG, Murphy SA, White JA, Kesaniemi YA, Pedersen TR, Brady AJ, Mitchel Y, et al. Atherothrombotic risk stratification and ezetimibe for secondary prevention. *J Am Coll Cardiol* 2017; 69(8):911–21.

27. Tsujita K, Sugiyama S, Sumida H, Shimomura H, Yamashita T, Yamanaga K, Komura N, Sakamoto K, Oka H, Nakao K, Nakamura S, Ishihara M, et al. Impact of dual lipid-lowering strategy with ezetimibe and atorvastatin on coronary plaque regression in patients with percutaneous coronary intervention: the multicenter randomized controlled PRECISE-IVUS trial. *J Am Coll Cardiol* 2015; 66(5):495–507.

28. Hougaard M, Hansen HS, Thayssen P, Antonsen L, Junker A, Veien K, Jensen LO. Influence of ezetimibe in addition to high-dose atorvastatin therapy on plaque composition in patients with ST-segment elevation myocardial infarction assessed by serial: Intravascular ultrasound with iMap: the OCTIVUS trial. *Cardiovasc Revasc Med* 2017; 18(2):110–7.

29. Seidah NG, Awan Z, Chretien M, Mbikay M. PCSK9: a key modulator of cardiovascular health. *Circ Res* 2014; 114(6):1022–36.

30. Bergeron N, Phan BA, Ding Y, Fong A, Krauss RM. Proprotein convertase subtilisin/kexin type 9 inhibition: a new therapeutic mechanism for reducing cardiovascular disease risk. *Circulation* 2015; 132(17):1648–66.

31. Leander K, Malarstig A, Van't Hooft FM, Hyde C, Hellenius ML, Troutt JS, Konrad RJ, Ohrvik J, Hamsten A, de Faire U. Circulating proprotein convertase subtilisin/kexin type 9 (PCSK9) predicts future risk of cardiovascular events independently of established risk factors. *Circulation* 2016; 133(13):1230–9.

32. Betteridge DJ. Cardiovascular endocrinology in 2012. PCSK9: an exciting target for reducing LDL-cholesterol levels. *Nat Rev Endocrinol* 2013; 9(2):76–8.

33. Farnier M. PCSK9 inhibitors. *Curr Opin Lipidol* 2013; 24(3):251–8.

34. Norata GD, Tibolla G, Catapano AL. Targeting PCSK9 for hypercholesterolemia. *Annu Rev Pharmacol Toxicol* 2014; 54:273–93.

35. Robinson JG, Farnier M, Krempf M, Bergeron J, Luc G, Averna M, Stroes ES, Langslet G, Raal FJ, El Shahawy M, Koren MJ, Lepor NE, et al. Efficacy and safety of alirocumab in reducing lipids and cardiovascular events. *N Engl J Med* 2015; 372(16):1489–99.

36. Robinson JG, Nedergaard BS, Rogers WJ, Fialkow J, Neutel JM, Ramstad D, Somaratne R, Legg JC, Nelson P, Scott R, Wasserman SM, Weiss R, et al. Effect of evolocumab or ezetimibe added to moderate- or high-intensity statin therapy on LDL-C lowering in patients with hypercholesterolemia: the LAPLACE-2 randomized clinical trial. *JAMA* 2014; 311(18):1870–82.

37. Blom DJ, Hala T, Bolognese M, Lillestol MJ, Toth PD, Burgess L, Ceska R, Roth E, Koren MJ, Ballantyne CM, Monsalvo ML, Tsirtsonis K, et al. A 52-week placebo-controlled trial of evolocumab in hyperlipidemia. *N Engl J Med* 2014; 370(19):1809–19.

38. Raal FJ, Stein EA, Dufour R, Turner T, Civeira F, Burgess L, Langslet G, Scott R, Olsson AG, Sullivan D, Hovingh GK, Cariou B, et al. PCSK9 inhibition with evolocumab (AMG 145) in heterozygous familial hypercholesterolaemia (RUTHERFORD-2): a randomised, double-blind, placebo-controlled trial. *Lancet* 2015; 385(9965):331–40.

39. Raal FJ, Honarpour N, Blom DJ, Hovingh GK, Xu F, Scott R, Wasserman SM, Stein EA, TESLA Investigators. Inhibition of PCSK9 with evolocumab in homozygous familial hypercholesterolaemia (TESLA Part B): a randomised, double-blind, placebo-controlled trial. *Lancet* 2015; 385(9965):341–50.

40. Raal FJ, Hovingh GK, Blom D, Santos RD,

Harada-Shiba M, Bruckert E, Couture P, Soran H, Watts GF, Kurtz C, Honarpour N, Tang L, et al. Long-term treatment with evolocumab added to conventional drug therapy, with or without apheresis, in patients with homozygous familial hypercholesterolaemia: an interim subset analysis of the open-label TAUSSIG study. *Lancet Diabetes Endocrinol* 2017; 5(4):280–90.

41. Sabatine MS, Giugliano RP, Wiviott SD, Raal FJ, Blom DJ, Robinson J, Ballantyne CM, Somaratne R, Legg J, Wasserman SM, Scott R, Koren MJ, et al. Efficacy and safety of evolocumab in reducing lipids and cardiovascular events. *N Engl J Med* 2015; 372(16):1500–9.

42. Sabatine MS, Giugliano RP, Keech AC, Honarpour N, Wiviott SD, Murphy SA, Kuder JF, Wang H, Liu T, Wasserman SM, Sever PS, Pedersen TR, et al. Evolocumab and clinical outcomes in patients with cardiovascular disease. *N Engl J Med* 2017; 376(18):1713–22.

43. Nissen SE, Stroes E, Dent-Acosta RE, Rosenson RS, Lehman SJ, Sattar N, Preiss D, Bruckert E, Ceska R, Lepor N, Ballantyne CM, Gouni-Berthold I, et al. Efficacy and tolerability of evolocumab vs ezetimibe in patients with muscle-related statin intolerance: the GAUSS-3 randomized clinical trial. *JAMA* 2016; 315(15):1580–90.

44. Koren MJ, Sabatine MS, Giugliano RP, Langslet G, Wiviott SD, Kassahun H, Ruzza A, Ma Y, Somaratne R, Raal FJ. Long-term low-density lipoprotein cholesterol-lowering efficacy, persistence, and safety of evolocumab in treatment of hypercholesterolemia: results up to 4 years from the open-label OSLER-1 extension study. *JAMA Cardiol* 2017; 2(6):598–607.

45. Toth PP, Descamps O, Genest J, Sattar N, Preiss D, Dent R, Djedjos C, Wu Y, Geller M, Uhart M, Somaratne R, Wasserman SM, et al. Pooled safety analysis of evolocumab in over 6000 patients from double-blind and open-label extension studies. *Circulation* 2017; 135(19):1819–31.

46. Fitzgerald K, White S, Borodovsky A, Bettencourt BR, Strahs A, Clausen V, Wijngaard P, Horton JD, Taubel J, Brooks A, Fernando C, Kauffman RS, et al. A Highly durable RNAi therapeutic inhibitor of PCSK9. *N Engl J Med* 2017; 376(1):41–51.

47. Ray KK, Landmesser U, Leiter LA, Kallend D, Dufour R, Karakas M, Hall T, Troquay RP, Turner T, Visseren FL, Wijngaard P, Wright RS, et al. Inclisiran in patients at high cardiovascular risk with elevated LDL cholesterol. *N Engl J Med* 2017; 376(15):1430–40.

CHAPTER 3

New Drugs for Hypertriglyceridemia

CHAPTER HIGHLIGHTS

- Hypertriglyceridemia has been recognized as a significant contributor to the development of cardiovascular diseases.
- Drugs for treating hypertriglyceridemia typically include fibrates and niacin as well as potent statins such as atorvastatin and rosuvastatin.
- Over the past decade or so, the United States Food and Drug Administration has approved several omega-3 fatty acid drugs for treating severe hypertriglyceridemia (≥ 500 mg/dl).
- These omega-3 fatty acid-based drugs include Lovaza, Vascepa, and Epanova, with Epanova being the newest member which was approved in 2014.

KEYWORDS | Docosahexaenoic acid; Eicosapentaenoic acid; Epanova; Hypertriglyceridemia; LDL cholesterol; Lovaza; n-3 Fatty acid; Omega-3 fatty acids; Triglyceride; Vascepa

CITATION | Li YR. Cardiovascular Medicine: New Therapeutic Drugs Approved by the US FDA (2013–2017). Cell Med Press, Raleigh, NC, USA. 2018. http://dx.doi.org/10.20455/ndcvd.2018.03

ABBREVIATIONS | DHA, docosahexaenoic acid; EPA, eicosapentaenoic acid; GPR120, G protein-coupled receptor 120; HDL, high-density lipoprotein; LDL, low-density lipoprotein; US FDA, the United States Food and Drug Administration; VLDL, very low-density lipoprotein

CHAPTER AT A GLANCE

1. INTRODUCTION

Hypertriglyceridemia is a common form of dyslipidemia. With regards to clinical trials and therapeutic drug development, low-density lipoprotein (LDL) cholesterol, a major risk factor for atherosclerotic cardiovascular diseases, has received much attention. The multiple new drugs approved by the United States Food and Drug Administration (US FDA) for treating hypercholesterolemia (see Chapter 2) attest to the above notion. In contrast, clinical studies and new drug development are relatively less intensive on hypertriglyceridemia. Indeed, specific drugs for treating hypertriglyceridemia are old and include primarily fibrates and niacin as well as certain potent statins (e.g., atorvastatin and rosuvastatin) (see Chapter 1).

Recent evidence including that from genetic studies supports an important role for hypertriglyceridemia in the development of cardiovascular diseases [1–3], stimulating efforts to develop novel therapeutics for this common lipid disorder [4–6]. In this context, since 2004, the US FDA has approved three new drugs containing omega-3 fatty acids for specifically treating severe hypertriglyceridemia. They are omega-3 fatty acid ethyl esters (Lovaza) (US FDA 2004; a generic form of omega-3 fatty acid ethyl esters, known as Omtryg, was also approved by the US FDA in 2004.), icosapent ethyl (Vascepa) (US FDA 2012), and omega-3-carboxylic acids (Epanova) (US FDA 2014).

This chapter describes the newest member of this drug class, i.e., Epanova for treating severe hypertriglyceridemia (triglycerides ≥500 mg/dl). It should be noted that the amounts of the effective omega-3 fatty acids in the over-the-counter products, such as fish oil supplements are typically much lower than those in the above US FDA-approved pharmaceutical preparations.

2. OMEGA-3 CARBOXYLIC ACIDS (EPANOVA)

2.1. Overview

Omega-3 fatty acids, also known as ω-3 fatty acids, constitute a series of essential unsaturated fatty acids that have a final carbon-carbon double bond in the n-3 position (also known as the ω position), that is, the third bond from the methyl end of the fatty acid. As such, omega-3 fatty acids are also referred to as n-3 fatty acids [7–9]. Nutritionally important omega-3 fatty acids include the plant-derived α-linolenic acid (ALA) and the marine-derived eicosapentaenoic acid (EPA) and docosahexaenoic acid (DHA), all of which are polyunsaturated [10, 11] (structures shown in **Figure 3.1**). The US FDA approval of Epanova was primarily based on a 12-week randomized controlled trial (EVOLVE) involving 199 patients whose triglyceride levels were between 500 and 2,000 mg/dl. Treatment with Epanova significantly reduces triglycerides, non-high-density lipoprotein (HDL) cholesterol, and very low-density lipoprotein (VLDL) cholesterol, but increases LDL cholesterol [12] (see Section 2.3 on the potential mechanism of LDL cholesterol elevation).

2.2. Chemistry and Pharmacokinetics

Epanova is a coated soft-gelatin capsule containing 1 gram of fish oil-derived free fatty acids, designated as omega-3-carboxylic acids,

FIGURE 3.1. Chemical structures of omega-3 fatty acids. The three main forms of omega-3 fatty acids are alpha-linolenic acid (ALA), eicosapentaenoic acid (EPA), and docosahexaenoic acid (DHA). Lovaza is a mixture of esters of EPA and DHA, whereas Vascepa is an ester of EPA. Different from Lovaza and Vascepa, Epanova is a mixture of free EPA and DHA.

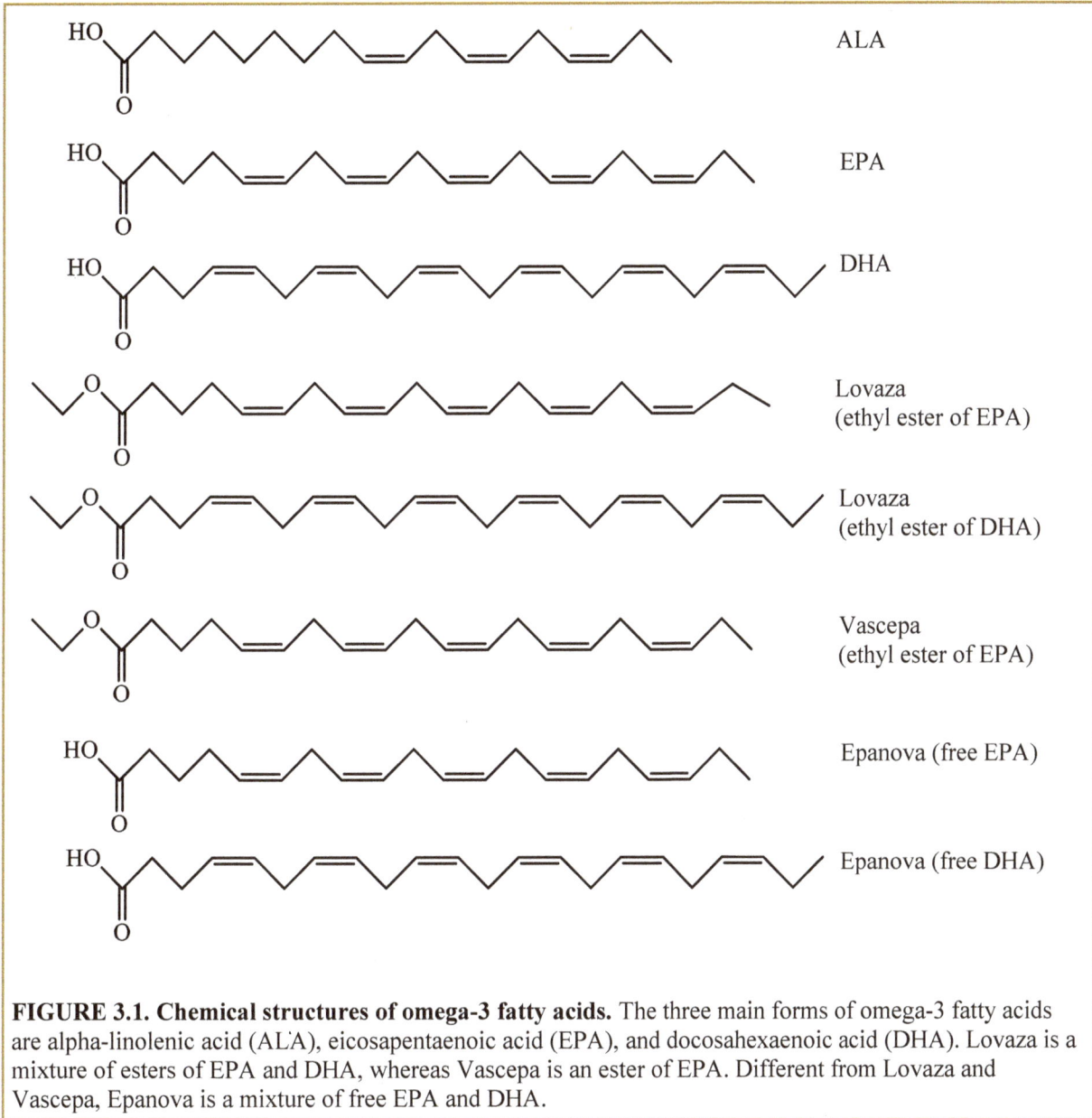

with at least 850 mg of polyunsaturated fatty acids, including multiple omega-3 fatty acids with EPA and DHA being the most abundant. The major chemical and pharmacokinetic properties of Epanova as well as Vascepa and Lovaza are summarized in **Table 3.1**.

2.3. Molecular Mechanisms and Pharmacological Effects

2.3.1. Molecular Mechanisms

The mechanism of action of Epanova remains to be established. Potential mechanisms of action are outlined on the next page and illustrated in **Figure 3.2**.

- Inhibition of acyl-CoA:1,2-diacylglycerol acyltransferase, an enzyme involved in triglyceride biosynthesis
- Increased mitochondrial and peroxisomal β-oxidation in the liver, leading to increased consumption of fatty acids and thereby reduced triglyceride biosynthesis
- Increased lipoprotein lipase activity, leading to augmented hydrolysis of triglycerides in VLDLs and chylomicrons. Both Epanova and Vascepa have been shown to reduce plasma apolipoprotein CIII (ApoC-III) [13, 14], an inhibitor of lipoprotein lipase.
- Epanova may also reduce the synthesis of triglycerides in the liver because EPA and DHA are poor substrates for the enzymes responsible for triglyceride synthesis, and EPA and DHA inhibit esterification of other fatty acids.

Recently, the G protein-coupled receptor 120 (GPR120) has been shown to function as an omega-3 fatty acid receptor/sensor to mediate the anti-inflammatory and insulin-sensitizing effects of these fatty acids [15–17] (**Figure 3.3**). However, it remains unknown if GPR120 is also involved in the triglyceride-lowering activity of Epanova as well as Vascepa and Lovaza.

TABLE 3.1. Major chemical and pharmacokinetic properties of the three n-3 fatty acid drugs

Property	Epanova	Vascepa	Lovaza
Active chemical entity	Free acids of EPA and DHA	Ethyl ester of EPA	Ethyl esters of EPA and DHA
Contents of EPA and DHA	≥850 mg fatty acids (≥425–510 mg EPA and ≥127.5–212.5 mg DHA) per 1 g capsule	1 g EPA per 1 g capsule	~465 mg EPA and ~375 mg DHA per 1 g capsule
Relative ratio of EPA to DHA	EPA (73%), DHA (27%)	EPA (100%), DHA (0%)	EPA (55%), DHA (45%)
Absorption	Readily absorbable due to the drug in free fatty acid form	The drug is an esterified form and needs to be de-esterified before absorption	The drug is an esterified form and needs to be de-esterified before absorption
t_{max}	5–8 h (EPA), 5–9 h (DHA)	5 h	Not known
Metabolism	Oxidation in the liver similar to fatty acids derived from dietary sources	Oxidation in the liver similar to fatty acids derived from dietary sources	Oxidation in the liver similar to fatty acids derived from dietary sources
$t_{1/2}$	37 h (EPA), 46 h (DHA)	89 h	Not known

Note: $t_{1/2}$, elimination half-life; t_{max}, the time when the maximum plasma concentration is reached.

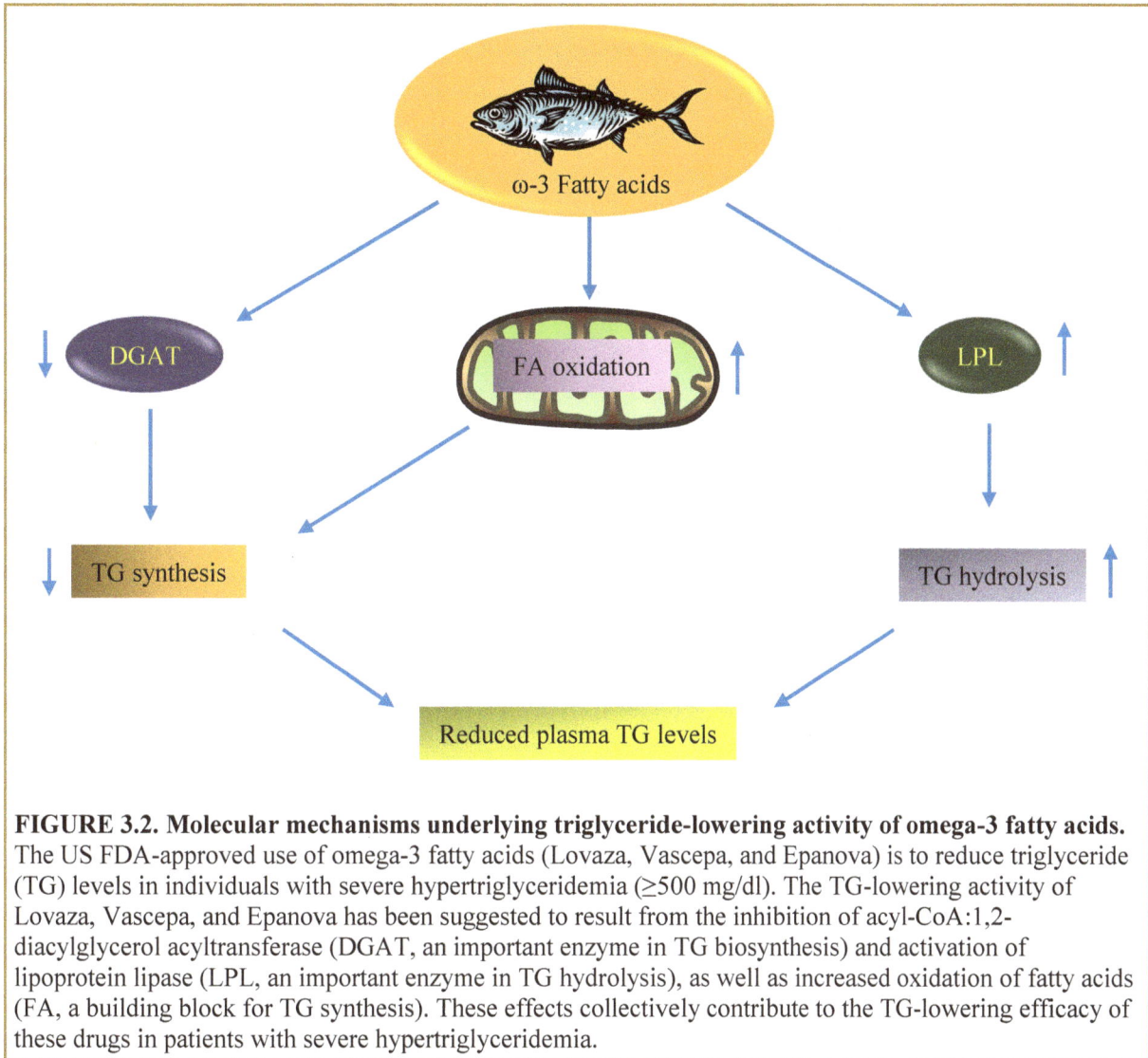

FIGURE 3.2. Molecular mechanisms underlying triglyceride-lowering activity of omega-3 fatty acids. The US FDA-approved use of omega-3 fatty acids (Lovaza, Vascepa, and Epanova) is to reduce triglyceride (TG) levels in individuals with severe hypertriglyceridemia ($\geq$500 mg/dl). The TG-lowering activity of Lovaza, Vascepa, and Epanova has been suggested to result from the inhibition of acyl-CoA:1,2-diacylglycerol acyltransferase (DGAT, an important enzyme in TG biosynthesis) and activation of lipoprotein lipase (LPL, an important enzyme in TG hydrolysis), as well as increased oxidation of fatty acids (FA, a building block for TG synthesis). These effects collectively contribute to the TG-lowering efficacy of these drugs in patients with severe hypertriglyceridemia.

2.3.2. Pharmacological Effects

Treatment with Epanova (2 g/day and 4 g/day) leads to 16–21% reduction in fasting triglyceride levels and 7–10% reduction in non-HDL cholesterol levels, and 14–21% reduction in VLDL cholesterol levels. However, the same treatment also increases LDL cholesterol levels by 13–15%. It is believed that the DHA component of the drug is responsible for the elevation of LDL cholesterol. It has been suggested that DHA may cause downregulation of the hepatocyte LDL receptors, thereby leading to reduced clearance of plasma LDL particles [18]. Because Vascepa does not contain DHA, treatment with this drug has been shown to reduce, rather than increase, LDL cholesterol [19]. On the other hand, treatment with Lovaza, a drug that contains both EPA and DHA, elevates LDL cholesterol. Comparison of the effects of the three omega-3 fatty acid drugs on lipid profiles is provided in **Table 3.2**.

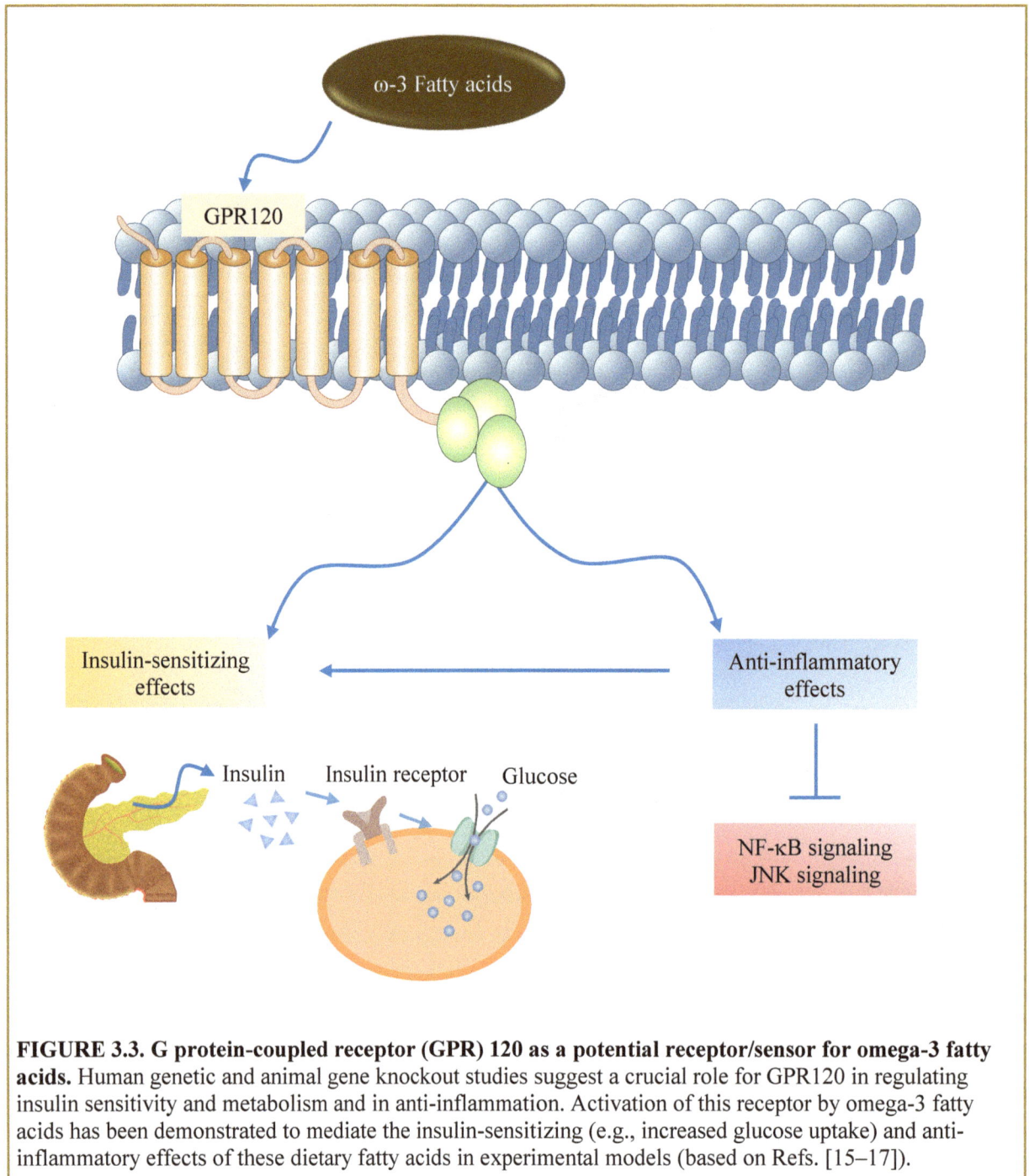

FIGURE 3.3. G protein-coupled receptor (GPR) 120 as a potential receptor/sensor for omega-3 fatty acids. Human genetic and animal gene knockout studies suggest a crucial role for GPR120 in regulating insulin sensitivity and metabolism and in anti-inflammation. Activation of this receptor by omega-3 fatty acids has been demonstrated to mediate the insulin-sensitizing (e.g., increased glucose uptake) and anti-inflammatory effects of these dietary fatty acids in experimental models (based on Refs. [15–17]).

2.4. Clinical Uses

2.4.1. Clinical Indications

Similar to Lovaza and Vascepa, Epanova is indicated as an adjunct to diet to reduce triglyceride levels in adult patients with severe hypertriglyceridemia (a plasma level of triglyceride ≥500 mg/dl).

TABLE 3.2. Effects of Epanova, Vascepa, and Lovaza on blood lipid profiles in patients with severe hypertriglyceridemia (≥500 mg/dl)

Drug	TG	TC	LDL-C	VLDL-C	Non-HDL-C	HDL-C
Epanova	−21	−9	+15	−21	−10	+4
Vascepa	−33	−16	−2	−29	−18	−4
Lovaza	−52	−8	+49	−41	−10	+9

Note: Data represent percentage changes from baseline versus placebo. The "−" and "+" denote decrease and increase, respectively. The dosage and duration of treatment: Epanova, 4 g daily, 12 weeks; Vascepa, 4 g daily, 12 weeks; Lovaza 4 g daily, 6 and 16 weeks. Data for Lovaza are combined from 2 clinical trials of 6 and 16 weeks of duration. HDL-C, high-density lipoprotein cholesterol; LDL-C, low-density lipoprotein cholesterol; Non-HDL-C, non-high-density lipoprotein cholesterol; TC, total cholesterol; TG, triglyceride; VLDL-C, very low-density lipoprotein cholesterol.

2.4.2. Limitations of Use

The effects of Epanova as well as Vascepa and Lovaza on the risk for pancreatitis in patients with severe hypertriglyceridemia have not been determined through rigorously designed clinical trials. Likewise, the effects of these drugs on cardiovascular mortality and morbidity in patients with severe hypertriglyceridemia remain to be established.

2.5. Therapeutic Dosages

Epanova is supplied as 1 g capsules. The recommended dosage is 2 g (2 capsules) or 4 g (4 capsules) once daily.

2.6. Adverse Effects and Drug Interactions

2.6.1. Adverse Effects

Epanova is well-tolerated. Its common adverse effects include diarrhea, nausea, abdominal pain or discomfort, and eructation. In some patients, Epanova increases LDL cholesterol levels (also see Section 2.7 for potential mechanisms). As such, LDL cholesterol levels should be monitored periodically during Epanova therapy.

2.6.2. Drug Interactions

Omega-3 fatty acids may prolong bleeding time. Patients receiving treatment with Epanova and other drugs affecting coagulation (e.g., antiplatelet drugs) should be monitored periodically.

2.6.3. Contraindications and FDA Pregnancy Category

▪ Epanova is contraindicated in patients with known hypersensitivity.
▪ FDA pregnancy category: C (see Chapter 2 for details on the FDA pregnancy category)

2.7. Comparison with Existing Members and New Development since the US FDA Approval

The chemical and pharmacokinetic properties of Epanova, Vascepa, and Lovaza are given in **Table 3.1**. One apparent difference between the Epanova and the other two is that the omega-3 fatty acids in both Vascepa and Lovaza are esterized and must be converted to the free forms in the body to become absorbable and pharmacologically active. In contrast, the EPA and DHA in Epanova are already in the free form, and as such, may have improved bioavailability compared to Vascepa and Lovaza.

As noted above, Epanova may increase LDL cholesterol in some patients, an effect shared by Lovaza, but not by Vascepa. It is believed that DHA is responsible for the LDL cholesterol elevation [18], but the exact mechanism of this action remains unclear. It has been suggested that DHA may reduce LDL receptor expression, thereby leading to decreased hepatic uptake of plasma LDL particles and consequent elevation of plasma LDL cholesterol [18]. Comparison of the effects of the three omega-3 fatty acid drugs on lipid profiles is provided in **Table 3.2**.

Over the past few years, the cardiovascular effects of omega-3 fatty acids have been investigated in several clinical trials, but with inconsistent results. For example, in a randomized controlled trial involving 12,513 patients with multiple cardiovascular risk factors, treatment with omega-3 fatty acids (1 g/day) did not reduce cardiovascular morbidity and mortality with a median of 5 years of follow-up [20]. On the other hand, in a randomized controlled trial (GISSI-HF) with 6,975 patients with chronic heart failure on standard therapy, supplementation with omega-3 fatty acids (1 g daily) for a median of 3.9 years led to a small, but statistically significant 8–9% reduction in mortality and admission to hospital for cardiovascular reasons [21].

More recently, in a multicenter, randomized controlled trial (OMEGA-REMODEL) with 358 patients presenting with acute myocardial infarction, treatment with a high dose (4 g daily) of omega-3 fatty acids was associated with reduction of adverse left ventricular remodeling, non-infarct myocardial fibrosis, and serum biomarkers of systemic inflammation beyond current guideline-based standard of care [22]. In a 2017 scientific advisory from the American Heart Association (AHA), upon reviewing the cumulative evidence from randomized controlled trials designed to assess the effect of omega-3 fatty acid supplementation on clinical cardiovascular events, it is concluded that omega-3 fatty acid supplement is a reasonable treatment for patients with prevalent coronary heart disease (such as a recent myocardial infarction) as well as patients with heart failure with reduced ejection fraction (HFrEF) [23] (**Figure 3.4**).

In addition to its role in cardiovascular diseases, the efficacy of omega-3 fatty acids in the intervention of other disorders has been also demonstrated in clinical trials. For example, a randomized controlled trial involving 736 pregnant women and their children (695) demonstrated that supplementation with omega-3 long-chain polyunsaturated fatty acids (2.4 g daily) in the third trimester of pregnancy reduced the absolute risk of persistent wheeze or asthma and infections of the lower respiratory tract in offspring by ~30% [24].

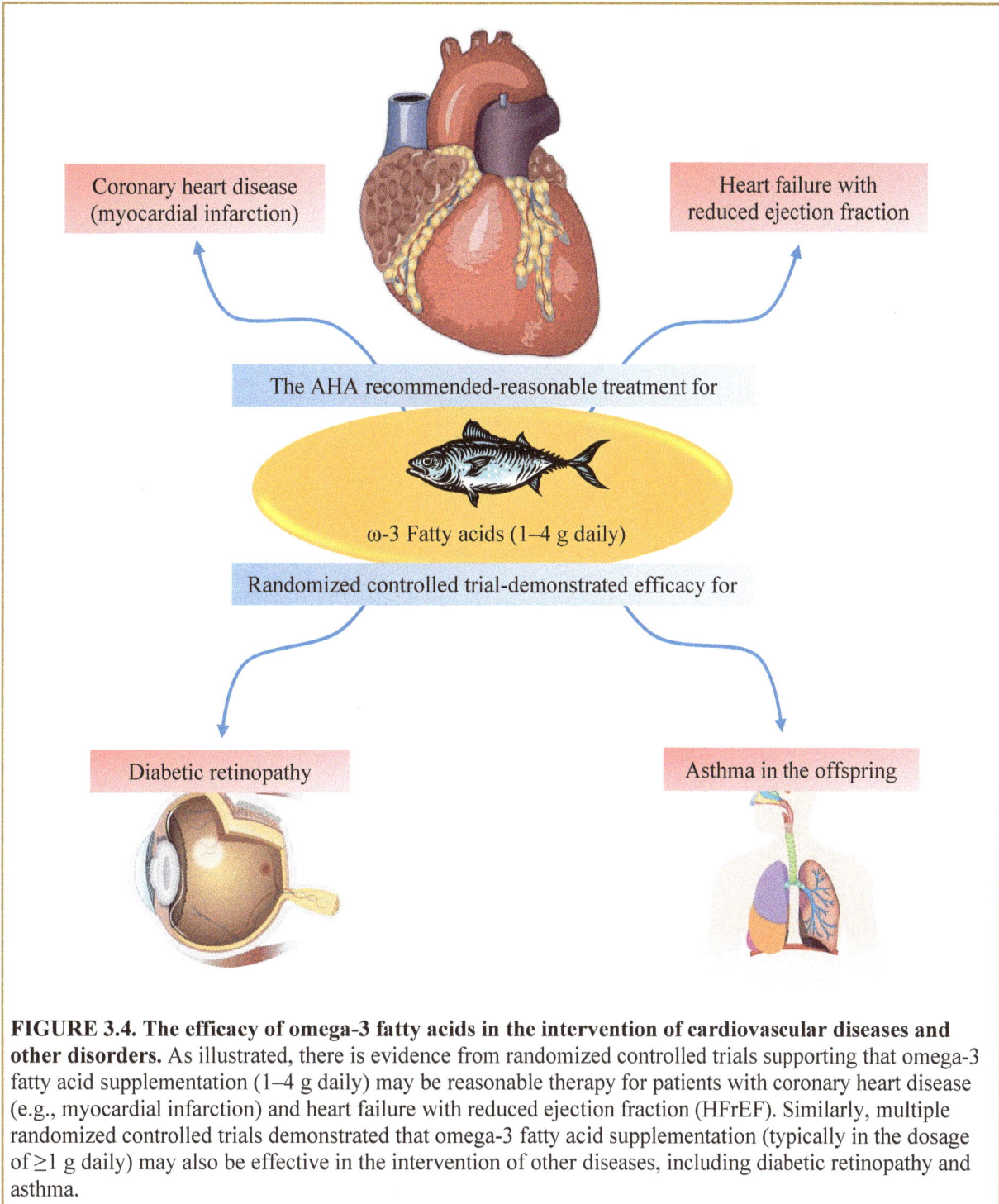

FIGURE 3.4. The efficacy of omega-3 fatty acids in the intervention of cardiovascular diseases and other disorders. As illustrated, there is evidence from randomized controlled trials supporting that omega-3 fatty acid supplementation (1–4 g daily) may be reasonable therapy for patients with coronary heart disease (e.g., myocardial infarction) and heart failure with reduced ejection fraction (HFrEF). Similarly, multiple randomized controlled trials demonstrated that omega-3 fatty acid supplementation (typically in the dosage of ≥1 g daily) may also be effective in the intervention of other diseases, including diabetic retinopathy and asthma.

Diabetic retinopathy is a devastating complication of individuals with type 2 diabetes mellitus. A randomized controlled trial involving 3,482 diabetic patients with a median follow-up of 6 years reported that in middle-aged and older individuals with type 2 diabetes, intake of at least 0.5 g/day of dietary omega-3 long-chain polyunsaturated fatty acids, easily achievable with 2 weekly servings of oily fish, was associated with a 48% decrease in the risk of sight-threatening diabetic retinopathy [25]. Hence, omega-3 fatty acids have a therapeutic value in multiple diseases (**Figure 3.4**). While the exact mechanisms underlying the clinical efficacy of omega-3 fatty acids remain to be established, it is possible that the anti-inflammatory activities of omega-3 fatty acids contribute, at least partially, to the clinical effectiveness. In this context, coronary heart disease, heart failure, asthma, and diabetes are all considered as inflammatory disorders [26–30].

3. SELF-ASSESSMENT QUESTIONS

3.1. Recently, the US FDA has approved an n-3 fatty acid-based pharmaceutical preparation for lowering blood triglycerides in patients with severe hypertriglyceridemia. Which of the following conditions will meet the criteria for the FDA-approved indication?

A. Blood HDL cholesterol <40 mg/dl and triglycerides >350 mg/dl
B. Blood LDL cholesterol >150 mg/dl and triglycerides <500 mg/dl
C. Blood triglycerides >300 mg/dl and HDL cholesterol >65 mg/dl
D. Blood triglycerides ≥500 mg/dl
E. Blood triglycerides between 250 and 450 mg/dl

3.2. Which of the following US FDA-approved drugs contains only eicosapentaenoic acid (EPA) as its active ingredient?

A. Epanova
B. Liptruzet
C. Lovaza
D. Omtryg
E. Vascepa

3.3. It has been demonstrated in clinical trials that some of the omega-3 fatty acid-based drugs may increase blood LDL cholesterol levels in some patients. Which of the following US FDA-approved drugs has the highest potential to cause elevation of LDL cholesterol?

A. Epanova
B. Liptruzet
C. Lovaza
D. Vascepa
E. Mipomersen

3.4. Which of the following has been shown to function as an omega-3 fatty acid receptor/sensor to mediate the anti-inflammatory and insulin-sensitizing effects of these fatty acids?

A. Cholesteryl ester transfer protein
B. Epidermal growth factor receptor
C. G protein-coupled receptor 120
D. Low-density lipoprotein receptor
E. Proprotein convertase subtilisin/kexin type 9

3.5. While the exact role of omega-3 fatty acids in cardiovascular medicine remains to be established, based on recent clinical trials reported in prestigious medical journals which of the following conditions is most likely to benefit from omega-3 fatty acid supplementation ($\geq$1 g daily)?

A. Heart failure with preserved ejection fraction
B. Heart failure with reduced ejection fraction
C. Ischemic stroke
D. Pulmonary hypertension
E. Ventricular fibrillation

ANSWERS AND EXPLANATIONS

3.1. The correct answer is D. Epanova is indicated as an adjunct to diet to reduce triglyceride levels in adult patients with severe hypertriglyceridemia ($\geq$500 mg/dl). This is currently the only indication approved by the US FDA for Epanova as well as Vascepa and Lovaza, and the approval was based on the demonstrated efficacy in this patient group.

3.2. The correct answer is E. Among the current US FDA-approved omega-3 fatty acid-based drugs, only Vascepa contains 100% eicosapentaenoic acid (EPA). The other drugs (Lovaza, Epanova, Omtryg) contain both EPA and docosahexaenoic acid (DHA) as active ingredients. Liptruzet is a fixed-dose combination of ezetimibe and atorvastatin.

3.3. The correct answer is C. Among the three omega-3 fatty acid-based drugs, Lovaza has the highest potential to cause elevation of LDL cholesterol, followed by Epanova. Vascepa (containing only EPA) does not increase LDL cholesterol. It is believed that the DHA component in the Lovaza as well as Epanova is responsible for the elevation of LDL cholesterol. Liptruzet is a fixed-dose combination of ezetimibe and atorvastatin that causes dramatic reduction of LDL cholesterol. Mipomersen is also an LDL cholesterol-lowering drug (refer to Chapter 2 for details on these cholesterol-lowering drugs).

3.4. The correct answer is C. However, it remains unknown if GPR120 also mediates the triglyceride-lowering activity of Epanova as well as Vascepa and Lovaza. Cholesteryl ester transfer protein (CETP) is the target of investigational drug, known as anacetrapib. Proprotein convertase subtilisin/kexin type 9 (PCSK9) is the molecular target of a new class of cholesterol-lowering drugs, known as PCSK9 inhibitors. Epidermal growth factor receptor is the molecular target of many new anticancer agents, such as gefitinib and erlotinib (for treating non-small cell lung cancer).

3.5. The correct answer is B. A well-known randomized controlled trial (GISSI-HF) with 6,975 patients with chronic heart failure on standard therapy demonstrated that supplementation with omega-3 fatty acids (1 g daily) for a median of 3.9 years led to a small, but statistically significant 8–9% reduction in mortality and admission to hospital for cardiovascular reasons. The evidence supporting a role for omega-3 fatty acids in the other disorders listed (e.g., heart failure with preserved ejection fraction, ischemic stroke, pulmonary hypertension, and ventricular fibrillation) is currently lacking.

REFERENCES

1. Jorgensen AB, Frikke-Schmidt R, Nordestgaard BG, Tybjaerg-Hansen A. Loss-of-function mutations in APOC3 and risk of ischemic vascular disease. *N Engl J Med* 2014; 371(1):32–41.

2. Dewey FE, Gusarova V, O'Dushlaine C, Gottesman O, Trejos J, Hunt C, Van Hout CV, Habegger L, Buckler D, Lai KM, Leader JB, Murray MF, et al. Inactivating variants in ANGPTL4 and risk of coronary artery disease. *N Engl J Med* 2016; 374(12):1123–33.

3. Dewey FE, Gusarova V, Dunbar RL, O'Dushlaine C, Schurmann C, Gottesman O, McCarthy S, Van Hout CV, Bruse S, Dansky HM, Leader JB, Murray MF, et al. Genetic and pharmacologic inactivation of ANGPTL3 and cardiovascular disease. *N Engl J Med* 2017; 377(3):211–21.

4. Nordestgaard BG, Varbo A. Triglycerides and cardiovascular disease. *Lancet* 2014; 384(9943):626–35.

5. Rosenson RS, Davidson MH, Hirsh BJ, Kathiresan S, Gaudet D. Genetics and causality of triglyceride-rich lipoproteins in atherosclerotic cardiovascular disease. *J Am Coll Cardiol* 2014; 64(23):2525–40.

6. Nordestgaard BG. Triglyceride-rich lipoproteins and atherosclerotic cardiovascular disease: new insights from epidemiology, genetics, and biology. *Circ Res* 2016; 118(4):547–63.

7. Albert CM, Campos H, Stampfer MJ, Ridker PM, Manson JE, Willett WC, Ma J. Blood levels of long-chain n-3 fatty acids and the risk of sudden death. *N Engl J Med* 2002; 346(15):1113–8.

8. Mozaffarian D, Rimm EB. Fish intake, contaminants, and human health: evaluating the risks and the benefits. *JAMA* 2006; 296(15):1885–99.

9. GISSI-Prevenzione Investigators (Gruppo Italiano per lo Studio della Sopravvivenza nell'Infarto miocardico). Dietary supplementation with n-3 polyunsaturated fatty acids and vitamin E after myocardial infarction: results of the GISSI-Prevenzione trial. *Lancet* 1999; 354(9177):447–55.

10. Chaddha A, Eagle KA. Cardiology patient page. omega-3 fatty acids and heart health. *Circulation* 2015; 132(22):e350–2.

11. De Caterina R. n-3 Fatty acids in cardiovascular disease. *N Engl J Med* 2011; 364(25):2439–50.

12. Kastelein JJ, Maki KC, Susekov A, Ezhov M, Nordestgaard BG, Machielse BN, Kling D, Davidson MH. Omega-3 free fatty acids for the treatment of severe hypertriglyceridemia: the Epanova for lowering very high triglycerides (EVOLVE) trial. *J Clin Lipidol* 2014; 8(1):94–106.

13. Ballantyne CM, Bays HE, Braeckman RA, Philip S, Stirtan WG, Doyle RT, Jr., Soni PN, Juliano RA. Icosapent ethyl (eicosapentaenoic acid ethyl ester): effects on plasma apolipoprotein C-III levels in patients from the MARINE and ANCHOR studies. *J Clin Lipidol* 2016; 10(3):635–45 e1.

14. Morton AM, Furtado JD, Lee J, Amerine W, Davidson MH, Sacks FM. The effect of omega-3 carboxylic acids on apolipoprotein CIII-containing lipoproteins in severe hypertriglyceridemia. *J Clin Lipidol* 2016; 10(6):1442–51 e4.

15. Oh DY, Talukdar S, Bae EJ, Imamura T, Morinaga H, Fan W, Li P, Lu WJ, Watkins SM, Olefsky JM. GPR120 is an omega-3 fatty acid receptor mediating potent anti-inflammatory and insulin-sensitizing effects. *Cell* 2010; 142(5):687–98.

16. Oh DY, Olefsky JM. Omega 3 fatty acids and GPR120. *Cell Metab* 2012; 15(5):564–5.

17. Oh DY, Walenta E, Akiyama TE, Lagakos WS, Lackey D, Pessentheiner AR, Sasik R, Hah N, Chi TJ, Cox JM, Powels MA, Di Salvo J, et al. A GPR120-selective agonist improves insulin resistance and chronic inflammation in obese mice. *Nat Med* 2014; 20(8):942–7.

18. Theobald HE, Chowienczyk PJ, Whittall R, Humphries SE, Sanders TA. LDL cholesterol-raising effect of low-dose docosahexaenoic acid in middle-aged men and women. *Am J Clin Nutr* 2004; 79(4):558–63.

19. Ballantyne CM, Braeckman RA, Bays HE, Kastelein JJ, Otvos JD, Stirtan WG, Doyle RT, Jr., Soni PN, Juliano RA. Effects of icosapent ethyl on lipoprotein particle concentration and size in statin-treated patients with persistent high triglycerides (the ANCHOR study). *J Clin Lipidol* 2015; 9(3):377–83.

20. Risk and Prevention Study Collaborative Group, Roncaglioni MC, Tombesi M, Avanzini F, Barlera S, Caimi V, Longoni P, Marzona I, Milani V, Silletta MG, Tognoni G, et al. n-3 Fatty acids in patients with multiple cardiovascular risk factors. *N Engl J Med* 2013; 368(19):1800–8.

21. Tavazzi L, Maggioni AP, Marchioli R, Barlera S, Franzosi MG, Latini R, Lucci D, Nicolosi GL, Porcu M, Tognoni G, GISSI-HF Investigators. Effect of n-3 polyunsaturated fatty acids in patients with chronic heart failure (the GISSI-HF trial): a randomised, double-blind, placebo-controlled trial. *Lancet* 2008; 372(9645):1223–30.

22. Heydari B, Abdullah S, Pottala JV, Shah R, Abbasi S, Mandry D, Francis SA, Lumish H, Ghoshhajra BB, Hoffmann U, Appelbaum E, Feng JH, et al. Effect of omega-3 acid ethyl esters on left ventricular remodeling after acute myocardial infarction: the OMEGA-REMODEL randomized clinical trial. *Circulation* 2016; 134(5):378–91.

23. Siscovick DS, Barringer TA, Fretts AM, Wu JH, Lichtenstein AH, Costello RB, Kris-Etherton PM, Jacobson TA, Engler MB, Alger HM, Appel LJ, Mozaffarian D, et al. Omega-3 polyunsaturated fatty acid (fish oil) supplementation and the prevention of clinical cardiovascular disease: a science advisory from the American Heart Association. *Circulation* 2017; 135(15):e867–e84.

24. Bisgaard H, Stokholm J, Chawes BL, Vissing NH, Bjarnadottir E, Schoos AM, Wolsk HM, Pedersen TM, Vinding RK, Thorsteinsdottir S, Folsgaard NV, Fink NR, et al. Fish oil-derived fatty acids in pregnancy and wheeze and asthma in offspring. *N Engl J Med* 2016; 375(26):2530–9.

25. Sala-Vila A, Diaz-Lopez A, Valls-Pedret C, Cofan M, Garcia-Layana A, Lamuela-Raventos RM, Castaner O, Zanon-Moreno V, Martinez-Gonzalez MA, Toledo E, Basora J, Salas-Salvado J, et al. Dietary marine omega-3 fatty acids and incident sight-threatening retinopathy in middle-aged and older individuals with type 2 diabetes: prospective investigation from the PREDIMED trial. *JAMA Ophthalmol* 2016; 134(10):1142–9.

26. Ridker PM, Everett BM, Thuren T, MacFadyen JG, Chang WH, Ballantyne C, Fonseca F, Nicolau J, Koenig W, Anker SD, Kastelein JJP, Cornel JH, et al. Antiinflammatory therapy with canakinumab for atherosclerotic disease. *N Engl J Med* 2017; 377(12):1119–31.

27. Harrington RA. Targeting inflammation in coronary artery disease. *N Engl J Med* 2017; 377(12):1197–8.

28. Westman PC, Lipinski MJ, Luger D, Waksman R, Bonow RO, Wu E, Epstein SE. Inflammation as a driver of adverse left ventricular remodeling after acute myocardial infarction. *J Am Coll Cardiol* 2016; 67(17):2050–60.

29. Niemann B, Rohrbach S, Miller MR, Newby DE, Fuster V, Kovacic JC. Oxidative stress and cardiovascular risk: obesity, diabetes, smoking, and pollution: part 3 of a 3-part series. *J Am Coll Cardiol* 2017; 70(2):230–51.

30. McCracken JL, Veeranki SP, Ameredes BT, Calhoun WJ. Diagnosis and management of asthma in adults: a review. *JAMA* 2017; 318(3):279–90.

UNIT II

SYSTEMIC HYPERTENSION

CHAPTER 4

Overview of Hypertension and Drug Therapy

CHAPTER HIGHLIGHTS

- Hypertension, if not specified, typically refers to systemic arterial hypertension. It is a major risk factor for myocardial infarction, stroke, heart failure, renal failure, and death.
- Hypertension is defined as systolic pressure ≥140 mm Hg and/or diastolic pressure ≥90 mm Hg. It is estimated to affect over 85 million American adults (one in every three adults) and one to two billion people worldwide.
- Dysregulation of the sympathetic nervous system and the renin-angiotensin-aldosterone system (RAAS) has been recognized as the key pathophysiology underlying the genesis and progression of hypertension, and as such, serves as the major target for antihypertensive therapy.
- The commonly used antihypertensive drugs include diuretics, sympatholytics (e.g., β-blockers), RAAS inhibitors, and direct vasodilators. Effective management of hypertension frequently requires combination of two or more antihypertensive drugs from different drug classes.

KEYWORDS | Antihypertensive drugs; Diuretics; Epidemiology; Hypertension; Molecular pathophysiology; Renin-angiotensin-aldosterone system inhibitors; Sympatholytics; Vasodilators

CITATION | *Li YR. Cardiovascular Medicine: New Therapeutic Drugs Approved by the US FDA (2013–2017). Cell Med Press, Raleigh, NC, USA. 2018. http://dx.doi.org/10.20455/ndcvd.2018.04*

ABBREVIATIONS | ACEI, angiotensin-converting enzyme inhibitor; ARB, angiotensin receptor blocker; CCB, calcium channel blocker; CKD, chronic kidney disease; DRI, direct renin inhibitor; HCT, hydrochlorothiazide; JNC7, the Seventh Report of the Joint National Committee on the Prevention, Detection, Evaluation, and Treatment of High Blood Pressure; OSA, obstructive sleep apnea; RAAS, renin-angiotensin-aldosterone system; ROS, reactive oxygen species; US FDA, the United States Food and Drug Administration

CHAPTER AT A GLANCE

1. INTRODUCTION

Hypertension is the most common condition seen in primary care settings. It is a major risk factor for myocardial infarction, stroke, heart failure, renal failure, and death, if not detected early and treated appropriately. Recent advances in risk factor identification, molecular pathophysiology, and evidence based therapies, especially pharmacological agents, have led to significant improvement of hypertension management. To set a stage for the subsequent discussion of the new antihypertensive drugs approved by the United States Food and Drug Administration (US FDA), this chapter provides an overview on several aspects of hypertension, including definition, epidemiology, pathophysiology, and mechanistically based drug therapy.

2. MOLECULAR MEDICINE OF HYPERTENSION

Hypertension, when not specified, typically refers to increased blood pressure in systemic circulation, and hence is also known as systemic arterial hypertension. In addition to systemic circulation, hypertension also occurs in pulmonary and portal circulations. Pulmonary hypertension, a less common form of hypertension, refers to an abnormal elevation in pulmonary artery pressure. It may be the result of left-sided heart failure, pulmonary parenchymal or vascular disease, thromboembolism, or a combination of these factors [5]. Pulmonary hypertension is the most common cause of right ventricular enlargement and failure (see Chapters 6 and 7 for details on pulmonary hypertension). This section defines systemic arterial hypertension and provides an overview of its epidemiology. As noted above, the term hypertension is used to refer to the systemic arterial hypertension throughout this chapter.

2.1. Definitions and Classifications

2.1.1. The JNC 7 Classification of Blood Pressure

Hypertension, also known as high blood pressure, is defined as systolic pressure ≥140 mm Hg and/or diastolic pressure ≥90 mm Hg. Based on the JNC7 (the Seventh Report of the Joint National Committee on the Prevention, Detection, Evaluation, and Treatment of High Blood Pressure), blood pressure is classified into 4 categories (**Table 4.1**). According to the JNC7, hypertension is further classified into two stages, i.e., stage 1 and stage 2.

2.1.2. Hypertension Crisis

Hypertension crisis is a term to refer to critical clinical conditions of severely elevated blood pressure. Hypertension crisis can present as hypertensive urgency or as hypertensive emergency. Hypertensive urgency is a situation where the blood pressure is severely elevated (≥180 mm Hg for systolic pressure or ≥110 mm Hg for diastolic pressure), but there is no associated organ damage. Individuals experiencing hypertensive urgency may or may not experience one or more

JNC

The major guidelines on hypertension management in the United States are issued by the Joint National Committee on Prevention, Detection, Evaluation, and Treatment of High Blood Pressure (JNC), a group coordinated by the National Heart, Lung, and Blood Institute. The first report, known as JNC1, was published in 1976. The seventh report, known as JNC7, is considered the most comprehensive guideline on hypertension management, which was initially published in 2003 and then updated in 2004. The long-awaiting JNC8 guideline was released in early 2014. Listed below is the history of the various versions of the JNC guidelines.
- JNC8: published in 2014
- JNC7: published in 2003
- JNC6: published in 1997
- JNC5: published in 1992
- JNC4: published in 1988
- JNC3: published in 1984
- JNC2: published in 1980
- JNC1: published in 1976

TABLE 4.1. The JNC7 classification of blood pressure

Blood pressure classification	Systolic blood pressure (mm Hg)	Diastolic blood pressure (mm Hg)
Normal	<120	and <80
Prehypertension	120–139	or 80–89
Stage 1 hypertension	140–159	or 90–99
Stage 2 hypertension	≥160	or ≥100

of these symptoms: severe headache, shortness of breath, nosebleeds, and severe anxiety.

The term hypertensive emergency refers to severely elevated blood pressure levels that are damaging organs, which can be manifested as stroke, myocardial infarction, renal failure, and loss of consciousness. Hypertensive emergencies generally occur at blood pressure levels exceeding 180 mm Hg (systolic) or 120 mm Hg (diastolic), but can also occur at even lower levels in patients whose blood pressure had not been previously high.

2.1.3. Primary and Secondary Hypertension

Based on the etiologies, hypertension is classified into primary and secondary hypertension. In 90–95% of hypertensive patients, a single reversible cause of the elevated blood pressure cannot be identified, and hence, the patients are said to have primary (or essential) hypertension. In the remaining 5–10% cases, a cause can be identified, and hence, the patients are said to have secondary hypertension. Some of the common causes of secondary hypertension are outlined below and the underlying mechanisms are given in **Table 4.2**. Other causes of secondary hypertension include thyroid disorder, sleep apnea, obesity, pregnancy, and medications.

- *Kidney diseases, especially chronic kidney disease*: Chronic kidney disease (CKD) refers to a condition of decreased kidney function shown by glomerular filtration rate (GFR) of less than 60 ml/min per 1.73 m^2, or markers of kidney damage, or both, of at least 3 months duration, regardless of the underlying cause [1]. On the one hand, diabetes and hypertension are the main causes of CKD in all high-income and middle-income countries, and also in many low-income nations. On the other hand, CKD is one of the most common causes of secondary hypertension [2, 3]. Thus, hypertension and CDK are two closely intertwined conditions that are risk factors for each other. Other kidney diseases that may also cause hypertension include renal artery stenosis, glomerular kidney disease, and polycystic kidney disease.
- *Primary aldosteronism*: Primary aldosteronism is a heterogeneous group of disorders characterized by hypertension and aldosterone overproduction relatively autonomous from the renin-angiotensin system. It is a frequent cause of secondary hypertension, even in

the general population of patients with hypertension [4, 5]. It is also a common cause of resistant hypertension [6].

■ *Cushing's syndrome*: Cushing's syndrome results from chronic exposure to excess glucocorticoids, which can be from either exogenous pharmacological doses of corticosteroids or from an endogenous source of cortisol [7]. Hypertension is one of the most distinguishing features of endogenous Cushing's syndrome, as it is present in most adult patients and in almost half of children and adolescent patients [8, 9].

■ *Obstructive sleep apnea (OSA)*: An apnea is the absence of inspiratory airflow for at least 10 seconds. OSA occurs when complete upper airway occlusion occurs (absent airflow, tongue falling backward) in the face of continued activity of inspiratory thoracic pump muscles. OSA affects 34% of men and 17% of women and is largely undiagnosed, and it is a cause of hypertension and associated with an increased incidence of stroke, heart failure, atrial fibrillation, and coronary heart disease [10]. More than 70% of patients with resistant hypertension have OSA, and effective treatment of OSA improves blood pressure [11, 12].

■ *Pheochromocytomas*: Pheochromocytomas are rare neuroendocrine tumors with a highly variable clinical presentation but most commonly presenting with episodes of headaches, sweating, palpitations, and hypertension [13].

TABLE 4.2. Major mechanisms of secondary hypertension

Cause	Major mechanism
Kidney diseases	Increased renin release due to decreased renal perfusion
Primary aldosteronism	Water and salt retention due to increased levels of aldosterone
Cushing's syndrome	Water and salt retention due to increased release of corticosteroids
Obstructive sleep apnea	Intermittent hypoxia leading to increased oxidative stress, systemic inflammation, and sympathetic activity
Pheochromocytomas	Release of catecholamines from the tumors of the adrenal chromaffin cells

2.2. Epidemiology and Health Impact of Hypertension

2.2.1. Epidemiology

Hypertension, or raised blood pressure, currently affects over 85 million American adults (one in three adults) [14] and is estimated to affect one to two billion people worldwide [15, 16]. Hypertension is the biggest single contributor to the global burden of disease and to global mortality [17]. Many risk factors for development of hypertension have been identified, including age, ethnicity, family history of hypertension and genetic factors, lower education and socioeconomic status, greater weight, lower physical activity, tobacco use,

psychosocial stressors, sleep apnea, and dietary factors (including dietary fats, higher sodium intake, lower potassium intake, and excessive alcohol intake) [17, 18].

Notably, the prevalence of hypertension in people of African heritage in the United States is among the highest in the world; 41% of the total African American population and 44% of African American women have hypertension. Moreover, a recent study reported that African Americans, compared with Caucasians, also appear to be more susceptible to stroke, given the same level of elevated blood pressure. African Americans have more hypertension and are less likely to have it controlled, and when it is not controlled they are at greater risk for incident stroke (relative to Caucasians with the same blood pressure levels) [19].

2.2.2. Health Impact

Hypertension remains the most common, readily identifiable, and reversible risk factor for myocardial infarction, stroke, heart failure, and kidney diseases [20, 21]. Hypertension exerts remarkable health impact at both individual and population levels. For example, a 50-year-old man of normal body mass with blood pressure of 146/86 mm Hg has:

- almost 3 times the risk of dying from a heart attack,
- almost 4 times the risk of dying from a stroke,
- about twice the risk of developing heart failure, and
- about 3 times the risk of developing kidney disease than if he had normal blood pressure (<120/80 mm Hg).

Similarly, a 40-year-old woman of normal body mass with blood pressure of 146/86 mm Hg has:

- more than 3 times the risk of dying from a heart attack,
- almost 4 times the risk of dying from a stroke,
- about 3 times the risk of developing heart failure, and
- about 3 times the risk of developing kidney disease than if she had normal blood pressure (<120/80 mm Hg).

Approximately 69% of people who have a first myocardial infarction, 77% of those who have a first stroke, and 74% of those who have congestive heart failure have blood pressure >140/90 mm Hg. Compared with hypertensive individuals at 50 years of age, people with untreated blood pressure <140/90 mm Hg survive on average 7 years longer without cardiovascular diseases [14, 22]. In addition to the >85 million hypertensive patients in the United States, more than 36% of the American adults have prehypertension. Although prehypertension is not hypertension, it is associated with stroke [23] and estimated to decrease life expectancy by approximately 5 years [24].

2.3. Pathophysiology of Hypertension

To understand the molecular pathophysiology of hypertension, it is necessary to review the physiology of blood pressure regulation.

2.3.1. Physiology of Blood Pressure Regulation

Blood pressure is the product of cardiac output and peripheral vascular resistance (**Figure 4.1**). Therefore, factors that affect either the cardiac output or the peripheral resistance, or both will impact blood pressure. As blood pressure is vital, its regulation is tightly controlled with the coordinated involvement of many organs and pathways. As described below, when blood pressure drops, several systems or pathways become activated to cause increased cardiac output and peripheral resistance, and thereby the consequent recovery of the blood pressure.

2.3.1.1. THE SYMPATHETIC NERVOUS SYSTEM

A decrease in blood pressure activates the baroreceptor reflex, causing increased activities of the sympathetic nervous system. The activation of the sympathetic nervous system results in recovery of blood pressure via the following 3 major mechanisms [25]:

- Increased heart rate and contractility, leading to augmented cardiac output
- Constriction of blood vessels, leading to increased peripheral vascular resistance
- Activation of β_1-adrenergic receptors on renal juxtaglomerular cells, causing increased release of renin and the subsequent activation of the renin-angiotensin-aldosterone system (see Section 2.3.1.2 below)

2.3.1.2. THE RENIN-ANGIOTENSIN-ALDOSTERONE SYSTEM

As noted above, activation of the sympathetic nervous system due to blood pressure drop increases the release of renin and the subsequent activation of the renin-angiotensin-aldosterone system (RAAS). Hence, activation of the sympathetic nervous system is always coupled with the concomitant activation of the RAAS. In addition, increased renin release also occurs as a result of the decreased renal arterial pressure (or renal perfusion pressure). When the RAAS becomes activated, the following events result, contributing to the recovery of blood pressure:

- Constriction of arterials caused by angiotensin II, leading to increased peripheral vascular resistance
- Increased water and salt retention due to increased levels of aldosterone, leading to increased blood volume and hence the cardiac output

2.3.1.3. THE VASOPRESSIN SYSTEM

A decrease in arterial pressure causes increased release of vasopressin via the baroreflex mechanism. This results in increased water retention and thereby the increased blood volume and cardiac output. The increased blood volume and cardiac output lead to elevation of blood pressure.

2.3.1.4. FLUID RETENTION BY THE KIDNEYS

A decrease in renal arterial pressure also causes less excretion of water and salt by the kidneys. This increases blood volume and cardiac output.

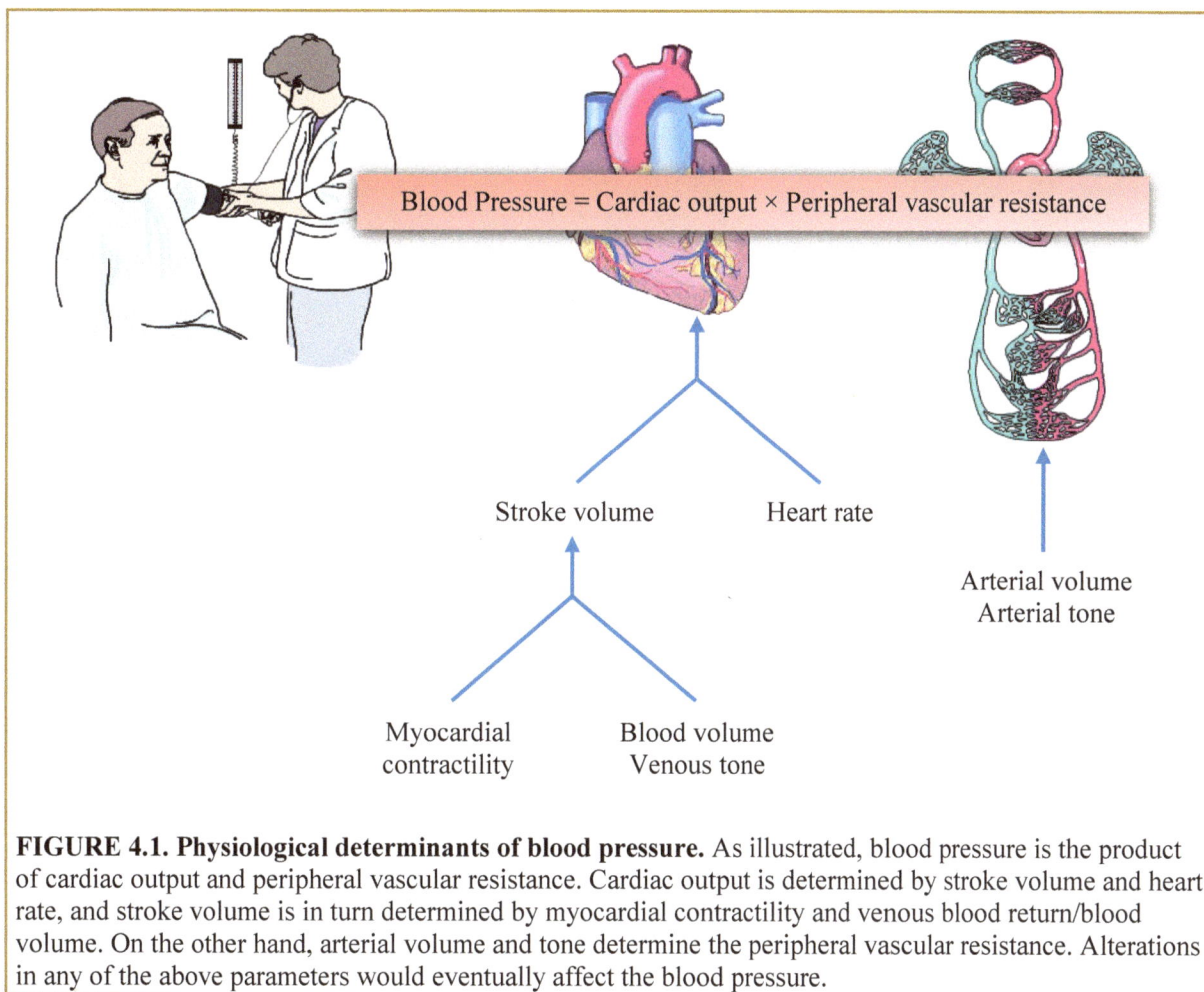

Blood Pressure = Cardiac output × Peripheral vascular resistance

Stroke volume   Heart rate

Arterial volume
Arterial tone

Myocardial
contractility

Blood volume
Venous tone

FIGURE 4.1. Physiological determinants of blood pressure. As illustrated, blood pressure is the product of cardiac output and peripheral vascular resistance. Cardiac output is determined by stroke volume and heart rate, and stroke volume is in turn determined by myocardial contractility and venous blood return/blood volume. On the other hand, arterial volume and tone determine the peripheral vascular resistance. Alterations in any of the above parameters would eventually affect the blood pressure.

2.3.2. Molecular Pathophysiology of Hypertension Development

2.3.2.1. OVERVIEW

As noted earlier, 90–95% hypertension cases are without identifiable causes. Mechanistic studies over the last decades have revealed a critical involvement of both the sympathetic nervous system and the RAAS in the genesis and progression of hypertension [25–28]. Indeed, these two systems serve as targets of many current antihypertensive drugs. In addition, endothelial dysfunction and oxidative stress also serve as important pathophysiological mechanisms of hypertension (**Figure 4.2**).

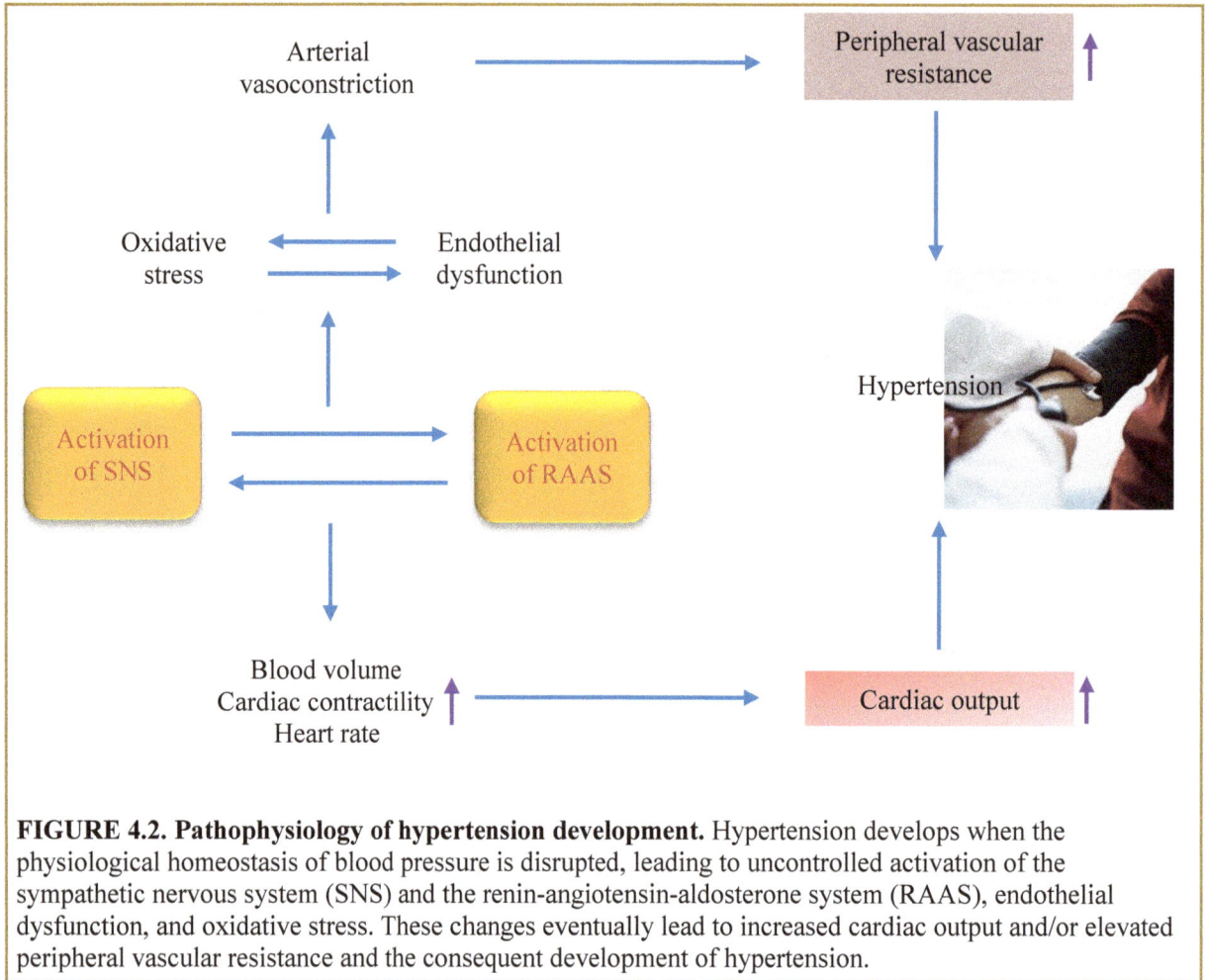

FIGURE 4.2. Pathophysiology of hypertension development. Hypertension develops when the physiological homeostasis of blood pressure is disrupted, leading to uncontrolled activation of the sympathetic nervous system (SNS) and the renin-angiotensin-aldosterone system (RAAS), endothelial dysfunction, and oxidative stress. These changes eventually lead to increased cardiac output and/or elevated peripheral vascular resistance and the consequent development of hypertension.

2.3.2.2. CROSS-TALK

Notably, the above mechanisms are closely related and there is extensive cross-talk between them. For example, as mentioned earlier, activation of the sympathetic nervous system causes activation of the RAAS. RAAS activation also increases the activity of the sympathetic nervous system. Activation of RAAS contributes to endothelial dysfunction and vascular remodeling. Endothelial dysfunction characterized by decreased nitric oxide bioavailability and increased formation of endothelin plays an important role in the development and progression of hypertension.

2.3.2.3. OXIDATIVE STRESS AS A POTENTIAL FINAL COMMON PATHWAY

Activation of the sympathetic nervous system and RAAS also results in increased formation of reactive oxygen species (ROS). On the one hand, ROS directly cause damage and dysfunction of endothelium. On the other hand, ROS, such as superoxide, react with nitric oxide, forming more reactive species, and at the same time decreasing the

Reactive oxygen species (ROS)
ROS is a term frequently encountered in biology and medicine. This term can be simply defined as oxygen-containing reactive species. It is a collective term to include superoxide ($O_2^{\cdot-}$), hydrogen peroxide (H_2O_2), hydroxyl radical ($OH^{\cdot}$), singlet oxygen ($^{1}O_2$), peroxyl radical ($LOO^{\cdot}$), alkoxyl radical ($LO^{\cdot}$), lipid hydroperoxide ($LOOH$), peroxynitrite ($ONOO^{-}$), hypochlorous acid ($HOCl$), and ozone (O_3), among others. ROS are double-edged swords exerting both physiological and pathophysiological effects.

bioavailability of nitric oxide, leading to endothelial dysfunction. In both experimental models and human subjects, administration of antioxidant compounds has been shown to have antihypertensive effects via decreasing ROS formation or increasing the levels of nitric oxide. Accordingly, antioxidant compounds are emerging therapeutic modalities for hypertension [29, 30].

TABLE 4.3. Historical overview of the development of drug therapy for hypertension

Time	Drug therapy of hypertension
1940s	Potassium thiocyanate Kempner diet (rice and fruits; low in calories, fat, protein, and sodium) Lumbodorsal sympathectomy
1950s	*Rauwolfia serpentina* (a plant containing a number of bioactive chemicals, including yohimbine, reserpine, ajmaline, deserpidine, rescinnamine, serpentinine) Ganglionic blockers Veratrum alkaloids Hydralazine Guanethidine Thiazide diuretics
1960s	α_2-Adrenergic receptor agonists Spironolactone β-Adrenergic receptor antagonists
1970s	α_1-Adrenergic receptor antagonists Angiotensin-converting enzyme inhibitors
1980s	Calcium channel blockers
1990s	Angiotensin receptor blockers Endothelin receptor blockers (for pulmonary hypertension)
2000s	Renin inhibitors (aliskiren)
2010s	Byvalson (a fixed-dose combination of nebivolol and valsartan)

Note: This table is primarily based on Ref. [31] with modifications.

3. OVERVIEW OF MECHANISTICALLY BASED DRUG THERAPY

3.1. Historical Overview

The treatment of hypertension has been one of medicine's major successes of the past half-century. Since the introduction of the thiazide diuretics in the late 1950s, many classes of antihypertensive drugs have been developed and approved for clinical use (**Table 4.3**) [31].

Five of these, namely, diuretics, β-blockers, angiotensin-converting enzyme inhibitors, calcium channel blockers, and angiotensin receptor blockers, now represent the primary treatment options for hypertension [32, 33].

3.2. Mechanistic Overview

As blood pressure is determined by cardiac output and peripheral vascular resistance, antihypertensive drugs regardless of their chemical classes achieve their blood pressure-lowering effects by eventually decreasing either cardiac output or peripheral vascular resistance, or both. As listed below and further described in **Table 4.4**, there are four major categories of antihypertensive agents.

- Diuretics
- Sympatholytics
- RAAS inhibitors
- Direct vasodilators

TABLE 4.4. Four major categories of antihypertensive drugs and their mechanisms of action

Drug category	Mechanism of action
Diuretics - Thiazides and related diuretics - Loop diuretics - Potassium-sparing diuretics (PSDs)	- Diuretics decrease plasma volume, leading to reduced cardiac output - Diuretics, especially thiazide diuretics reduce peripheral resistance - PSDs eplerenone and spironolactone block aldosterone receptors - PSDs amiloride and triamterene inhibit Na^+ reabsorption by apical membrane Na^+ channel in the collecting duct
Sympatholytics - α-Blockers - β-Blockers - Centrally acting drugs	- Blockage of peripheral α-receptors causes peripheral vasodilation and decreased peripheral vascular resistance - Blockage of $β_1$-receptors decreases heart rate and stroke volume, leading to decreased cardiac output - Blockage of $β_1$-receptors decreases renin release, leading to decreased activation of RAAS - Centrally acting drugs decrease the sympathetic outflow from the brain to peripheral tissues, leading to decreased peripheral vascular resistance and reduced activation of RAAS
RAAS inhibitors - Angiotensin-converting enzyme inhibitors (ACEIs) - Angiotensin receptor blockers (ARBs) - Renin inhibitors - Aldosterone receptor blockers	- ACEIs decrease the formation of angiotensin II, and reduce angiotensin II-mediated vasoconstriction and aldosterone production - ARBs suppress the effects of angiotensin II on vasculature by blocking the angiotensin II type 1 receptors - Renin inhibitors decrease the conversion of angiotensinogen to angiotensin I, thereby leading to decreased activity of RAAS - Aldosterone receptor blockers block the actions of aldosterone
Direct vasodilators - Calcium channel blockers (CCBs) - Other direct vasodilators	- CCBs cause vasodilation, decreasing peripheral vascular resistance - Some CCBs also suppress cardiac contractility, decreasing cardiac output - Other direct vasodilators cause vasodilation, reducing peripheral vascular resistance

3.3. Overview of the US FDA-Approved Antihypertensive Drugs

The commonly used antihypertensive agents, their initial US FDA approval data, and major indications are listed in **Tables 4.5–4.9**. Effective management of hypertension, especially stage 2 hypertension frequently needs combination of two or more drugs from different drug classes that act via different mechanisms. Some of the fixed-dose combination drugs are given in **Tables 4.10** and **4.11**.

TABLE 4.5. Diuretics in treating hypertension

Diuretics	FDA approval date	Major indication
Thiazide and thiazide-like diuretics		
Chlorthalidone (Hygroton)	Prior to January 1, 1982	Hypertension; edema
Chlorothiazide (Diuril)	Prior to January 1, 1982	Hypertension; edema
Hydrochlorothiazide (Esidrix)	Prior to January 1, 1982	Hypertension; edema
Indapamide (Lozol)	July 1983	Hypertension; edema
Metolazone (Mykrox)	Prior to January 1, 1982	Hypertension; edema
Loop diuretics		
Bumetanide (Bumex)	February 1983	Edema; (hypertension is not listed as a US FDA-approved indication)
Ethacrynic acid (Edecrin)	Prior to January 1, 1982	Edema; (hypertension is not listed as a US FDA-approved indication)
Furosemide (Lasix)	Prior to January 1, 1982	Edema; hypertension (e.g., malignant hypertension and volume-based hypertension in patients with advanced kidney disease)
Torsemide (Demadex)	August 1993	Edema; hypertension (e.g., malignant hypertension and volume-based hypertension in patients with advanced kidney disease)
Potassium-sparing diuretics		
Amiloride (Midamor)	Prior to January 1, 1982	As adjunctive treatment with thiazide diuretics or other kaliuretic diuretic agents in congestive heart failure or hypertension to prevent hypokalemia
Triamterene (Dyrenium)	Prior to January 1, 1982	Edema
Eplerenone (Inspra)	September 2002	Heart failure; hypertension
Spironolactone (Aldactone)	Prior to January 1, 1982	Primary hyperaldosteronism; hypertension; edema; hypokalemia; heart failure

Note: Loop diuretics are not useful in treating chronic hypertension due to lack of outcome data. However, these drugs may be useful under certain conditions, such as malignant hypertension and volume-based hypertension in patients with advanced kidney disease to achieve a rapid blood pressure reduction.

TABLE 4.6. RAAS inhibitors for treating hypertension

RAAS Inhibitor	FDA approval date	Major indication
ACE inhibitors		
Benazepril (Lotensin)	June 1991	Hypertension
Captopril (Capoten)	Prior to January 1, 1982	Hypertension; heart failure; left ventricular dysfunction after myocardial infarction; diabetic nephropathy
Enalapril (Vasotec)	February 1988	Hypertension; heart failure; asymptomatic left ventricular dysfunction
Enalaprilat (Vasotec injection)	February 1988	Hypertension when oral therapy is not practical
Fosinopril (Monopril)	May 1991	Hypertension; heart failure
Lisinopril (Prinivil)	December 1987	Hypertension; heart failure; acute myocardial infarction
Moexipril (Univasc)	April 1995	Hypertension
Perindopril (Aceon)	December 1993	Hypertension; stable coronary artery disease
Quinapril (Accupril)	November 1991	Hypertension; heart failure
Ramipril (Altace)	January 1991	Hypertension
Trandolapril (Mavik)	April 1996	Hypertension; heart failure post myocardial infarction; left ventricular dysfunction post myocardial infarction
Angiotensin AT1 receptor blockers (ARBs)		
Azilsartan (Edarbi)	February 2011	Hypertension
Candesartan (Atacand)	June 1998	Hypertension; heart failure
Eprosartan (Teveten)	December 1997	Hypertension
Irbesartan (Avapro)	September 1997	Hypertension; diabetic nephropathy
Losartan (Cozaar)	April 1995	Hypertension; hypertensive patients with left ventricular hypertrophy
Olmesartan (Benicar)	April 2002	Hypertension
Telmisartan (Micardis)	November 1998	Hypertension
Valsartan (Diovan)	December 1996	Hypertension; heart failure
Direct renin inhibitors (DRIs)		
Aliskiren (Tekturna)	March 2007	Hypertension

Note: Aliskiren is the first-in-class and currently the only member of the direct renin inhibitor drug class approved by the US FDA. It is also the second newest member of the RAAS inhibitors. Azilsartan is currently the newest member of the RAAS inhibitors, which was approved by the US FDA in 2011. The aldosterone receptor antagonists eplerenone and spironolactone, which are not listed here (see potassium-sparing diuretics in Table 4.5.), are also classified as RAAS inhibitors.

TABLE 4.7. Calcium channel blockers (CCBs) for treating hypertension

Drug	FDA approval date	Major indication
Dihydropyridine CCBs		
Amlodipine (Norvasc)	December 1987	Hypertension; chronic stable angina and vasospastic angina
Felodipine (Plendil)	July 1991	Hypertension
Isradipine (DynaCirc)	December 1990	Hypertension
Nicardipine (Cardene)	December 1988	Hypertension; chronic stable angina
Nifedipine (Adalat)	Prior to January 1, 1982	Hypertension; chronic stable angina and vasospastic angina
Nisoldipine (Sular)	February 1995	Hypertension
Nondihydropyridine CCBs		
Diltiazem (Cardizem)	November 1982	Hypertension; chronic stable angina and vasospastic angina; cardiac arrhythmias
Verapamil (Calan)	Prior to January 1, 1982	Hypertension; chronic stable angina and vasospastic angina; cardiac arrhythmias

Note: Nimodipine (not listed here) is indicated for the improvement of neurological outcome by reducing the incidence and severity of ischemic deficits in patients with subarachnoid hemorrhage from ruptured intracranial berry aneurysms. It is not indicated for treating hypertension.

TABLE 4.8. β-Blockers for treating hypertension

Drug	FDA approval date	Major indication
Classical β-blockers		
Atenolol (Tenormin)	Prior to January 1, 1982	Hypertension; angina pectoris; acute myocardial infarction
Betaxolol (Kerlone)	August 1985	Hypertension
Bisoprolol (Zebeta)	July 1992	Hypertension; heart failure
Metoprolol (Mopressor, Toprol-XL)	Prior to January 1, 1982	Hypertension; angina pectoris; myocardial infarction; heart failure
Nadolol (Corgard)	Prior to January 1, 1982	Hypertension; angina pectoris
Propranolol (Inderal)	Prior to January 1, 1982	Hypertension; angina pectoris; cardiac arrhythmias; myocardial infarction; migraine; essential tremor; hypertrophic subaortic stenosis
Timolol (Blocadren)	Prior to January 1, 1982	Hypertension; myocardial infarction; migraine; elevated intraocular pressure (topical ophthalmic drops)

TABLE 4.8. (*continued*)

Drug	FDA approval date	Major indication
β-Blockers with intrinsic sympathomimetic activity		
Acebutolol (Sectral)	December 1984	Hypertension; ventricular arrhythmias
Penbutolol (Levatol)	December 1987	Hypertension
Pindolol (Visken)	September 1982	Hypertension
β-Blockers with α-blocking activity		
Carvedilol (Coreg)	September 1995	Hypertension; heart failure; left ventricular dysfunction following myocardial infarction
Labetalol (Normodyne)	August 1984	Hypertension
β-Blockers with nitric oxide-mediated vasodilatory activity		
Nebivolol (Bystolic)	December 2007	Hypertension

Note: Only the extended release form of metoprolol (metoprolol succinate extended-release) is indicated in treating heart failure with reduced ejection fraction (HFrEF).

TABLE 4.9. Other drugs for treating hypertension

Drug	FDA approval date	Major indication
Non-selective α-blockers		
Phenoxybenzamine (Dibenzyline)	Prior to January 1, 1982	Treatment of pheochromocytoma to control episodes of hypertension
Phentolamine (Regitine)	Prior to January 1, 1982	Treatment of pheochromocytoma to control episodes of hypertension
α₁-Selective blockers		
Doxazosin (Cardura)	November 1990	Benign prostatic hyperplasia; hypertension
Prazosin (Minipress)	Prior to January 1, 1982	Hypertension
Terazosin (Hytrin)	August 1987	Benign prostatic hyperplasia; hypertension
Centrally acting drugs (α₂ agonists)		
Clonidine (Catapres)	Prior to January 1, 1982	Hypertension; severe pain; attention deficit hyperactivity disorder
Guanabenz (Wytensin)	September 1982	Hypertension
Guanfacine (Tenex)	October 1986	Hypertension; attention deficit hyperactivity disorder
Methyldopa	Prior to January 1, 1982	Hypertension (including hypertension crisis when given parenterally)

TABLE 4.9. (*continued*)

Drug	FDA approval date	Major indication
Direct vasodilators		
Fenoldopam (Corlopam)	September 1997	Hypertension crisis
Hydralazine (Apresoline)	Prior to January 1, 1982	Hypertension (including severe hypertension)
Minoxidil (Loniten)	Prior to January 1, 1982	Moderate to severe hypertension
Sodium Nitroprusside (Nitropress)	Prior to January 1, 1982	Hypertension crisis; acute heart failure

Note: α_1-Selective blockers are not preferred drugs for chronic treatment of hypertension because of their adverse effects as well as the availability of other more effective drugs.

TABLE 4.10. Diuretic-based fixed-dose combination of two drugs (with one being a diuretic) for treating hypertension

Fixed-dose combination	FDA approval date	Major indication
An ACE inhibitor plus a diuretic		
Benazepril/hydrochlorothiazide (Lotensin HCT)	May 1992	Hypertension
Captopril/hydrochlorothiazide (Capozide)	October 1984	Hypertension
Enalapril/hydrochlorothiazide (Vaseretic)	October 1986	Hypertension
Fosinopril/hydrochlorothiazide (Monopril HCT)	November 1994	Hypertension
Lisinopril/hydrochlorothiazide (Prinzide)	February 1989	Hypertension
Moexipril/hydrochlorothiazide (Uniretic)	June 1997	Hypertension
Quinapril/hydrochlorothiazide (Accuretic)	December 1999	Hypertension
An ARB plus a diuretic		
Candesartan/hydrochlorothiazide (Atacand HCT)	September 2000	Hypertension
Eprosartan/hydrochlorothiazide (Teveten HCT)	November 2001	Hypertension
Irbesartan/hydrochlorothiazide (Avalide)	September 1997	Hypertension
Losartan/hydrochlorothiazide (Hyzaar)	April 1995	Hypertension
Olmesartan/hydrochlorothiazide (Benicar HCT)	June 2003	Hypertension
Telmisartan/hydrochlorothiazide (Micardis HCT)	November 2000	Hypertension
Valsartan/hydrochlorothiazide (Diovan HCT)	March 1998	Hypertension
A β-blocker plus a diuretic		
Atenolol/chlorthalidone (Tenoretic)	June 1984	Hypertension
Bisoprolol/hydrochlorothiazide (Ziac)	March 1993	Hypertension

TABLE 4.10. (*continued*)

Fixed-dose combination	FDA approval date	Major indication
A β-blocker plus a diuretic (continued)		
Metoprolol/hydrochlorothiazide (Lopressor HCT)	December 1984	Hypertension
Nadolol/bendroflumethiazide (Corzide)	May 1983	Hypertension
Propranolol/hydrochlorothiazide (Inderide)	July 1985	Hypertension
Timolol/hydrochlorothiazide (Timolide)	Prior to January 1, 1982	Hypertension
A centrally acting drug plus a diuretic		
Clonidine/chlorthalidone (Clorpres)	February 1987	Hypertension
Methyldopa/hydrochlorothiazide (Aldoril)	Prior to January 1, 1982	Hypertension
A diuretic plus a diuretic		
Amiloride/hydrochlorothiazide (Moduretic)	Prior to January 1, 1982	Hypertension
Spironolactone/hydrochlorothiazide (Aldactazide)	December 1982	Hypertension
Triamterene/hydrochlorothiazide (Dyazide)	Prior to January 1, 1982	Hypertension

Note: Diuretics are the most common component drugs in fixed-dose combination drugs.

TABLE 4.11. Other fixed-dose combination drugs for treating hypertension

Fixed-dose combination	FDA approval date	Major indication
A β-blocker plus an ARB		
Nebivolol/valsartan (Byvalson)	June 2016	Hypertension
A CCB plus an ACEI		
Amlodipine/benazepril (Lotrel)	March 1995	Hypertension
Amlodipine/peridopril (Prestalia)	January 2015	Hypertension
Enalapril/felodipine (Lexxel)	January 1997	Hypertension
Enalapril/diltiazem (Teczem)	October 1996	Hypertension
Trandolapril/verapamil (Tarka)	October 1996	Hypertension
A CCB plus an ARB		
Amlodipine/telmisartan (Twynsta)	October 2009	Hypertension
Amlodipine/valsartan (Exforge)	June 2007	Hypertension
Amlodipine/omelsartan (Azor)	September 2007	Hypertension
A CCB plus a DRI		
Amlodipine/aliskiren (Tekamlo)	August 2010	Hypertension

TABLE 4.11. (*continued*)

Fixed-dose combination	FDA approval date	Major indication
A CCB plus an ARB (or a DRI) plus a diuretic (3-drug combination)		
Amlodipine/aliskiren/hydrochlorothiazide (Amturnide)	December 2010	Hypertension
Amlodipine/olmesartan/hydrochlorothiazide (Tribenzor)	July 2010	Hypertension
Amlodipine/valsartan/hydrochlorothiazide (Exforge HCT)	April 2009	Hypertension

4. SELF-ASSESSMENT QUESTIONS

4.1. A 42-year-old man presents to the physician's office complaining of frequent headache and dizziness. His blood pressure is about 150/90 mm Hg upon repeated measurements. He is otherwise healthy except that his body mass index is 28. Which of the following is the best diagnosis of his condition?

A. Hypertension emergency
B. Prehypertension
C. Pulmonary hypertension
D. Stage 1 hypertension
E. Stage 2 hypertension

4.2. Hypertension currently affects over 85 million US adults. Among the US populations, which of the following has the highest prevalence of hypertension?

A. Asian males
B. Black females
C. Black males
D. Hispanic females
E. White females

4.3. A 39-year-old female is diagnosed with primary aldosteronism. Her blood pressure is consistently in the range of 140–150/90–100 mm Hg. She is otherwise healthy. Which of the following is most likely responsible for her high blood pressure?

A. Decreased activation of renal β_1 adrenergic receptors
B. Decreased heart rate
C. Increased myocardial contraction
D. Increased renal perfusion
E. Increased water and salt retention

4.4. A 45-year-old man is brought to the emergency department because of severe headache, shortness of breath, and anxiety. Blood pressure is about 190/110 mm Hg upon repeated measurements. He is otherwise normal without evidence of organ damage. Which of the following best describes the patient's condition?

A. Hypertension emergency
B. Hypertension urgency
C. Pulmonary hypertension
D. Secondary hypertension
E. Stage 1 hypertension

4.5. A recent meta-analysis of prospective studies (762,393 participants from 19 prospective cohort studies) shows a clear association between blood pressure ≥120/80 mm Hg and stroke, with significantly increased risk even in the 120–129/80–84 mm Hg range. Which of the following best describes the conclusion of this meta-analysis?

A. Control of prehypertension is unlikely associated with decreased risk of stroke
B. Hypertension or high blood pressure increases the risk of stroke
C. Increase of blood pressure within the normal range is associated with increased risk of stroke
D. Prehypertension is associated with increased risk of stroke
E. Stroke increases the risk of prehypertension

4.6. A 52-year-old patient with resistant hypertension is put on a drug to control his blood pressure. A few days later, he develops hyperkalemia. Which of the following is most likely the drug prescribed?

A. Amlodipine
B. Chlorthalidone
C. Furosemide
D. Metoprolol
E. Spironolactone

4.7. A 38-year-old man with stage 1 hypertension is being treated with an antihypertensive drug that acts via blocking the angiotensin-II AT1 receptors. Which of the following is mostly likely the drug that the patient is receiving?

A. Amlodipine
B. Captopril
C. Chlorthalidone
D. Losartan
E. Verapamil

4.8. A 28-year-old female is diagnosed with pheochromocytoma. A decision is made to put her on a drug therapy to control her hypertensive episodes before the surgical removal of her tumor. Which of the following is most likely the molecular target of the antihypertensive drug therapy?

A. Aldosterone receptor
B. α-Adrenergic receptor
C. Angiotensin II receptor type 1
D. Angiotensin-converting enzyme
E. β-Adrenergic receptor

4.9. Although it has been traditionally believed that combination of a β-blocker and an angiotensin receptor blocker (ARB) or an angiotensin-converting enzyme inhibitor (ACEI) may lead to unfavorable clinical response in hypertensive patients, the US FDA recently approved a fixed-dose combination of a β-blocker and an ARB for treating hypertension. Which of the following is this newly approved fixed-dose combination drug?

A. Atenolol/losartan
B. Bisoprolol/azilsartan
C. Metoprolol/irbesartan
D. Nebivolol/valsartan
E. Pindolol/candesartan

4.10. A hypertensive patient with benign prostatic hyperplasia is treated with a drug to improve his lower urinary tract symptom (LUTS). Before he experiences a significant improvement in his LUTS, he notices that his elevated blood pressure is back to normal. Which of the following is most likely the molecular target of the drug therapy?

A. Aldosterone receptor
B. α_1-Adrenergic receptor
C. α_2-Adrenergic receptor
D. β_1-Adrenergic receptor
E. Voltage-dependent calcium channel

ANSWERS AND EXPLANATIONS

4.1. The correct answer is D. JNC7 stage 1 hypertension is defined as systolic blood pressure of 140–159 mm Hg and/or diastolic blood pressure of 90–99 mm Hg.

4.2. The correct answer is B. The prevalence of hypertension in blacks in the US is among the highest in the world; 41% of the total black population and 44% of black women have hypertension.

4.3. The correct answer is E. Increased aldosterone results in increased water and salt retention, thereby leading to increased blood pressure.

4.4. The correct answer is B. Hypertensive urgency is a situation where the blood pressure is severely elevated (>180 mm Hg for systolic pressure or >110 mm Hg for diastolic pressure), but there is no associated organ damage (which would otherwise occur in hypertensive emergency). Individuals experiencing hypertensive urgency may or may not experience one or more of these symptoms: severe headache, shortness of breath, nosebleeds, and severe anxiety.

4.5. The correct answer is D. The JNC7 defines prehypertension as systolic blood pressure of 120–139 mm Hg and/or diastolic blood pressure of 80–89 mm Hg.

4.6. The correct answer is E. Among the drugs listed, only spirono-lactone, a potassium-sparing diuretic and an aldosterone receptor antagonist causes hyperkalemia. Chlorthalidone and furosemide are diuretics that cause hypokalemia. The calcium channel blocker amlodipine and the β-blocker metoprolol do not cause significant changes in serum potassium.

4.7. The correct answer is D. Among the drugs listed, only losartan, an angiotensin receptor blocker, reduces blood pressure via blocking the AT1 receptors. Amlodipine and verapamil are calcium channel blockers. Captopril is an angiotensin-converting enzyme inhibitor, whereas chlorthalidone is a thiazide diuretic.

4.8. The correct answer is B. The drugs of choice for controlling the hypertensive episodes in patients with pheochromocytoma are the non-selective α-blockers, phenoxybenzamine and phentolamine. These drugs potently block both α_1- and α_2-receptors.

4.9. The correct answer is D. Nebivolol/valsartan is the only fixed-dose combination of a β-blocker and an angiotensin receptor blocker approved by the US FDA. Nebivolol is a unique β-blocker that also causes nitric oxide production in the vasculature.

4.10. The correct answer is B. The patient is most likely being treated with an α_1-blocker to improve his LUTS. α_1-Blockers also reduce blood pressure via causing vasodilation. It should be noted that α_1-blockers are primarily used in the treatment of benign prostatic hyperplasia and are not preferred drugs for treating chronic hypertension due to the availability of other more effective antihypertensive drugs.

REFERENCES

1. Webster AC, Nagler EV, Morton RL, Masson P. Chronic kidney disease. *Lancet* 2017; 389(10075):1238–52.
2. Razzak M. Hypertension: understanding baroreflex dysfunction in chronic kidney disease. *Nat Rev Nephrol* 2014; 10(3):124.
3. Pimenta E, Oparil S. Management of hypertension in the elderly. *Nat Rev Cardiol* 2012; 9(5):286–96.
4. Tomaschitz A, Pilz S, Ritz E, Obermayer-Pietsch B, Pieber TR. Aldosterone and arterial hypertension. *Nat Rev Endocrinol* 2010; 6(2):83–93.
5. Monticone S, Burrello J, Tizzani D, Bertello C, Viola A, Buffolo F, Gabetti L, Mengozzi G, Williams TA, Rabbia F, Veglio F, Mulatero P. Prevalence and clinical manifestations of primary aldosteronism encountered in primary care practice. *J Am Coll Cardiol* 2017; 69(14):1811–20.
6. Vongpatanasin W. Resistant hypertension: a review of diagnosis and management. *JAMA* 2014; 311(21):2216–24.
7. Lacroix A, Feelders RA, Stratakis CA, Nieman LK. Cushing's syndrome. *Lancet* 2015; 386(9996):913–27.
8. Cicala MV, Mantero F. Hypertension in Cushing's syndrome: from pathogenesis to treatment. *Neuroendocrinology* 2010; 92 Suppl 1:44–9.
9. Goodman RL. Diagnosis and differential diagnosis of Cushing's syndrome. *N Engl J Med* 2017; 377(2):e3.
10. Javaheri S, Barbe F, Campos-Rodriguez F, Dempsey JA, Khayat R, Javaheri S, Malhotra A, Martinez-Garcia MA, Mehra R, Pack AI, Polotsky VY, Redline S, et al. Sleep apnea: types, mechanisms, and clinical cardiovascular consequences. *J Am Coll Cardiol* 2017; 69(7):841–58.

11. Martinez-Garcia MA, Capote F, Campos-Rodriguez F, Lloberes P, Diaz de Atauri MJ, Somoza M, Masa JF, Gonzalez M, Sacristan L, Barbe F, Duran-Cantolla J, Aizpuru F, et al. Effect of CPAP on blood pressure in patients with obstructive sleep apnea and resistant hypertension: the HIPARCO randomized clinical trial. *JAMA* 2013; 310(22):2407–15.

12. Sanchez-de-la-Torre M, Khalyfa A, Sanchez-de-la-Torre A, Martinez-Alonso M, Martinez-Garcia MA, Barcelo A, Lloberes P, Campos-Rodriguez F, Capote F, Diaz-de-Atauri MJ, Somoza M, Gonzalez M, et al. Precision medicine in patients with resistant hypertension and obstructive sleep apnea: blood pressure response to continuous positive airway pressure treatment. *J Am Coll Cardiol* 2015; 66(9):1023–32.

13. Lenders JW, Eisenhofer G, Mannelli M, Pacak K. Phaeochromocytoma. *Lancet* 2005; 366(9486):665–75.

14. Benjamin EJ, Blaha MJ, Chiuve SE, Cushman M, Das SR, Deo R, de Ferranti SD, Floyd J, Fornage M, Gillespie C, Isasi CR, Jimenez MC, et al. Heart disease and stroke statistics–2017 update: a report from the American Heart Association. *Circulation* 2017; 135(10):e146–e603.

15. ICD Risk Factor Collaboration. Worldwide trends in blood pressure from 1975 to 2015: a pooled analysis of 1479 population-based measurement studies with 19.1 million participants. *Lancet* 2017; 389(10064):37–55.

16. Mills KT, Bundy JD, Kelly TN, Reed JE, Kearney PM, Reynolds K, Chen J, He J. Global disparities of hypertension prevalence and control: a systematic analysis of population-based studies from 90 countries. *Circulation* 2016; 134(6):441–50.

17. Poulter NR, Prabhakaran D, Caulfield M. Hypertension. *Lancet* 2015; 386(9995):801–12.

18. Sacks FM, Campos H. Dietary therapy in hypertension. *N Engl J Med* 2010; 362(22):2102–12.

19. Howard G, Lackland DT, Kleindorfer DO, Kissela BM, Moy CS, Judd SE, Safford MM, Cushman M, Glasser SP, Howard VJ. Racial differences in the impact of elevated systolic blood pressure on stroke risk. *JAMA Intern Med* 2013; 173(1):46–51.

20. Forouzanfar MH, Liu P, Roth GA, Ng M, Biryukov S, Marczak L, Alexander L, Estep K, Hassen Abate K, Akinyemiju TF, Ali R, Alvis-Guzman N, et al. Global burden of hypertension and systolic blood pressure of at least 110 to 115 mm Hg, 1990–2015. *JAMA* 2017; 317(2):165–82.

21. Blacher J, Levy BI, Mourad JJ, Safar ME, Bakris G. From epidemiological transition to modern cardiovascular epidemiology: hypertension in the 21st century. *Lancet* 2016; 388(10043):530–2.

22. Go AS, Mozaffarian D, Roger VL, Benjamin EJ, Berry JD, Blaha MJ, Dai S, Ford ES, Fox CS, Franco S, Fullerton HJ, Gillespie C, et al. Heart disease and stroke statistics–2014 update: a report from the American Heart Association. *Circulation* 2014; 129(3):e28–e292.

23. Huang Y, Cai X, Li Y, Su L, Mai W, Wang S, Hu Y, Wu Y, Xu D. Prehypertension and the risk of stroke: a meta-analysis. *Neurology* 2014; 82(13):1153–61.

24. Schunkert H. Pharmacotherapy for prehypertension: mission accomplished? *N Engl J Med* 2006; 354(16):1742–4.

25. Guyenet PG. The sympathetic control of blood pressure. *Nat Rev Neurosci* 2006; 7(5):335–46.

26. Paulis L, Unger T. Novel therapeutic targets for hypertension. *Nat Rev Cardiol* 2010; 7(8):431–41.

27. Grassi G, Mark A, Esler M. The sympathetic nervous system alterations in human hypertension. *Circ Res* 2015; 116(6):976–90.

28. Te Riet L, van Esch JH, Roks AJ, van den Meiracker AH, Danser AH. Hypertension: renin-angiotensin-aldosterone system alterations. *Circ Res* 2015; 116(6):960–75.

29. Drummond GR, Selemidis S, Griendling KK, Sobey CG. Combating oxidative stress in vascular disease: NADPH oxidases as therapeutic targets. *Nat Rev Drug Discov* 2011; 10(6):453–71.

30. Dikalova AE, Itani HA, Nazarewicz RR, McMaster WG, Flynn CR, Uzhachenko R, Fessel JP, Gamboa JL, Harrison DG, Dikalov SI. Sirt3 impairment and SOD2 hyperacetylation in vascular oxidative stress and hypertension. *Circ Res* 2017; 121(5):564–74.

31. Chobanian AV. Shattuck Lecture. The hypertension parado: more uncontrolled disease despite improved therapy. *N Engl J Med* 2009; 361(9):878–87.

32. Chobanian AV, Bakris GL, Black HR, Cushman WC, Green LA, Izzo JL, Jr., Jones DW, Materson BJ, Oparil S, Wright JT, Jr., Roccella EJ, National Heart, Lung, and Blood Institute, et

al. The Seventh Report of the Joint National Committee on Prevention, Detection, Evaluation, and Treatment of High Blood Pressure: the JNC 7 report. *JAMA* 2003; 289(19):2560–72.

33. James PA, Oparil S, Carter BL, Cushman WC, Dennison-Himmelfarb C, Handler J, Lackland DT, LeFevre ML, MacKenzie TD, Ogedegbe O, Smith SC, Jr., Svetkey LP, et al. 2014 Evidence-based guideline for the management of high blood pressure in adults: report from the panel members appointed to the Eighth Joint National Committee (JNC 8). *JAMA* 2014; 311(5):507–20.

CHAPTER 5

New Drugs for Systemic Hypertension

CHAPTER HIGHLIGHTS

- Fixed-dose combination of two antihypertensive agents from different drug classes has become a standard therapy that leads to a greater reduction in blood pressure and lower rates of adverse reactions than would increasing the monotherapy dose.
- Over the past five years, the United States Food and Drugs Administration (US FDA) has approved two new fixed-dose combination drugs for treating systemic hypertension. They are Prestalia (perindopril/amlodipine) and Byvalson (nebivolol/valsartan).
- The approval of Byvalson by the US FDA represents a major change in combinational antihypertensive therapy. In this context, combination of a β-blocker and a renin-angiotensin-aldosterone system (RAAS) inhibitor (e.g., an angiotensin receptor blocker) had long been regarded to cause less additive effects.

KEYWORDS | Amlodipine; Angiotensin receptor blocker; Angiotensin-converting enzyme inhibitor; Antihypertensive drug; β-Blocker; Calcium channel blocker; Fixed-dose combination; Nebivolol; Perindopril; Prestalia; Systemic hypertension; Valsartan

CITATION | *Li YR. Cardiovascular Medicine: New Therapeutic Drugs Approved by the US FDA (2013–2017). Cell Med Press, Raleigh, NC, USA. 2018. http://dx.doi.org/10.20455/ndcvd.2018.05*

ABBREVIATIONS | ACE, angiotensin-converting enzyme; COX-2, cyclooxygenase-2; CYP, cytochrome P450; FDC, fixed-dose combination; NSAID, nonsteroidal anti-inflammatory drug; RAAS, renin-angiotensin-aldosterone system; US FDA, the United States Food and Drug Administration

CHAPTER AT A GLANCE

1. INTRODUCTION

Combining two or more antihypertensive drugs from different drug classes is more likely to lead to a greater reduction in blood pressure and lower rates of adverse reactions than would increasing the monotherapy dose. Indeed, many hypertensive patients need two drugs to achieve adequate blood pressure control. The two-drug combination therapy may commence either as separate entities or as a fixed-dose combination (FDC). Recently, the United States Food and Drug Administration (US FDA) has approved two FDC drugs for treating systemic hypertension. They are Prestalia (perindopril/amlodipine) and Byvalson (nebivolol/valsartan), approved in January 2015 and June 2016, respectively.

2. FIXED-DOSE COMBINATION OF PERINDOPRIL AND AMLODIPINE (PRESTALIA)

2.1. Overview

Prestalia is a combination of perindopril arginine, an angiotensin-converting enzyme (ACE) inhibitor, and amlodipine besylate, a dihydropyridine calcium channel blocker. The US FDA approval of Prestalia was based on a 6-week randomized controlled trial (PATH) in 837 subjects. The study demonstrated that the fixed-dose combination of perindopril arginine with amlodipine (14/10 mg) in a single pill lowered both systolic and diastolic blood pressure more significantly than monotherapy with either perindopril erbumine (16 mg) or amlodipine besylate (10 mg), with a reduction in adverse effects (especially ankle edema), compared to amlodipine alone [1]. A low strength of Prestalia (3.5/2.5 mg) was also studied in a randomized controlled trial involving 1,581 hypertensive patients. At week 8, Prestalia 3.5/2.5 mg produced statistically significantly greater reductions in blood pressure than the monotherapy with either perindopril arginine 3.5 mg or amlodipine 2.5 mg.

2.2. Chemistry and Pharmacokinetics

The structures of perindopril arginine and amlodipine besylate are shown in **Figure 5.1**. The new salt form (perindopril arginine) is more stable and has a longer shelf-life than perindopril erbumine. Following administration of Prestalia, the peak plasma concentration of perindopril, perindoprilat (an active metabolite of perindopril), and amlodipine occurs at approximately 1, 4, and 6–12 h, respectively. The half-life of perindopril is ~1.3 h. Elimination of perindoprilat is multiphasic and shows a terminal elimination half-life of about

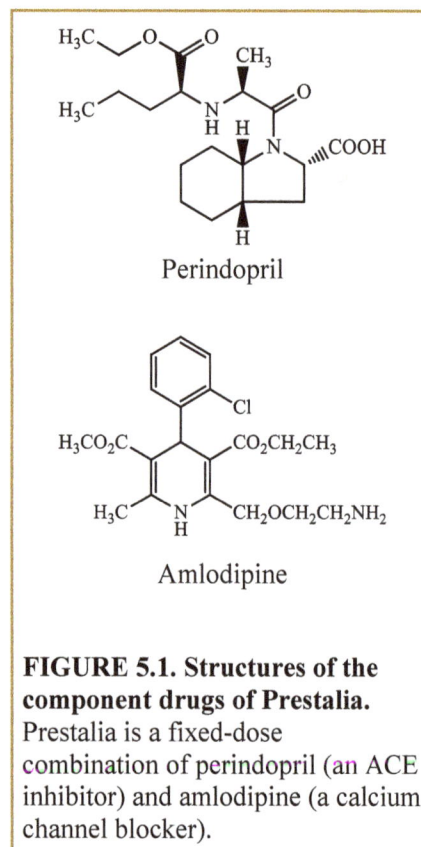

FIGURE 5.1. Structures of the component drugs of Prestalia. Prestalia is a fixed-dose combination of perindopril (an ACE inhibitor) and amlodipine (a calcium channel blocker).

120 h, resulting from slow dissociation of perindoprilat from plasma and tissue ACE binding sites. Amlodipine elimination is also biphasic with a terminal elimination half-life of ~30–50 h. The major pharmacokinetic properties of the component drugs of Prestalia are provided in **Table 5.1**. The reader may refer to Ref. [2] for detailed description of the pharmacokinetics and other aspects of perindopril and amlodipine.

TABLE 5.1. Pharmacokinetic properties of the component drugs of Prestalia

Property	Perindopril	Amlodipine
Oral bioavailability	75%	64–90%
t_{max}	1 h (perindopril); 4 h (perindoprilat)	6–12 h
Effect of food on absorption	Minimal	No effects
Plasma protein binding	60% (perindopril); 10–20% (perindoprilat)	90%
Vd	Not available	21 L/kg bw
Metabolism	Hydrolysis by hepatic esterases; glucuronidation	Hepatic metabolism by cytochrome P450 (CYP) 3A4
Elimination	Urine (nearly exclusively)	Urine (major)
Clearance	219–362 ml/min	Not available
$t_{1/2}$	1.3 h (perindopril); 120 h (terminal elimination half-life of perindoprilat)	30–50 h (terminal elimination half-life)

Note: bw, body weight; $t_{1/2}$, elimination half-life; t_{max}, the time when the maximum plasma concentration is reached; Vd, volume of distribution.

2.3. Molecular Mechanisms and Pharmacological Effects

2.3.1. Molecular Mechanisms

Perindopril, a prodrug, is hydrolyzed to perindoprilat, which inhibits ACE, reducing the formation of angiotensin II, leading to decreased vasoconstriction and decreased aldosterone secretion. In addition, perindopril increases bradykinin, a vasodilating molecule, contributing to the reduction of blood pressure (**Figure 5.2**).

Amlodipine is a dihydropyridine calcium channel blocker that inhibits the transmembrane influx of calcium ions through the L-type voltage-dependent calcium channels (VDCC), into vascular smooth muscle cells. In vascular smooth muscle cells, influx of extracellular calcium ions through the L-type VDCC causes further release of calcium ions from sarcoplasmic reticulum, a phenomenon known as calcium-induced calcium release. The increased cytosolic calcium ions bind to calmodulin (CaM) to form a calcium-CaM complex. The calcium-CaM complex then activates myosin light chain kinase, which in turn causes phosphorylation of myosin light chain. The phosphorylated myosin light chain interacts with actin to form actin-myosin cross-bridges, thereby leading to smooth muscle cell contraction. By blocking the L-type VDCC in vascular smooth muscle cells, amlodipine treatment results in smooth muscle relaxation and the subsequent vasodilation (**Figure 5.3**).

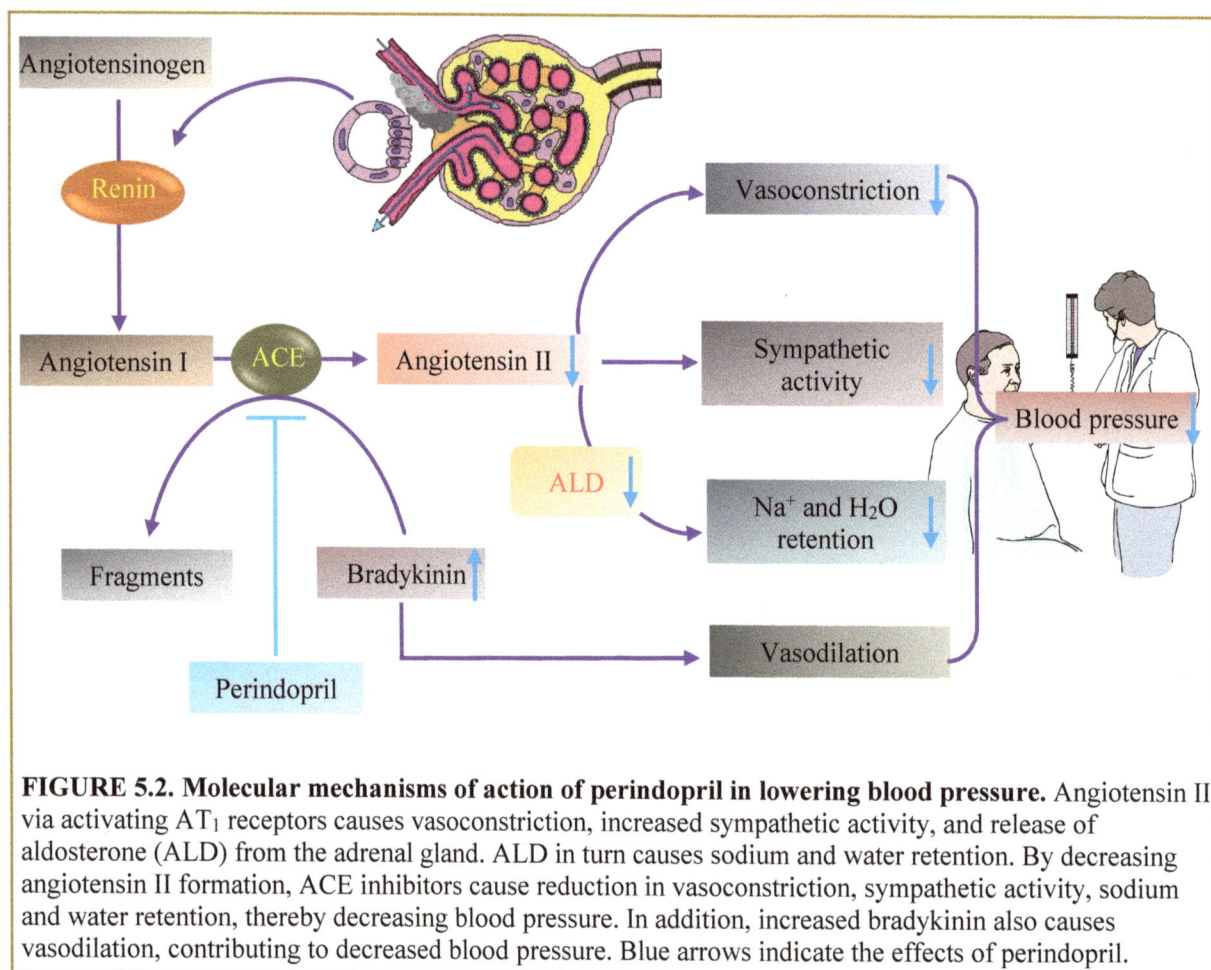

FIGURE 5.2. Molecular mechanisms of action of perindopril in lowering blood pressure. Angiotensin II via activating AT_1 receptors causes vasoconstriction, increased sympathetic activity, and release of aldosterone (ALD) from the adrenal gland. ALD in turn causes sodium and water retention. By decreasing angiotensin II formation, ACE inhibitors cause reduction in vasoconstriction, sympathetic activity, sodium and water retention, thereby decreasing blood pressure. In addition, increased bradykinin also causes vasodilation, contributing to decreased blood pressure. Blue arrows indicate the effects of perindopril.

2.3.2. Pharmacological Effects

Hypertensive patients treated with Prestalia are more likely to reach a target blood pressure than the monotherapy with perindopril or amlodipine. It is estimated that a patient with a baseline blood pressure of 170/105 mm Hg has approximately a 26% likelihood of achieving a goal of <140 mm Hg (systolic) and 31% likelihood of achieving <90 mm Hg (diastolic) on perindopril erbumine 16 mg. The likelihood of achieving these same goals on amlodipine 10 mg is approximately 40% (systolic) and 46% (diastolic). These likelihoods rise to 50% (systolic) and 65% (diastolic) with Prestalia 14/10 mg.

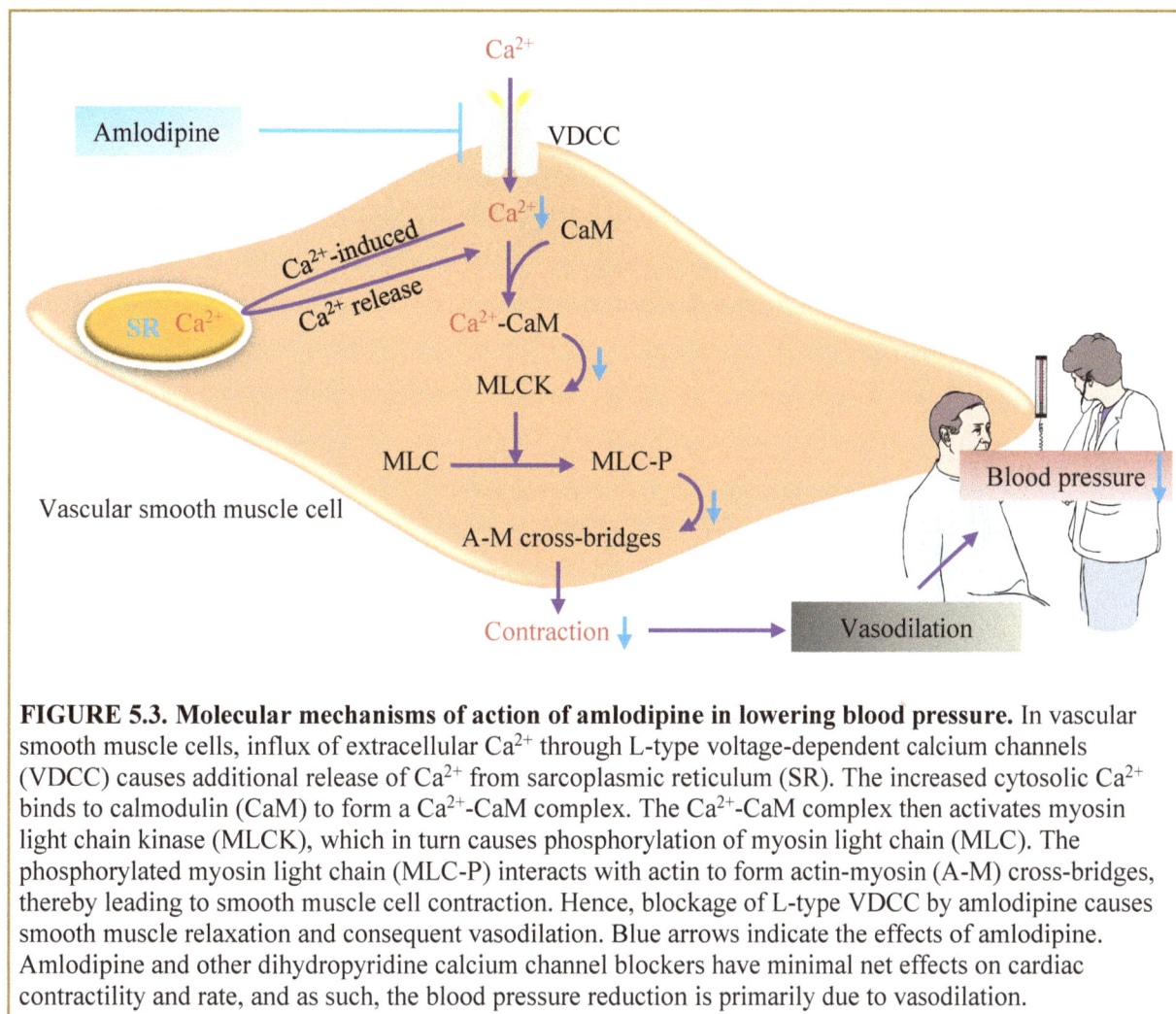

FIGURE 5.3. Molecular mechanisms of action of amlodipine in lowering blood pressure. In vascular smooth muscle cells, influx of extracellular Ca^{2+} through L-type voltage-dependent calcium channels (VDCC) causes additional release of Ca^{2+} from sarcoplasmic reticulum (SR). The increased cytosolic Ca^{2+} binds to calmodulin (CaM) to form a Ca^{2+}-CaM complex. The Ca^{2+}-CaM complex then activates myosin light chain kinase (MLCK), which in turn causes phosphorylation of myosin light chain (MLC). The phosphorylated myosin light chain (MLC-P) interacts with actin to form actin-myosin (A-M) cross-bridges, thereby leading to smooth muscle cell contraction. Hence, blockage of L-type VDCC by amlodipine causes smooth muscle relaxation and consequent vasodilation. Blue arrows indicate the effects of amlodipine. Amlodipine and other dihydropyridine calcium channel blockers have minimal net effects on cardiac contractility and rate, and as such, the blood pressure reduction is primarily due to vasodilation.

2.4. Clinical Uses

Prestalia is indicated for the treatment of hypertension in patients whose blood pressure cannot be adequately controlled with monotherapy, or as initial therapy in patients who are likely to need multiple drugs to achieve their blood pressure goals.

2.5. Therapeutic Dosages

The dosage forms and strengths of Prestalia are listed below.

- Oral: tablets of 3.5/2.5, 7/5, and 14/10 mg (perindopril arginine/ amlodipine)

The recommended starting dose of Prestalia is 3.5/2.5 mg once daily. Dosage is adjusted according to blood pressure goals. In general, the patient should wait 1–2 weeks between titration steps. The maximum recommended dose is 14/10 mg once daily.

2.6. Adverse Effects and Drug Interactions

2.6.1. Adverse Effects

Prestalia is generally well-tolerated. Common adverse effects include peripheral edema, cough, headache, and dizziness. The adverse effects match with those caused by the individual drug component. For example, edema, headache, and dizziness are adverse effects of amlodipine. On the other hand, cough (dry cough) is a common adverse effect of ACE inhibitor therapy. It is of note that the rate of peripheral edema (e.g., ankle edema) with Prestalia is much lower than that with amlodipine monotherapy [3].

2.6.2. Drug Interactions

The pharmacokinetics of perindopril and amlodipine are not altered when the drugs are co-administered. Drug interactions are caused by the individual component, amlodipine or perindopril [2].

2.6.2.1. PERINDOPRIL

The major drug interactions for perindopril are outlined below.

- *Potassium supplements and potassium-sparing diuretics*: increased risk of hyperkalemia
- *Lithium*: increased serum lithium levels, leading to lithium toxicity
- *Injectable gold (sodium aurothiomalate)*: Concomitant use may cause nitritoid reactions, such as flushing, nausea, vomiting, or hypotension. This, however, occurs rarely.
- *Nonsteroidal anti-inflammatory drugs (NSAIDs)*: risk of renal impairment and loss of antihypertensive effect. Co-administration of NSAIDS, including selective cyclooxygenase-2 (COX-2) inhibitors, with ACE inhibitors, including perindopril, may result in deterioration of renal function, including possible acute renal failure. The antihypertensive effects of ACE inhibitors, including perindopril, may be attenuated by NSAIDS, including selective COX-2 inhibitors.
- *Dual inhibition of the RAAS*: increased risk of renal impairment, hypotension, and hyperkalemia. Co-administration of aliskiren with Prestalia should be avoided in patients with diabetes. Use of aliskiren with Prestalia should also be avoided in patients with renal impairment (glomerular filtration rate <60 ml/min).

2.6.2.2. AMLODIPINE

The major drug interactions for amlodipine are outlined below.

- *Simvastatin*: Co-administration of simvastatin with Prestalia leads to increased exposure to simvastatin (by ~77%). When co-administered with Prestalia, the dosage of simvastatin should not go beyond 20 mg daily.
- *Cyclosporine*: Co-administration of Prestalia with cyclosporine leads to increased exposure to cyclosporine (by ~40%).

- *CYP3A4 inhibitors*: Co-administration of Prestalia with CYP3A4 inhibitors (e.g., diltiazem, itraconazole) may increase exposure to amlodipine and the risk of hypotension and edema.

2.6.3. Contraindications and FDA Pregnancy Category

- Prestalia is contraindicated in patients with hereditary or idiopathic angioedema, with or without previous ACE inhibitor treatment, and in patients who are hypersensitive to perindopril, to any other ACE inhibitors, or to amlodipine.
- Do not co-administer aliskiren with ACE inhibitors, including Prestalia, in patients with diabetes due to increased risk of renal impairment, hypotension, and hyperkalemia as demonstrated by the ALTITUDE trial [4].
- FDA pregnancy category: D. When pregnancy is detected, Prestalia should be discontinued as soon as possible. Drugs, including Prestalia, that act directly on the RAAS can cause injury and death to the developing fetus.

2.7. Comparison with Existing Members and New Development since the US FDA Approval

In addition to Prestalia, several FDC drugs of ACE inhibitors and calcium channel blockers have also been approved by the US FDA over the past two decades (see Chapter 4). These include Lotrel (benazepril/amlodipine) (approved in 1995), Teczem (enalapril/diltiazem) (approved in 1996), Lexxel (enalapril/felodipine) (approved in 1997), and Tarka (trandolapril/verapamil) (approved in 2010). In addition, FDC drugs of angiotensin receptor blockers and calcium channel blockers are also available for treating hypertension, which include Azor (amlodipine/olmesartan) (approved in 2007), Exforge (amlodipine/valsartan) (approved in 2007), and Twynsta (amlodipine/telmisartan) (approved in 2009) (see Chapter 4).

Currently, comparative studies of Prestalia with other FDC drugs of ACE inhibitors and calcium channel blockers are lacking. There are, however, randomized controlled trials comparing Prestalia with Azor and Exforge. In this context, one study involving 1,757 hypertensive patients suggested that Prestalia produced greater reductions in blood pressure, and better and quicker rates of control of hypertension than the combination of amlodipine and valsartan [5]. On the other hand, another study showed that the FDC drug Azor (amlodipine/olmesartan) was superior to the combination of perindopril and amlodipine in reducing central systolic blood pressure in hypertensive patients with diabetes [6].

3. FIXED-DOSE COMBINATION OF NEBIVOLOL AND VALSARTAN (BYVALSON)

3.1. Overview

Combination between β-blockers and renin-angiotensin-aldosterone system (RAAS) inhibitors is believed to be less effective based on some early clinical trials primarily on traditional β-blockers (e.g., atenolol, propranolol) [7] and a concern that an overlapping mechanism of action between the two classes of drugs (i.e., inhibition of renin release by β-blockers) would cause less additive effects on blood pressure reduction. This notion has been challenged recently. In fact, the US FDA in 2015 approved Byvalson, a fixed-dose combination of nebivolol, a vasodilatory $β_1$-selective antagonist and $β_3$ agonist, and valsartan, an angiotensin receptor blocker. The approval of Byvalson was based on a randomized controlled trial involving 4,118 hypertensive patients. At week 8, the fixed-dose combination of nebivolol and valsartan (20 and 320 mg/day) group had significantly greater reduction in diastolic blood pressure from baseline than monotherapy with either nebivolol (40 mg/day) or valsartan (320 mg/day). The tolerability of the fixed-dose combination was comparable to that of the monotherapy [8].

3.2. Chemistry and Pharmacokinetics

Byvalson is available as tablets for oral administration. Each tablet contains 5.45 mg of nebivolol hydrochloride, which is equivalent to 5 mg of nebivolol free base, and 80 mg of valsartan (structures shown in **Figure 5.4**). Following oral administration of Byvalson, peak plasma nebivolol and valsartan concentrations are reached ~1–6 h and ~2–4 h post-dosing, respectively. The rate and extent of absorption of nebivolol and valsartan from Byvalson are the same as when administered separately. The major pharmacokinetic properties of the component drugs are given in **Table 5.2**.

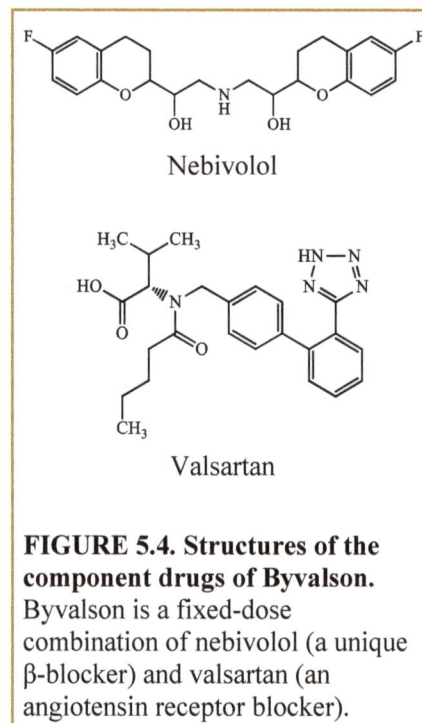

FIGURE 5.4. Structures of the component drugs of Byvalson. Byvalson is a fixed-dose combination of nebivolol (a unique β-blocker) and valsartan (an angiotensin receptor blocker).

TABLE 5.2. Pharmacokinetic properties of the component drugs of Byvalson

Property	Nebivolol	Valsartan
Oral bioavailability	Not known	25%
Effect of food on absorption	No effect	Decrease
t_{max}	1–6 h	2–4 h
Plasma protein binding	98%	95%
Vd	Not available	0.243 L/kg bw
Metabolism	Direct glucuronidation; CYP2D6	Unknown; minor involvement of CYP2C9
Elimination	Urine and feces	Feces (major); urine (minor)
Clearance	Not available	33.3 ml/min
$t_{1/2}$	12 h in CYP2D6 extensive metabolizers (most people), and 19 h in poor metabolizers	6 h

Note: bw, body weight; $t_{1/2}$, elimination half-life; t_{max}, the time when the maximum plasma concentration is reached; Vd, volume of distribution.

3.3. Molecular Mechanisms and Pharmacological Effects

3.3.1. Molecular Mechanisms

The mechanisms of action of the antihypertensive response of nebivolol have not been definitively established. Factors that may be involved include: (1) decreased heart rate, (2) decreased myocardial contractility, (3) decreased sympathetic activity, (4) suppression of renin activity, and (5) vasodilation and decreased peripheral vascular resistance. Notably, nebivolol activates β_3 receptors in cardiovascular tissues, leading to increased production of nitric oxide, a vasodilator and cardiovascular protector [9, 10] (**Figure 5.5**).

Valsartan blocks the vasoconstriction and aldosterone-secreting effects of angiotensin II by selectively blocking the binding of angiotensin II to the AT1 receptors in many tissues, such as vascular smooth muscle and the adrenal gland (**Figure 5.6**). Nebivolol/valsartan combination prevents valsartan-induced increases in plasma renin. While both nebivolol and valsartan monotherapy cause reduction of plasma aldosterone, combination of nebivolol and valsartan results in additive effects. The additive effects in aldosterone reduction could contribute, at least partly, to the more effective blood pressure-lowering activity of Byvalson.

3.3.2. Pharmacological Effects

Valsartan increases plasma renin activity (PRA) by 54–73%, whereas nebivolol results in a 51–65% reduction in PRA. Nebivolol in combination with valsartan reduces PRA by 17–39%. Nebivolol, valsartan, and Byvalson all decrease plasma aldosterone levels [11]. Administration of Byvalson to patients with essential hypertension leads to a significant reduction of sitting and standing diastolic and systolic blood pressure. Decreases in pulse rate from baseline also occur in the Byvalson and nebivolol treatment groups [8].

3.4. Clinical Uses

Byvalson is indicated for the treatment of hypertension to lower blood pressure. Byvalson may be used alone or in combination with other antihypertensive agents.

3.5. Therapeutic Dosages

The dosage forms and strengths of Byvalson are listed below.

- Oral: tablets containing 5 mg of nebivolol and 80 mg of valsartan

As initial therapy and in patients whose blood pressure is not adequately controlled on valsartan 80 mg or nebivolol 10 mg, the recommended dose of Byvalson is 5 mg/80 mg (nebivolol/valsartan) once daily. Maximum antihypertensive effects are attained within 2–4 weeks. Increasing the dose of Byvalson does not result in any meaningful further blood pressure reduction [8], which could be attributed to the flat dose responses for both nebivolol and valsartan.

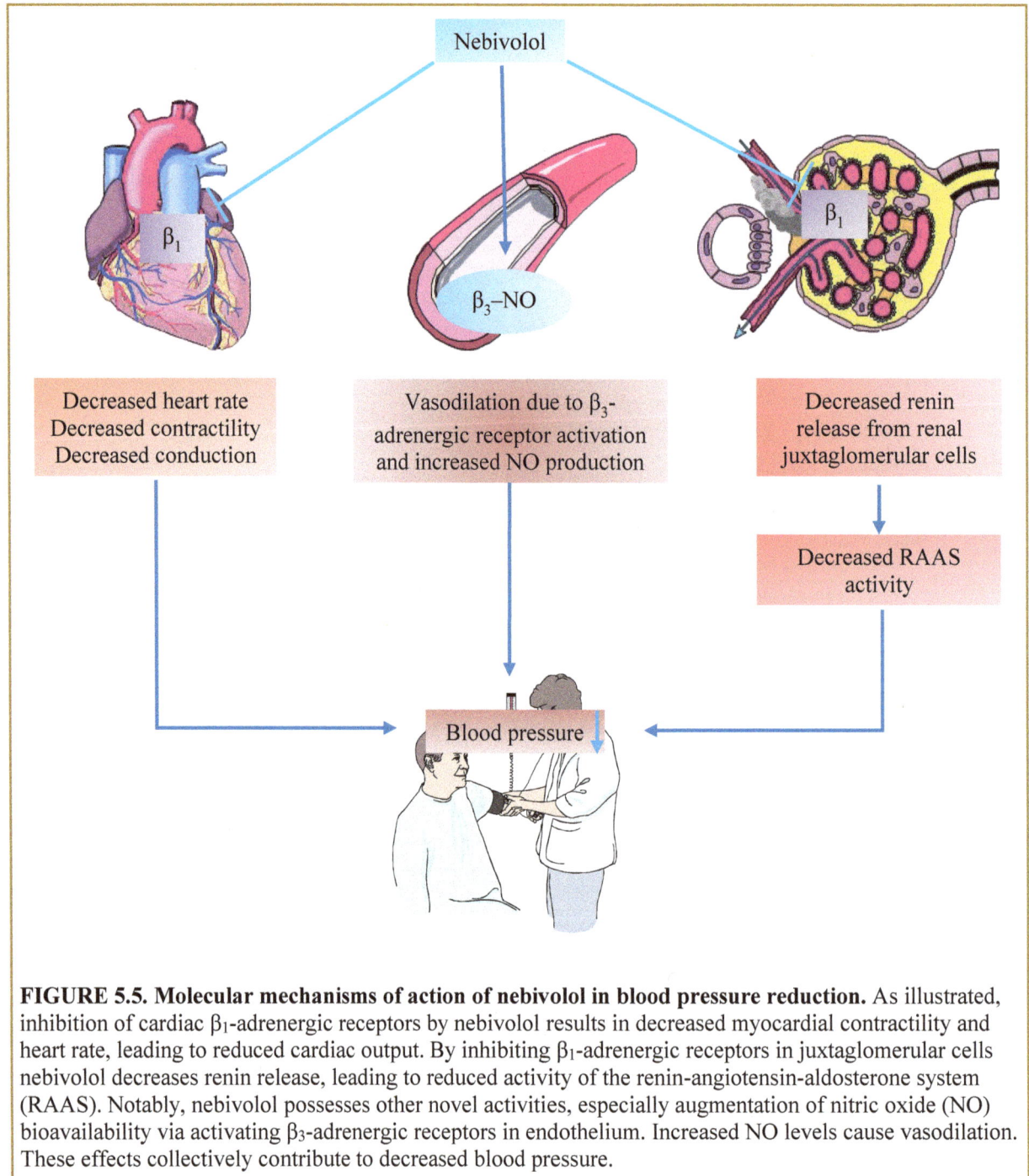

FIGURE 5.5. Molecular mechanisms of action of nebivolol in blood pressure reduction. As illustrated, inhibition of cardiac β_1-adrenergic receptors by nebivolol results in decreased myocardial contractility and heart rate, leading to reduced cardiac output. By inhibiting β_1-adrenergic receptors in juxtaglomerular cells nebivolol decreases renin release, leading to reduced activity of the renin-angiotensin-aldosterone system (RAAS). Notably, nebivolol possesses other novel activities, especially augmentation of nitric oxide (NO) bioavailability via activating β_3-adrenergic receptors in endothelium. Increased NO levels cause vasodilation. These effects collectively contribute to decreased blood pressure.

3.6. Adverse Effects and Drug Interactions

3.6.1. Adverse Effects

Like monotherapy with nebivolol and valsartan, Byvalson is generally well-tolerated [12]. The adverse effects of Byvalson are characteristic of the component drugs. The most common adverse effects of nebivolol and valsartan include headache, dizziness, and fatigue. Valsartan may also increase blood potassium levels due to its inhibition of aldosterone production.

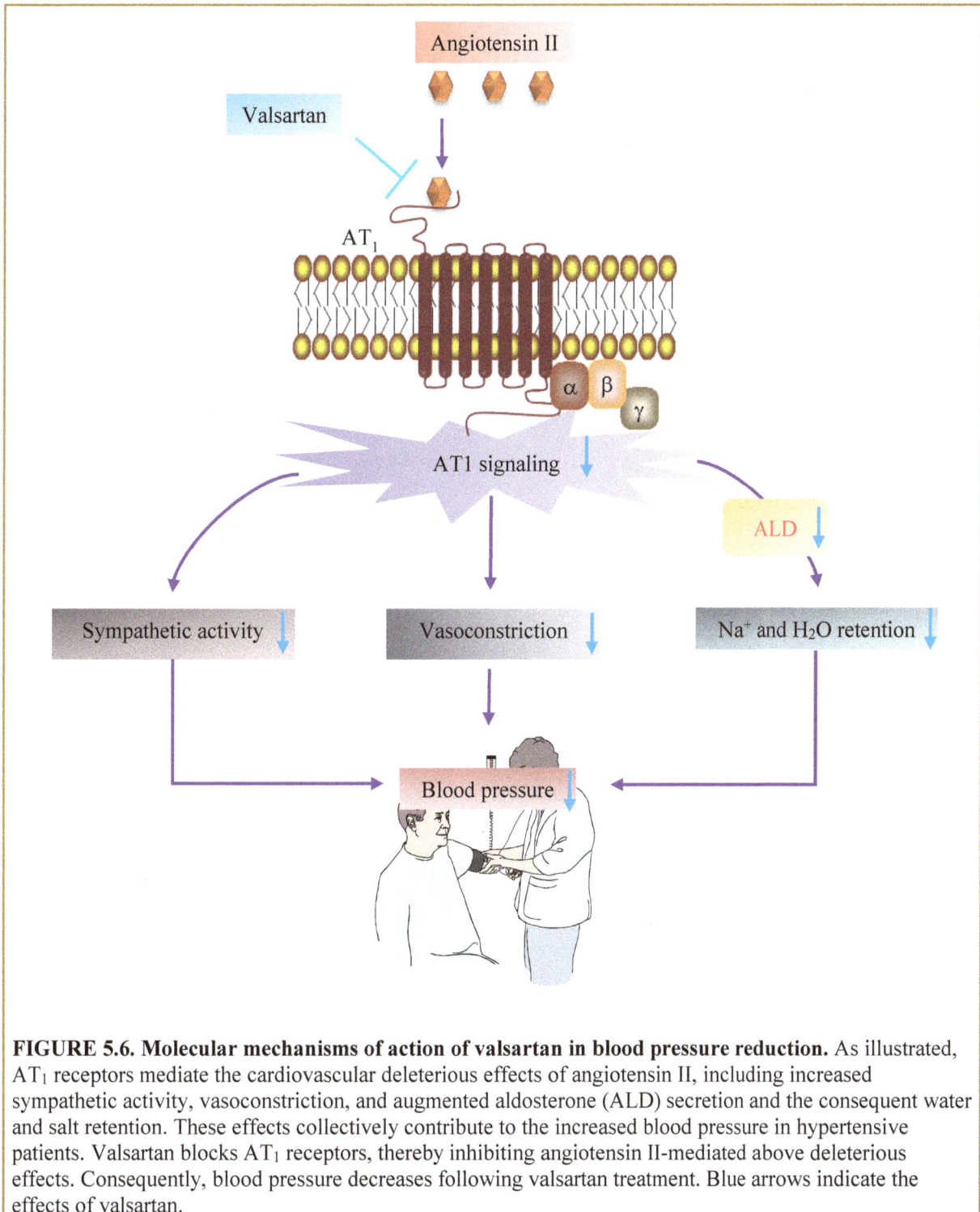

FIGURE 5.6. Molecular mechanisms of action of valsartan in blood pressure reduction. As illustrated, AT_1 receptors mediate the cardiovascular deleterious effects of angiotensin II, including increased sympathetic activity, vasoconstriction, and augmented aldosterone (ALD) secretion and the consequent water and salt retention. These effects collectively contribute to the increased blood pressure in hypertensive patients. Valsartan blocks AT_1 receptors, thereby inhibiting angiotensin II-mediated above deleterious effects. Consequently, blood pressure decreases following valsartan treatment. Blue arrows indicate the effects of valsartan.

3.6.2. Drug Interactions

Up to date, no drug interaction studies have been conducted with Byvalson. Hence, this section describes the drug interactions of the individual drug components. It is assumed that the drug interactions associated with nebivolol and valsartan would be applicable to Byvalson treatment.

3.6.2.1. NEBIVOLOL

Nebivolol may cause significant drug interactions. The major drug interactions associated with nebivolol include the following:

- *CYP2D6 inhibitors*: As noted earlier, nebivolol is metabolized by hepatic CYP2D6. CYP2D6 enzyme inhibitors (e.g., quinidine, propafenone, fluoxetine, paroxetine) increase nebivolol levels, and as such, concomitant use of nebivolol with any of the above drugs should be avoided.
- *Hypotensive drugs*: Concomitant use of nebivolol with other β-blockers should be avoided. In the presence of the antihypertensive reserpine or clonidine, nebivolol may produce excessive reduction of sympathetic activity.
- *Digitalis glycosides*: Concomitant use of nebivolol and digoxin increases the risk of bradycardia, as both drugs slow atrioventricular (AV) conduction and decrease heart rate.
- *Calcium channel blockers*: Nebivolol can exacerbate the effects of myocardial depressants or inhibitors of AV conduction, such as certain calcium channel blockers (e.g., diltiazem, verapamil) or antiarrhythmic agents (e.g., disopyramide).

3.6.2.2. VALSARTAN

The clinically significant drug interactions associated with valsartan include the following:

- *Agents increasing serum potassium*: Valsartan reduces aldosterone levels, which may lead to potassium retention (recall: aldosterone causes sodium retention and potassium secretion). Concomitant use of valsartan with potassium-sparing diuretics or potassium supplements may lead to hyperkalemia.
- *NSAIDs, including COX-2 inhibitors*: Concomitant use with NSAIDs including COX-2 inhibitors may lead to increased risk of renal impairment and loss of the antihypertensive effectiveness of valsartan.
- *Use with other RAAS inhibitors*: Dual inhibition of the RAAS may lead to increased risk of renal impairment, hypotension, and hyperkalemia. Co-administration of aliskiren (a direct renin inhibitor) with Byvalson should be avoided in patients with diabetes mellitus and in patients with renal impairment (glomerular filtration rate <60 ml/min) due to increased harm.
- *Lithium*: Increases in serum lithium concentrations and lithium toxicity have been reported during concomitant administration of lithium with angiotensin receptor blockers, including valsartan.

3.6.3. Contraindications and FDA Pregnancy Category

3.6.3.1. CONTRAINDICATIONS

The contraindications of Byvalson are outlined below.

- Severe bradycardia
- Heart block greater than first degree
- Patients with cardiogenic shock
- Decompensated cardiac failure
- Sick sinus syndrome (unless a permanent pacemaker is in place.)
- Patients with severe hepatic impairment
- Hypersensitivity to any component of this product
- Do not co-administer aliskiren with Byvalson in patients with diabetes due to the increased risk of adverse effect (see above).

3.6.3.2. FDA PREGNANCY CATEGORY

- D. When pregnancy is detected, Byvalson should be discontinued as soon as possible. Drugs, including Byvalson, that act directly on the RAAS can cause injury and death to the developing fetus.

3.7. Comparison with Existing Members and New Development since the US FDA Approval

Byvalson is the first and the only fixed-dose combination of a β-blocker and an angiotensin receptor blocker currently available in the United States. While studies comparing Byvalson with other fixed-dose combination drugs are currently lacking, nebivolol has been shown to exert novel beneficial effects on the cardiovascular system as compared with other β-blockers. As noted earlier, activation of $β_3$ receptors by nebivolol in endothelial cells causes increased production of nitric oxide, leading to vasodilation and improvement of endothelial dysfunction in essential hypertension [10, 13–15].

Recently, nebivolol is also found to improve endothelial dysfunction, pulmonary vascular remodeling, and right heart function in pulmonary hypertension [16], and to ameliorate myocardial ischemia-reperfusion injury via endothelial nitric oxide synthase and neuronal nitric oxide synthase activation [9]. These novel beneficial effects of nebivolol would likely make Byvalson a promising therapy for effective blood pressure reduction in hypertensive patients with other concomitant cardiovascular diseases. In this regard, recent evidence points to that in patients at high risk for cardiovascular events, intensive blood pressure control is associated with improved cardiovascular outcomes [17–21].

4. SELF-ASSESSMENT QUESTIONS

4.1. The PATH study, a 6-week randomized controlled trial in 837 subjects revealed that the fixed-dose combination of perindopril arginine with amlodipine (14/10 mg) in a single pill lowered both systolic and diastolic blood pressure more effectively than monotherapy with either perindopril erbumine (16 mg) or amlodipine besylate (10 mg). Compared to amlodipine alone, the combination therapy also led to a reduction in which of the following adverse effects?

A. Ankle edema
B. Dizziness
C. Dry cough
D. Headache
E. Hypotension

4.2. Prestalia, a fixed-dose combination of perindopril and amlodipine results in a peak plasma concentration of perindoprilat at 4 h following oral administration. The elimination of perindoprilat shows a long terminal elimination half-life resulting from slow dissociation of perindoprilat from plasma and tissue angiotensin-converting enzyme binding sites. Which of the following is most likely the terminal elimination half-life of perindoprilat?

A. 30 h
B. 60 h
C. 120 h
D. 240 h
E. 480 h

4.3. A 35-year-old man is diagnosed with stage 2 hypertension. He is prescribed a recently approved fixed-dose combination drug to effectively control his blood pressure. However, he experiences persistent dry cough following treatment with the new drug. Which of the following is most likely the combination?

A. Ezetimibe/atorvastatin
B. Losartan/hydrochlorothiazide
C. Metoprolol/hydrochlorothiazide
D. Nebivolol/valsartan
E. Perindopril/amlodipine

4.4. A 46-year-old man with a family history of hypertension presents to a physician's office complaining of headache and dizziness. Repeated measurements of his blood pressure reveal a systolic pressure of 145–150 mm Hg and a diastolic pressure of 88–93 mm Hg. A decision is made to put him on a newly approved fixed-dose combination (FDC) drug that likely improves the endothelial function by increasing nitric oxide bioavailability. Which of the following is most likely the FDC drug?

A. Amlodipine/aliskiren/hydrochlorothiazide
B. Nadolol/bendroflumethiazide
C. Nebivolol/valsartan
D. Perindopril/amlodipine
E. Trandolapril/verapamil

4.5. A 52-year-old Caucasian woman is treated with Byvalson (5 mg/80 mg, once daily) to control her elevated blood pressure. Which of the following will most likely occur in this patient following the drug treatment?

A. Decreased plasma renin activity
B. Decreased vascular nitric oxide production
C. Increased heart rate
D. Increased plasma aldosterone levels
E. Increased plasma renin activity

ANSWERS AND EXPLANATIONS

4.1. The correct answer is A. Clinical studies have demonstrated that the rate of ankle edema with Prestalia treatment is much lower than that with amlodipine monotherapy.

4.2. The correct answer is C. Elimination of perindoprilat is multiphasic and shows a terminal elimination half-life of 120 h.

4.3. The correct answer is E. Persistent dry cough is a common and characteristic adverse effect of perindopril and other angiotensin-converting enzyme inhibitors. The other drugs listed are not associated with dry cough.

4.4. The correct answer is C. Among the drugs listed, only nebivolol has been established to augment endothelial nitric oxide production causing vasodilation.

4.5. The correct answer is A. Valsartan increases plasma renin activity (PRA) by 54–73%, whereas nebivolol results in a 51–65% reduction in PRA. Nebivolol in combination with valsartan reduces PRA by 17–39%. Byvalson increases nitric oxide production, decreases heart rate, and reduces plasma aldosterone levels.

REFERENCES

1. Elliott WJ. Perindopril arginine + amlodipine for the treatment of hypertension in the USA. *Expert Opin Pharmacother* 2015; 16(14):2217–29.
2. Li YR. *Cardiovascular Diseases: From Molecular Pharmacology to Evidence-Based Therapeutics.* John Wiley & Sons, New Jersey, USA. 2015.
3. Elliott WJ, Whitmore J, Feldstein JD, Bakris GL. Efficacy and safety of perindopril arginine + amlodipine in hypertension. *J Am Soc Hypertens* 2015; 9(4):266–74.
4. Parving HH, Brenner BM, McMurray JJ, de Zeeuw D, Haffner SM, Solomon SD, Chaturvedi N, Persson F, Desai AS, Nicolaides M, Richard A, Xiang Z, et al. Cardiorenal end points in a trial of aliskiren for type 2 diabetes. *N Engl J Med* 2012; 367(23):2204–13.
5. Mancia G, Asmar R, Amodeo C, Mourad JJ, Taddei S, Gamba MA, Chazova IE, Puig JG. Comparison of single-pill strategies first line in hypertension: perindopril/amlodipine versus valsartan/amlodipine. *J Hypertens* 2015; 33(2):401–11.
6. Ruilope LM, SEVITENSION Study Investigators. Fixed-combination olmesartan/amlodipine was superior to perindopril + amlodipine in reducing central systolic blood pressure in hypertensive patients with diabetes. *J Clin Hypertens (Greenwich)* 2016; 18(6):528–35.
7. Wiysonge CS, Opie LH. β-Blockers as initial therapy for hypertension. *JAMA* 2013; 310(17):1851–2.
8. Giles TD, Weber MA, Basile J, Gradman AH,

Bharucha DB, Chen W, Pattathil M, NAC-MD-01 Study Investigators. Efficacy and safety of nebivolol and valsartan as fixed-dose combination in hypertension: a randomised, multicentre study. *Lancet* 2014; 383(9932):1889–98.

9. Aragon JP, Condit ME, Bhushan S, Predmore BL, Patel SS, Grinsfelder DB, Gundewar S, Jha S, Calvert JW, Barouch LA, Lavu M, Wright HM, et al. Beta3-adrenoreceptor stimulation ameliorates myocardial ischemia-reperfusion injury via endothelial nitric oxide synthase and neuronal nitric oxide synthase activation. *J Am Coll Cardiol* 2011; 58(25):2683–91.

10. Dessy C, Saliez J, Ghisdal P, Daneau G, Lobysheva, II, Frerart F, Belge C, Jnaoui K, Noirhomme P, Feron O, Balligand JL. Endothelial beta3-adrenoreceptors mediate nitric oxide-dependent vasorelaxation of coronary microvessels in response to the third-generation beta-blocker nebivolol. *Circulation* 2005; 112(8):1198–205.

11. Giles TD, Bakris G, Oparil S, Weber MA, Li H, Mallick M, Bharucha DB, Chen C, Ferguson WG, NAC-MD-01 Study Investigators. Correlations of plasma renin activity and aldosterone concentration with ambulatory blood pressure responses to nebivolol and valsartan, alone and in combination, in hypertension. *J Am Soc Hypertens* 2015; 9(11):845–54.

12. Neutel JM, Giles TD, Punzi H, Weiss RJ, Li H, Finck A. Long-term safety of nebivolol and valsartan combination therapy in patients with hypertension: an open-label, single-arm, multicenter study. *J Am Soc Hypertens* 2014; 8(12):915–20.

13. Tzemos N, Lim PO, MacDonald TM. Nebivolol reverses endothelial dysfunction in essential hypertension: a randomized, double-blind, crossover study. *Circulation* 2001; 104(5):511–4.

14. Kalinowski L, Dobrucki LW, Szczepanska-Konkel M, Jankowski M, Martyniec L, Angielski S, Malinski T. Third-generation beta-blockers stimulate nitric oxide release from endothelial cells through ATP efflux: a novel mechanism for antihypertensive action. *Circulation* 2003; 107(21):2747–52.

15. Mason RP, Kalinowski L, Jacob RF, Jacoby AM, Malinski T. Nebivolol reduces nitroxidative stress and restores nitric oxide bioavailability in endothelium of black Americans. *Circulation* 2005; 112(24):3795–801.

16. Perros F, Ranchoux B, Izikki M, Bentebbal S, Happe C, Antigny F, Jourdon P, Dorfmuller P, Lecerf F, Fadel E, Simonneau G, Humbert M, et al. Nebivolol for improving endothelial dysfunction, pulmonary vascular remodeling, and right heart function in pulmonary hypertension. *J Am Coll Cardiol* 2015; 65(7):668–80.

17. Group SR, Wright JT, Jr., Williamson JD, Whelton PK, Snyder JK, Sink KM, Rocco MV, Reboussin DM, Rahman M, Oparil S, Lewis CE, Kimmel PL, et al. A randomized trial of intensive versus standard blood-pressure control. *N Engl J Med* 2015; 373(22):2103–16.

18. Emdin CA, Rahimi K, Neal B, Callender T, Perkovic V, Patel A. Blood pressure lowering in type 2 diabetes: a systematic review and meta-analysis. *JAMA* 2015; 313(6):603–15.

19. Xie X, Atkins E, Lv J, Bennett A, Neal B, Ninomiya T, Woodward M, MacMahon S, Turnbull F, Hillis GS, Chalmers J, Mant J, et al. Effects of intensive blood pressure lowering on cardiovascular and renal outcomes: updated systematic review and meta-analysis. *Lancet* 2016; 387(10017):435–43.

20. Ettehad D, Emdin CA, Kiran A, Anderson SG, Callender T, Emberson J, Chalmers J, Rodgers A, Rahimi K. Blood pressure lowering for prevention of cardiovascular disease and death: a systematic review and meta-analysis. *Lancet* 2016; 387(10022):957–67.

21. Williamson JD, Supiano MA, Applegate WB, Berlowitz DR, Campbell RC, Chertow GM, Fine LJ, Haley WE, Hawfield AT, Ix JH, Kitzman DW, Kostis JB, et al. Intensive vs standard blood pressure control and cardiovascular disease outcomes in adults aged ≥75 years: a randomized clinical trial. *JAMA* 2016; 315(24):2673–82.

UNIT III

PULMONARY HYPERTENSION

CHAPTER 6

Overview of Pulmonary Hypertension and Drug Therapy

CHAPTER HIGHLIGHTS

- Pulmonary hypertension is a substantial global health issue associated with high mortality. This term refers to 5 groups of disorders, i.e., pulmonary arterial hypertension (PAH), pulmonary hypertension owing to left heart disease, pulmonary hypertension owing to lung diseases and/or hypoxia, chronic thromboembolic pulmonary hypertension, and pulmonary hypertension with unclear multifactorial mechanisms.
- Among the 5 groups of pulmonary hypertension, PAH has received the most attention regarding the molecular pathophysiology and mechanistically based drug therapy.
- Drugs for PAH target three main signaling pathways that are central in the control of pulmonary vasomotor tone and vascular cell proliferation. They are prostacyclin, endothelin 1, and nitric oxide pathways.
- The targeted drugs for PAH are classified into 5 groups, namely, endothelin receptor antagonists, phosphodiesterase type 5 inhibitors, soluble guanylate cyclase stimulators, prostacyclin analogues, and prostacyclin IP receptor agonists.

KEYWORDS | Calcium channel blocker; Endothelin receptor antagonist; Epidemiology; Molecular pathophysiology; Phosphodiesterase type 5 inhibitor; Prostacyclin analogue; Prostacyclin IP receptor agonist; Pulmonary arterial hypertension; Pulmonary hypertension; Soluble guanylate cyclase stimulator

CITATION | Li YR. *Cardiovascular Medicine: New Therapeutic Drugs Approved by the US FDA (2013–2017). Cell Med Press, Raleigh, NC, USA. 2018. http://dx.doi.org/10.20455/ndcvd.2018.06*

ABBREVIATIONS | ACCF, the American College of Cardiology Foundation; AHA, the American Heart Association; ALK1, activin receptor-like kinase type 1; BMPR2, bone morphogenic protein receptor type II; CAV1, caveolin-1; CCB, calcium channel blocker; CHEST, the American College of Chest Physicians; CTEPH, chronic thromboembolic pulmonary hypertension; EIF2AK4, eukaryotic translation initiation factor 2 alpha kinase 4; ENG, endoglin; ERA, endothelin receptor antagonist; ERS, the European Respiratory Society; ESC, the European Society of Cardiology; HIV, human immunodeficiency virus; KCNK3, potassium channel subfamily K member 3; PAH, pulmonary arterial hypertension; PAPm, mean pulmonary artery pressure; PDE5, phosphodiesterase type 5; PH-LHD, pulmonary hypertension due to left heart disease; sGC, soluble guanylate cyclase; SMAD9, mothers against decapentaplegic homolog 9; US FDA, the United States Food and Drug Administration; WHO, the World Health Organization

CHAPTER AT A GLANCE

1. INTRODUCTION

Pulmonary hypertension is a substantial global health issue associated with significant mortality [1, 2]. It can be a severe disease with a markedly decreased exercise tolerance and heart failure. All age groups are affected with rapidly growing burdens in elderly people, particularly in countries with aging populations. Recent advances in risk factor identification, molecular pathophysiology, and mechanistically based therapies, especially targeted drugs, have led to significant improvement of pulmonary hypertension management. To lay a foundation for the subsequent discussion of the new anti-pulmonary hypertensive drugs approved by the United States Food and Drug Administration (US FDA), this chapter provides an overview on several aspects of pulmonary hypertension, including definitions, classifications, epidemiology, pathophysiology, and mechanistically based drug therapy.

2. MOLECULAR MEDICINE OF PULMONARY HYPERTENSION

2.1. Definitions and Classifications

2.1.1. Definitions

The term pulmonary hypertension has been defined in various ways in the literature. For example, pulmonary hypertension may be defined as an abnormal increase in blood pressure in the pulmonary artery, pulmonary vein, or pulmonary capillaries, together known as the lung vasculature, leading to shortness of breath, dizziness, fainting, and other symptoms, all of which are exacerbated by exertion [3]. A concise and more widely adopted definition is that pulmonary hypertension refers to a mean pulmonary artery pressure (PAPm) ≥25 mm Hg at rest, measured during right heart catheterization [4]. It is considered that currently there is still insufficient evidence to add an exercise criterion to this definition of pulmonary hypertension [4].

Available data have shown that the normal PAPm at rest is 14 ± 3 mm Hg with an upper limit of normal of approximately 20 mm Hg. The clinical significance of a PAPm between 21 and 24 mm Hg is unclear. Patients presenting with a pulmonary artery pressure in this range should be carefully followed when they are at risk for developing pulmonary arterial hypertension (PAH, see below), such as patients with connective tissue disease or family members of patients with heritable PAH [4, 5].

Right heart catheterization

Right heart catherization is also known as pulmonary artery catheterization. It is considered the gold standard for diagnosis of pulmonary hypertension. During the procedure, a cardiologist places a thin, flexible tube (catheter) into the patient's jugular or femoral vein. The catheter is then threaded into the right ventricle and pulmonary artery. Right heart catheterization allows the direct measurement of the pressure in the main pulmonary arteries and right ventricle. It also allows the indirect estimation of the left atrial pressure via measuring pulmonary artery wedge pressure (PAWP). The catheter has a lumen (port) that opens at the tip of the catheter distal to the balloon. This port is connected to a pressure transducer. Just behind the tip of the catheter is a small balloon that can be inflated with air. When properly positioned in a branch of the pulmonary artery, the distal port measures pulmonary artery pressure (PAP; ~25/10 mm Hg; systolic/diastolic pressure). The mean PAP (PAPm) can be calculated as following: PAPm = (systolic PAP + 2 × diastolic PAP) ÷ 3 (based primarily on *Cardiovascular Physiology Concepts* [RE Klabunde], 2nd edition. Lippincott Williams & Wilkins, Baltimore, MD, USA. 2012).

As described next, pulmonary hypertension is classified into various groups, with PAH as the most notable one. The term PAH describes a subpopulation of patients with pulmonary hypertension characterized hemodynamically by the presence of pre-capillary pulmonary hypertension including an end-expiratory pulmonary artery wedge pressure (PAWP) ≤15 mm Hg and a pulmonary vascular resistance >3 Wood units in the absence of other causes of pre-capillary pulmonary hypertension, such as pulmonary hypertension due to lung diseases, chronic thromboembolic pulmonary hypertension, or other rare diseases [4].

2.1.2. Classifications

Based on the presence of identified causes or risk factors, the World Health Organization (WHO) in the 1970s classified pulmonary hypertension into two categories: primary pulmonary hypertension and secondary pulmonary hypertension. Research over the last several decades has established that pulmonary hypertension is a complex, multidisciplinary disorder, and consequently, the past two decades have witnessed the evolvement of the classification schemes of this disease, both clinically and functionally.

In 1998, a clinical classification scheme of 5 groups was established to individualize different categories of pulmonary hypertension sharing similar pathological findings, similar hemodynamic characteristics, and similar management. They are: (1) Group 1, pulmonary arterial hypertension; (2) Group 2, pulmonary hypertension due to left heart disease; (3) Group 3, pulmonary hypertension due to chronic lung disease and/or hypoxia; (4) Group 4, chronic thromboembolic pulmonary hypertension; and (5) Group 5, pulmonary hypertension due to unclear multifactorial mechanisms [6]. Subsequently, this clinical classification scheme has further matured and become accepted and been widely used in the clinical practice, guideline development, and regulatory approval of the labeling of new drugs for pulmonary hypertension [7, 8]. **Table 6.1** shows the most recently updated WHO clinical classification of pulmonary hypertension [7, 8].

In addition to the above clinical classification, the WHO has also developed a functional classification scheme to help determine how limited a patient with pulmonary hypertension is in his/her ability to do the activities of daily living (**Table 6.2**). In general, patients with more severe pulmonary hypertension tend to have a higher functional class. Like the clinical classification scheme, this functional classification scheme is also used in the clinical practice and guideline development, as well as regulatory approval of the labeling of new anti-pulmonary hypertensive drugs.

2.2. Epidemiology

2.2.1. Pulmonary Hypertension as a Whole

The exact prevalence of pulmonary hypertension in the United States and the world is unknown. This may be partially due to the heterogenic nature of the disease etiology. A recent surveillance in the

> **Pulmonary artery wedge pressure**
> PAWP, an indicator of left atrial pressure, is also known as pulmonary artery occlusive pressure (PAOP) or pulmonary capillary wedge pressure (PCWP). To measure PAWP, the catheter balloon (see Right heart catheterization box on p. 96) is inflated, which occludes the branch of the pulmonary artery. When this occurs, the pressure in the distal port rapidly falls, and reaches a stable lower value after a few seconds, that is very similar to left atrial pressure (mean pressure normally 8–10 mm Hg) (based primarily on *Cardiovascular Physiology Concepts* [RE Klabunde], 2nd edition. Lippincott Williams & Wilkins, Baltimore, MD, USA. 2012).

TABLE 6.1. The updated WHO clinical classification of pulmonary hypertension

1. Pulmonary arterial hypertension
1.1 Idiopathic PAH
1.2 Heritable PAH
  1.2.1 BMPR2
  1.2.2 ALK1, ENG, SMAD9, CAV1, KCNK3
  1.2.3 Unknown
1.3 Drug and toxin induced
1.4 Associated with:
  1.4.1 Connective tissue disease
  1.4.2 HIV infection
  1.4.3 Portal hypertension
  1.4.4 Congenital heart diseases
  1.4.5 Schistosomiasis
1′. Pulmonary veno-occlusive disease and/or pulmonary capillary hemangiomatosis
1′.1 Idiopathic
1′.2 Heritable
  1′.2.1 EIF2AK4 mutation
  1′.2.2 Other mutations
1′.3 Drugs, toxins, and radiation induced
1′.4 Associated with:
  1′.4.1 Connective tissue disease
  1′.4.2 HIV infection
1″. Persistent pulmonary hypertension of the newborn

2. Pulmonary hypertension owing to left heart disease
2.1 Left ventricular systolic dysfunction
2.2 Left ventricular diastolic dysfunction
2.3 Valvular disease
2.4 Congenital/acquired left heart inflow/outflow tract obstruction and congenital cardiomyopathies

3. Pulmonary hypertension owing to lung diseases and/or hypoxia
3.1 Chronic obstructive pulmonary disease
3.2 Interstitial lung disease
3.3 Other pulmonary diseases with mixed restrictive and obstructive pattern
3.4 Sleep-disordered breathing
3.5 Alveolar hypoventilation disorders
3.6 Chronic exposure to high altitude
3.7 Developmental lung diseases

4. Chronic thromboembolic pulmonary hypertension

5. Pulmonary hypertension with unclear multifactorial mechanisms
5.1 Hematologic disorders: chronic hemolytic anemia, myeloproliferative disorders, splenectomy
5.2 Systemic disorders: sarcoidosis, pulmonary histiocytosis, lymphangioleiomyomatosis
5.3 Metabolic disorders: glycogen storage disease, Gaucher disease, thyroid disorders
5.4 Others: tumoral obstruction, fibrosing mediastinitis, chronic renal failure, segmental pulmonary
   hypertension

Note: ALK1, activin receptor-like kinase type 1; BMPR2, bone morphogenic protein receptor type II; CAV1, caveolin-1; EIF2AK4, eukaryotic translation initiation factor 2 alpha kinase 4; ENG, endoglin; HIV, human immunodeficiency virus; KCNK3, potassium channel subfamily K member 3; SMAD9, mothers against decapentaplegic homolog 9. This table is based on Refs. [7, 8].

TABLE 6.2. The WHO functional classification of pulmonary hypertension

Class I	Patients with pulmonary hypertension but without resulting limitation of physical activity. Ordinary physical activity does not cause undue dyspnea or fatigue, chest pain or near syncope
Class II	Patients with pulmonary hypertension resulting in slight limitation of physical activity. They are comfortable at rest. Ordinary physical activity causes undue dyspnea or fatigue, chest pain or near syncope
Class III	Patients with pulmonary hypertension resulting in marked limitation of physical activity. They are comfortable at rest. Less than ordinary activity causes undue dyspnea or fatigue, chest pain or near syncope
Class IV	Patients with pulmonary hypertension with inability to carry out any physical activity without symptoms. These patients manifest signs of right heart failure. Dyspnea and/or fatigue may even be present at rest. Discomfort is increased by any physical activity

United States reported that from 2001/2002 to 2009/2010, the age-adjusted rate of hospitalizations associated with pulmonary hypertension increased by 44%, from 91 per 100,000 discharges to 131 per 100,000 discharges. Notably, the increase was much larger in females than in males. The total estimated number of pulmonary hypertension hospitalizations in 2010 was between 471,864 and 728, 983 depending on the criteria used [9]. The same report also showed that the death rate for pulmonary hypertension as a contributing cause of death was 5.5 per 100,000 in 2001 and 6.5 per 100,000 in 2010 in the United States [9].

Like that in the United States, the global prevalence of pulmonary hypertension remains poorly determined. It is believed that the prevalence of pulmonary hypertension varies in the different regions of the world, being affected by various factors, including genetic and environmental factors. In this context, in the UK, a prevalence of 97 cases per million with a female-to-male ratio of 1.8 has been reported [5]. On the other hand, a prevalence of 3,260 cases per million (or 0.326%) was reported in an Australian cohort [10]. A more recent review of literature suggested a pulmonary hypertension prevalence of about 1% of the global population, which may increase to up to 10% in individuals aged more than 65 years [2].

2.2.2. Different Groups of Pulmonary Hypertension

Comparative epidemiological data on the prevalence of the different groups of pulmonary hypertension are not widely available. It is generally believed that Groups 1, 2, and 4 are the most common forms [5, 11, 12]. In this context, the prevalence of PAH (Group 1) in the general population is estimated to be 15–60 cases per million individuals [12, 13]. Pulmonary hypertension is common in patients with chronic heart failure, and up to 60% of patients with severe left ventricular systolic dysfunction and up to 70% of patients with heart failure with preserved ejection fraction may present with pulmonary hypertension (Group 2) [5]. In view of the increasingly high prevalence of chronic heart failure, Group 2 pulmonary hypertension may be the most common form among the five groups. While Groups 1, 2, and 4 are among the most common forms of pulmonary hypertension, over the past two decades PAH has received the greatest attention with regard to understanding the molecular pathophysiology and developing new drug therapy. Hence, the remaining sections of this this chapter focus primarily on PAH.

2.2.3. Subtypes and Risk Factors of PAH

2.2.3.1. SUBTYPES

The subtypes of PAH (see **Table 6.1**) vary among different regions. For example, in the Western countries, idiopathic and connective tissue disease-associated PAH are the most common subtypes of PAH. On the other hand, congenital heart disease-associated PAH is the most common subtype in China, whereas infection (e.g., schistosomiasis)-associated PAH is common in Brazil (reviewed in [12]).

2.2.3.2. RISK FACTORS

A number of risk factors for the development of PAH have been identified and are defined as any factor or condition that is suspected to play a predisposing or facilitating role in the development of the disease. Risk factors are classified as "definite", "likely", "possible", or "unlikely", based on the strength of their association with pulmonary hypertension and their probable causal role [5, 7, 8]. A "definite" association is defined as an epidemic, such as occurred with appetite suppressants in the 1960s, or large, multicenter epidemiological studies demonstrating an association between a drug (or condition) and PAH. A "likely" association is considered if a single-center case-control study or multiple case series demonstrate an association or if clinical and hemodynamic recovery occurs after stopping exposure, such as occurred in dasatinib-induced PAH. A "possible" association can be suspected, for example, for drugs with similar mechanisms of action as those in the "definite" or "likely" category but which have not yet been studied, such as drugs used to treat attention deficit disorder. Lastly, an "unlikely" association is defined as one in which a drug (or condition) has been studied in epidemiological studies and an association with PAH has not been demonstrated. "Definite" clinical associations are listed in **Table 6.1**, and the risk level of different drugs and toxins are given in **Table 6.3** [5, 7, 8].

2.3. Pathophysiology of PAH

Our understanding of the pathophysiology of PAH has undergone a paradigm shift in the past 10–15 years. Once a condition thought to be dominated by increased vasoconstrictor tone and thrombosis, PAH is now regarded as a vasculopathy in which structural changes/vascular remodeling driven by endothelial cell dysfunction, excessive vascular smooth muscle cell growth, vascular inflammation, as well as oxidative stress with recruitment and infiltration of circulating cells, play a major role. The disease pathophysiology involves perturbations of a number of molecular mechanisms, including pathways

TABLE 6.3. The risk levels of drugs and toxins in PAH

Definite risk factor	Likely risk factor	Possible risk factor	Unlikely risk factor
Aminorex Benfluorex Dexfenfluramine Fenfluramine SSRIs Toxic rapeseed oil	Amphetamines Dasatinib Methamphetamines L-Tryptophan	Amphetamine-like drugs Chemotherapeutic agents Cocaine Interferon α and β Phenylpropanolamine St. John's wort	Cigarette smoking Estrogen Oral contraceptives

Note: Selective serotonin reuptake inhibitors (SSRIs) have been demonstrated as a risk factor for the development of persistent pulmonary hypertension in the newborn in pregnant women exposed to SSRIs (especially after 20 weeks of gestation). The list is in alphabetical order and not indicative of relative importance. This table is based on Refs. [5, 7, 8].

involving growth factors, cytokines, metabolic and mitochondrial signaling, elastases and proteases, and ion channels, as well as germline mutations. These molecular alterations converge to produce excessive vasoconstriction and a pro-proliferative, apoptosis-resistant phenotype in pulmonary vasculature. In fact, currently approved drugs for treating PAH target three main signaling pathways that are central in the control of pulmonary vasomotor tone and vascular cell proliferation. They are endothelin 1, nitric oxide, and prostacyclin pathways [12, 14, 15] (**Figure 6.1**). Further elucidation of the molecular pathophysiology of PAH as well as other forms of pulmonary hypertension would increase our ability to develop more effective therapeutic modalities for combating this global health issue.

3. OVERVIEW OF MECHANISTICALLY BASED DRUG THERAPY

As noted earlier, among the various forms of pulmonary hypertension, PAH has received the most extensive attention with regard to developing novel pharmacological treatment. Hence, this section focuses on discussing the pharmacological agents for treating PAH. Drug therapies of other groups of pulmonary hypertension are also briefly described where applicable.

3.1. Overview of Mechanistically Based Drug Therapy of PAH

3.1.1. Overall Drug Treatments for PAH

Several classes of drugs have been used to treat PAH with the emphasis on ameliorating pulmonary vasoconstriction and thereby the improvement of patients' symptoms. Although the mainstay of therapy has focused on the use of vasodilators, management of PAH also involves other drugs, such as diuretics, anticoagulants, and digoxin. The pharmacological treatments for PAH are grouped into non-vasodilating therapies and vasodilating drug treatments (**Table 6.4**).

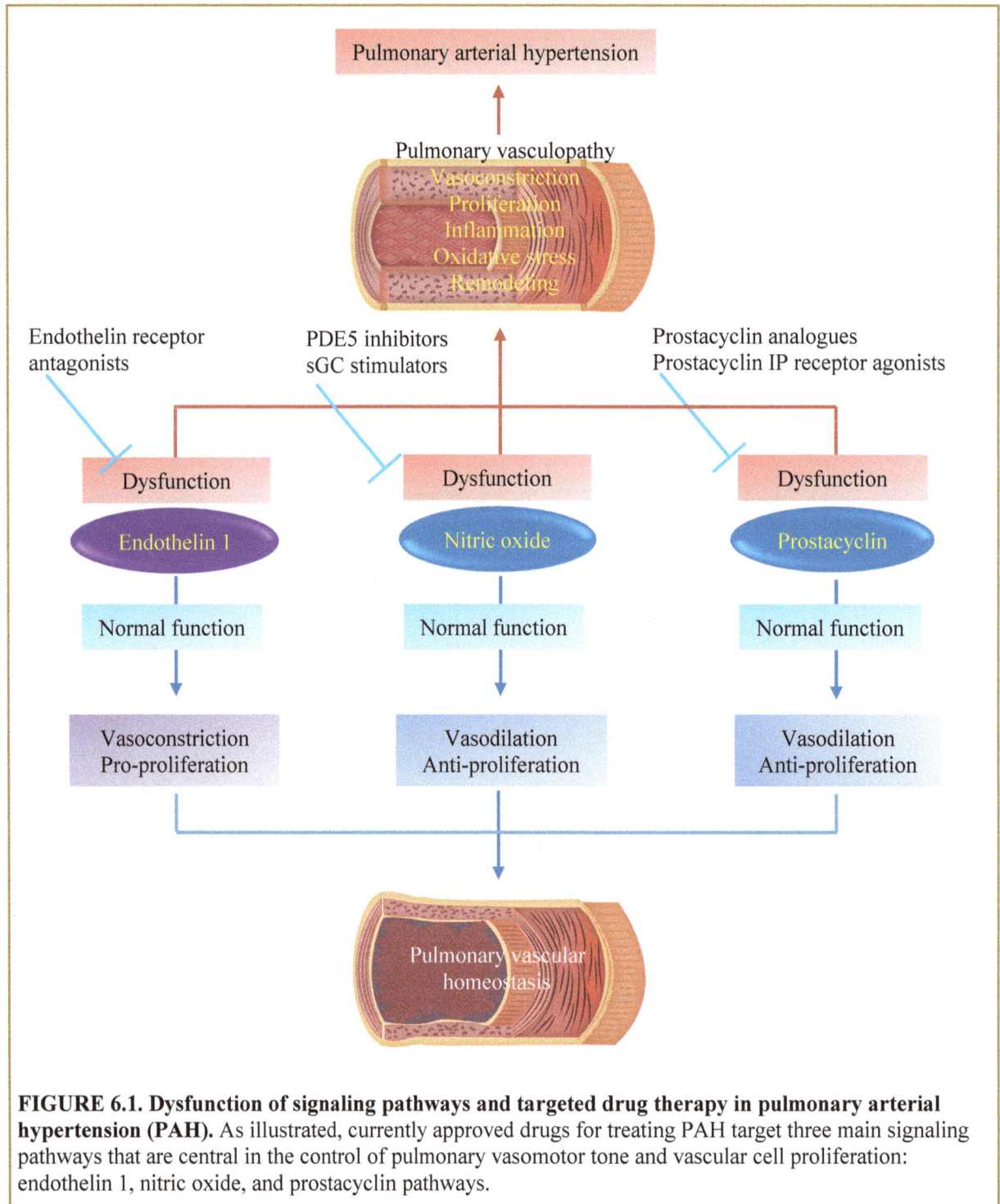

FIGURE 6.1. Dysfunction of signaling pathways and targeted drug therapy in pulmonary arterial hypertension (PAH). As illustrated, currently approved drugs for treating PAH target three main signaling pathways that are central in the control of pulmonary vasomotor tone and vascular cell proliferation: endothelin 1, nitric oxide, and prostacyclin pathways.

3.1.2. Overview of Guideline-Based Treatment Strategies for PAH

Guidelines and treatment algorithms on the management of pulmonary hypertension in both adults and pediatric patients have become available, and provide evidence-based treatment strategies for PAH

TABLE 6.4. Drug treatment of pulmonary arterial hypertension (PAH)

Drug treatment	Pharmacological effects and other comments
Non-vasodilating therapies	
Anticoagulants	▪ Suppression of thrombin, a contributor to disease progression ▪ Improvement of survival
Diuretics	▪ Relief of symptoms due to PAH-associated right ventricular failure and systemic venous congestion
Oxygen	▪ Improvement of hypoxemia
Digoxin	▪ Improvement of PAH-associated right ventricular dysfunction by increasing myocardial contractility
Vasodilating Drugs	
Calcium channel blockers (CCBs)	▪ Reduction of pulmonary artery pressure due to vasodilating activity ▪ The most commonly used CCBs include long acting nifedipine, diltiazem, and amlodipine ▪ Due to its potential negative inotropic effects (suppressing myocardial contractility), verapamil should be avoided
Endothelin receptor antagonists (ERAs)	▪ Endothelin (ET)-1 is a vasoconstrictor and a smooth muscle mitogen that may contribute to the development of PAH ▪ Blockage of ET receptors improves the symptoms of PAH patients, and several ERAs have become available for treating PAH ▪ Currently there are 3 US FDA-approved ERAs: ambrisentan, bosentan, and macitentan. Ambrisentan is a selective blocker of ET_A receptors and bosentan and macitentan are blockers of ET_A and ET_B receptors (see Box on the next page for more description)
Phosphodiesterase type 5 (PDE5) inhibitors	▪ Inhibition of PDE5 produces pulmonary vasodilation by promoting an enhanced and sustained level of cyclic guanosine monophosphate (cGMP), an identical effect to that of inhaled nitric oxide ▪ Both sildenafil and tadalafil have been approved for treating PAH in addition to their use in treating erectile dysfunction
Soluble guanylate cyclase stimulators	▪ Soluble guanylate cyclase (sGC) stimulators directly stimulate sGC and also sensitize nitric oxide-mediated activation of sGC, leading to increased cGMP ▪ Riociguat is the first-in-class member and currently the only member of the class approved by the US FDA
Prostacyclin analogues	▪ PAH patients show inadequate production of prostacyclin, a vasodilator with antiproliferative activities ▪ Administration of prostacyclin analogues has been a mainstay of PAH therapy for more than a decade ▪ There are currently three US FDA-approved prostacyclin drugs: epoprostenol, iloprost, and treprostinil
Prostacyclin IP receptor agonists	▪ This represents the newest class of anti-PAH drugs. These drugs are non-prostanoids and activate prostacyclin IP receptors causing vasodilation and suppression of vascular cell proliferation ▪ Selexipag is the first-in-class member and currently the only member of the class approved by the US FDA

and other groups of pulmonary hypertension [5, 16–22]. The most notable guidelines include: (1) the ACCF/AHA 2009 expert consensus document on pulmonary hypertension [20]; (2) the 2014 CHEST guideline and expert panel report on pharmacologic therapy for pulmonary hypertension in adults [21]; and (3) the 2015 ESC/ERS guideline for the diagnosis and treatment of pulmonary hypertension [5]. All the three guidelines provide detailed recommendations, which in principle are also largely similar, on the management of PAH as well as other types of pulmonary hypertension. The major recommended treatment strategies by each of the three guidelines are summarized below, and the reader is advised to refer to the original guideline documents for detailed recommendations.

3.1.2.1. THE ACCF/AHA 2009 GUIDELINE

The ACCF/AHA 2009 guideline document was developed by the American College of Cardiology Foundation (ACCF) Task Force on Expert Consensus Documents, and was cosponsored by the American Heart Association (AHA). The major recommended treatment strategies for PAH in this guideline document are outlined below [16, 20].

- Oral anticoagulation is proposed for most patients; diuretic treatment and supplemental oxygen are indicated in cases of fluid retention and hypoxemia, respectively.
- High doses of CCBs are indicated only in the minority of patients who respond to acute vasoreactivity testing.
- Nonresponders to acute vasoreactivity testing or responders who remain in the WHO functional class III (see **Table 6.2**), should be considered candidates for treatment with either an oral PDE5 inhibitor or an oral endothelin receptor antagonist.
- Continuous intravenous administration of epoprostenol remains the treatment of choice in the WHO functional class IV patients.
- Combination therapy is recommended for patients treated with PAH monotherapy who remain in the WHO functional class III.
- Atrial septostomy and lung transplantation are indicated for refractory patients or where medical treatment is unavailable.

3.1.2.2. THE 2014 CHEST GUIDELINE

The American College of Chest Physicians (CHEST) released the publication of "Pharmacologic therapy for pulmonary arterial hypertension in adults: CHEST guideline and expert panel report" in 2014, which represents the most recent efforts of the CHEST to deliver updated evidence-based recommendations on the management of PAH. The 2014 CHEST guideline contains 79 recommendations and expert consensus statements to aid clinicians in the management of PAH using the latest drug therapies for adults with the condition [21].

3.1.2.3. THE 2015 ESC/ERS GUIDELINE

The 2015 ESC/ERS guideline is the most recent document, issued by the European Society of Cardiology (ESC) and the European Respiratory Society (ERS), on the diagnosis and treatment of pulmonary

Endothelin and endothelin receptors

Endothelin (ET) is an important factor involved in regulating vascular tone and other vascular processes. In humans, there are 3 endothelins, ET-1, ET-2, and ET-3, with ET-1 being the main endothelin secreted by endothelial cells. ET-1 acts by binding to its receptors, ET_A and ET_B, in vascular cells. Abnormal activation of ET_A and ET_B receptors by ET-1 on vascular cells causes vasoconstriction, smooth muscle cell proliferation, and vascular inflammatory responses, which collectively contribute to the development of various forms of cardiovascular disorders, including pulmonary hypertension.

Atrial septostomy

Atrial septostomy is a procedure where a small hole is made (using a cardiac catheter) in the wall between the left and right atria of the heart. Atrial septostomy can be useful in people with advanced pulmonary hypertension because it reduces pressure in the right side of the heart.

hypertension, with a large portion of it devoted to PAH. In view of the increasingly complex nature of the disease, treatment of PAH patients cannot be considered as a mere prescription of drugs, but should be composed of a comprehensive strategy that includes the initial evaluation of severity and the subsequent response to treatment. The 2015 ESC/ERS guideline classifies the current treatment strategy for PAH patients into the following three main steps [5].

- The initial approach includes general measures (physical activity and supervised rehabilitation, pregnancy, birth control and post-menopausal hormonal therapy, elective surgery, infection prevention, psychosocial support, adherence to treatments, genetic counselling and travel), supportive therapy (oral anticoagulants, diuretics, oxygen, digoxin), referral to expert centers and acute vasoreactivity testing for the indication of chronic CCB therapy.
- The second step includes initial therapy with a high-dose CCB in vasoreactive patients or drugs approved for PAH in non-vasoreactive patients according to the prognostic risk of the patient and the grade of recommendation and level of evidence for each individual compound or combination of compounds.
- The third part is related to the response to the initial treatment strategy; in the case of an inadequate response, the role of combinations of approved drugs (see **Tables 6.4** and **6.5**) and lung transplantation are proposed.

3.1.3. Overview of the US FDA-Approved Drugs for Targeted Therapies of PAH

As introduced above, presently, a total of 10 specific drugs from five classes targeting the three main dysfunctional signaling pathways in PAH (see **Figure 6.1** for the 3 signaling pathways) have been approved by the US FDA. These include: (1) three ERAs (bosentan, macitentan, and ambrisentan); (2) two PDE5 inhibitors (sildenafil and tadalafil); (3) one soluble guanylate cyclase stimulator (riociguat); (4) three prostacyclin analogues (epoprostenol, treprostinil, and iloprost); and (5) the most recently approved prostacyclin IP receptor agonist selexipag. The initial FDA approval date and the major indications of each of the above 10 drugs are given in **Table 6.5**.

3.2. Overview of Mechanistically Based Drug Therapy for Other Forms of Pulmonary Hypertension

3.2.1. Group 2 (Pulmonary Hypertension due to Left Heart Disease)

Although the exact prevalence of pulmonary hypertension due to left heart disease (PH-LHD) remains unknown, it is arguably the most common form of pulmonary hypertension and it consists of three main subtypes: (1) pulmonary hypertension due to left ventricular systolic dysfunction; (2) pulmonary hypertension due to left ventricular diastolic dysfunction; and (3) pulmonary hypertension due to valvular disease [11, 23]. The primary goal of therapy in PH-LHD must be to improve global management of the underlying condition

TABLE 6.5. The US FDA-approved drugs for treating pulmonary arterial hypertension (PAH) via targeting three dysfunctional signaling pathways

Drug	FDA approval date	Major indication
Endothelin receptor antagonists		
Ambrisentan (Letairis)	June 2007	PAH
Bosentan (Tracleer)	November 2001	PAH in adults and pediatric patients aged ≥3 years
Macitentan (Opsumit)	October 2013	PAH
Phosphodiesterase type 5 inhibitors		
Sildenafil (Revatio)	June 2005	PAH
Tadalafil (Adcirca)	May 2009	PAH
Soluble guanylate cyclase stimulators		
Riociguat (Adempas)	October 2013	PAH; CTEPH
Prostacyclin analogues		
Epoprostenol (Flolan)	September 1995	PAH
Iloprost (Ventavis)	December 2004	PAH
Treprostinil (Orenitram, Remodulin, Tyvaso)	May 2002	PAH
Prostacyclin IP receptor agonists		
Selexipag (Uptravi)	December 2015	PAH

Note: CTEPH, chronic thromboembolic pulmonary hypertension (also see Section 3.2.3). Riociguat is the only one, among the 10 US FDA-approved drugs, that is indicated for both PAH and CTEPH. The three dysfunctional signaling pathways are endothelin 1-, nitric oxide-, and prostacyclin-mediated signaling.

prior to considering specific measures to treat pulmonary hypertension. This includes repair of valvular heart disease when indicated and aggressive therapy for heart failure with reduced systolic function. At present, the use of drugs approved for PAH is generally not recommended for PH-LDH, due to the lack of evidence supporting an efficacy in this form of pulmonary hypertension [11, 22].

3.2.2. Group 3 (Pulmonary Hypertension Associated with Lung Diseases)

Currently there is no specific therapy for pulmonary hypertension associated with lung diseases. Patients with lung diseases and pulmonary hypertension who are hypoxemic should receive long-term oxygen therapy, adapting the general recommendations for chronic obstructive pulmonary disease (COPD). Treatment of the underlying lung disease should be optimized. The use of drugs approved for PAH is not recommended for patients with pulmonary hypertension due to lung diseases [5].

Chronic obstructive pulmonary disease (COPD)

COPD is a common, preventable, and treatable disease that is characterized by persistent respiratory symptoms and airflow limitation that is due to airway and/or alveolar abnormalities usually caused by significant exposure to noxious particles or gases. COPD is currently the 4th leading cause of death in the world, and it is projected to be the 3rd leading cause of death by 2020 (based on *Global Initiatives for Chronic Obstructive Lung Disease: 2017 Report*).

3.2.3. Group 4 (Chronic Thromboembolic Pulmonary Hypertension)

Chronic thromboembolic pulmonary hypertension (CTEPH) results from obstructive pulmonary arterial remodeling as a consequence of major pulmonary vessel thromboembolism. Pulmonary thromboendarterectomy, a surgical treatment, is the treatment of choice for CTEPH. Optimal medical treatment for CTEPH consists of anticoagulants and diuretics, and oxygen in cases of heart failure or hypoxemia. Riociguat is recommended for the treatment of adults with persistent/recurrent CTEPH, after surgical treatment, or inoperable CTEPH. Off-label use of drugs approved for PAH may be considered in symptomatic patients with inoperable CTEPH [5, 24].

3.2.4. Group 5 (Pulmonary Hypertension with Unclear and/or Multifactorial Mechanisms)

Pulmonary hypertension with unclear and/or multifactorial mechanisms includes several disorders with multiple patho-etiologies. A common feature of these diseases is that the mechanisms of pulmonary hypertension are poorly understood and may include pulmonary vasoconstriction, proliferative vasculopathy, extrinsic compression, intrinsic occlusion, high-output cardiac failure, vascular obliteration, and left heart failure as causes. As such, these patients need careful diagnosis, and the treatment is tailored for specific diagnosis/etiology. The general notion is to treat the lung (the underling patho-etiologies), not the pulmonary pressure. Currently, there is no evidence supporting the use of drugs approved for PAH in the treatment of Group 5 pulmonary hypertension [5].

> **Pulmonary thromboendarterectomy (PTE)**
> PTE, also known as pulmonary endarterectomy (PEA), is a surgical procedure to remove the thromboembolic materials from the pulmonary arteries in the lungs. It is the treatment of choice to relieve pulmonary artery obstruction in patients with CTEPH. For up to two-third of patients, removal of the blood clots through PTE surgery can potentially cure this type of pulmonary hypertension.

4. SELF-ASSESSMENT QUESTIONS

4.1. Pulmonary hypertension is a term that includes five groups of disorders, collectively representing a substantial global health issue associated with high mortality. Which of the following groups has received the greatest attention with regard to targeted drug therapy?

A. Chronic thromboembolic pulmonary hypertension
B. Pulmonary arterial hypertension
C. Pulmonary hypertension owing to left heart disease
D. Pulmonary hypertension owing to lung diseases and/or hypoxia
E. Pulmonary hypertension with unclear multifactorial mechanisms

4.2. Among the 5 groups of pulmonary hypertension, which group is associated with left heart disease and arguably the most common form of pulmonary hypertension?

A. Group 1
B. Group 2
C. Group 3
D. Group 4
E. Group 5

4.3. Exposure to a number of drugs has been demonstrated to be associated with the development of pulmonary arterial hypertension (PAH). Which of the following is a definite risk factor for the development of PAH?

A. Benfluorex
B. Dasatinib
C. Interferon alpha
D. Interferon beta
E. Oral contraceptive

4.4. Five classes of drugs targeting 3 specific signaling pathways underlying the pathophysiology of pulmonary arterial hypertension (PAH) have been approved by the US FDA in recent years. Which of the following anti-PAH drugs is also approved by the US FDA for treating the Group 4 pulmonary hypertension (i.e., chronic thromboembolic pulmonary hypertension)?

A. Bosentan
B. Iloprost
C. Riociguat
D. Selexipag
E. Sildenafil

4.5. Which of the following drugs is the active ingredient of pharmaceutical preparations for treating both pulmonary arterial hypertension and erectile dysfunction?

A. Abrisentan
B. Epoprosteno
C. Riociguat
D. Selexipag
E. Tadalafil

ANSWERS AND EXPLANATIONS

4.1. The correct answer is B. Although Groups 1, 2, and 4 are among the most common forms of pulmonary hypertension, over the past decades PAH has received the greatest attention with regard to the molecular pathophysiology and drug therapy. Indeed, the US FDA-approved drugs for pulmonary hypertension are primarily for treating PAH (see **Table 6.5**).

4.2. The correct answer is B. Group 2 pulmonary hypertension is also known as pulmonary hypertension due to left heart disease (PH-LHD). While its exact prevalence remains unknown, PH-LHD is arguably the most common form of pulmonary hypertension and it consists of three main subtypes: (1) pulmonary hypertension due to left ventricular systolic dysfunction; (2) pulmonary hypertension due to left ventricular diastolic dysfunction; and (3) pulmonary hypertension due to valvular disease.

4.3. The correct answer is A. Exposure to certain drugs and toxins is associated with pulmonary arterial hypertension (PAH), and such associations are classified into definite, likely, possible, and unlikely, based on the strength of their association with PAH and their probable causal role in the disease process. The following agents are under the definite risk factor category: aminorex, benfluorex, dexfenfluramine, fenfluramine, selective serotonin reuptake inhibitors, and toxic rapeseed oil. Dasatinib is classified as a likely risk factor, while interferon alpha and beta are considered possible risk factors. Oral contraceptives are classified as unlikely risk factors.

4.4. The correct answer is C. Riociguat is a soluble guanylate cyclase stimulator approved by the US FDA for treating both pulmonary arterial hypertension (PAH) and chronic thromboembolic pulmonary hypertension. PAH is the only indication approved by the US FDA for the other drugs listed.

4.5. The correct answer is E. Both sildenafil and tadalafil, drugs initially approved for treating erectile dysfunction, are also approved by the US FDA for treating pulmonary arterial hypertension (PAH). Please note that the trade names, formulations, and strengths are different for these two drugs in treating erectile dysfunction versus PAH.

REFERENCES

1. Shah SJ. Pulmonary hypertension. *JAMA* 2012; 308(13):1366–74.
2. Hoeper MM, Humbert M, Souza R, Idrees M, Kawut SM, Sliwa-Hahnle K, Jing ZC, Gibbs JS. A global view of pulmonary hypertension. *Lancet Respir Med* 2016; 4(4):306–22.
3. Li YR. *Cardiovascular Diseases: From Molecular Pharmacology to Evidence-Based Therapeutics*. John Wiley & Sons, New Jersey, USA. 2015.
4. Hoeper MM, Bogaard HJ, Condliffe R, Frantz R, Khanna D, Kurzyna M, Langleben D, Manes A, Satoh T, Torres F, Wilkins MR, Badesch DB. Definitions and diagnosis of pulmonary hypertension. *J Am Coll Cardiol* 2013; 62(25 Suppl):D42–50.
5. Galie N, Humbert M, Vachiery JL, Gibbs S, Lang I, Torbicki A, Simonneau G, Peacock A, Vonk Noordegraaf A, Beghetti M, Ghofrani A, Gomez Sanchez MA, et al. 2015 ESC/ERS guidelines for the diagnosis and treatment of pulmonary hypertension: the Joint Task Force for the Diagnosis and Treatment of Pulmonary Hypertension of the European Society of Cardiology (ESC) and the European Respiratory Society (ERS): endorsed by: Association for European Paediatric and Congenital Cardiology (AEPC), International Society for Heart and Lung Transplantation (ISHLT). *Eur Heart J* 2016; 37(1):67–119.
6. Simonneau G, Galie N, Rubin LJ, Langleben D, Seeger W, Domenighetti G, Gibbs S, Lebrec D, Speich R, Beghetti M, Rich S, Fishman A. Clinical classification of pulmonary hypertension. *J Am Coll Cardiol* 2004; 43(12 Suppl S):5S–12S.
7. Simonneau G, Robbins IM, Beghetti M, Channick RN, Delcroix M, Denton CP, Elliott CG, Gaine SP, Gladwin MT, Jing ZC, Krowka MJ, Langleben D, et al. Updated clinical classification of pulmonary hypertension. *J Am Coll Cardiol* 2009; 54(1 Suppl):S43–54.
8. Simonneau G, Gatzoulis MA, Adatia I, Celermajer D, Denton C, Ghofrani A, Gomez Sanchez MA, Krishna Kumar R, Landzberg M, Machado RF, Olschewski H, Robbins IM, et al. Updated clinical classification of pulmonary hypertension. *J Am Coll Cardiol* 2013; 62(25 Suppl):D34–41.
9. George MG, Schieb LJ, Ayala C, Talwalkar A, Levant S. Pulmonary hypertension surveillance: United States, 2001 to 2010. *Chest* 2014; 146(2):476–95.
10. Strange G, Playford D, Stewart S, Deague JA, Nelson H, Kent A, Gabbay E. Pulmonary hypertension: prevalence and mortality in the

Armadale echocardiography cohort. *Heart* 2012; 98(24):1805–11.

11. Hoeper MM, McLaughlin VV, Dalaan AM, Satoh T, Galie N. Treatment of pulmonary hypertension. *Lancet Respir Med* 2016; 4(4):323–36.

12. Lau EMT, Giannoulatou E, Celermajer DS, Humbert M. Epidemiology and treatment of pulmonary arterial hypertension. *Nat Rev Cardiol* 2017; 14(10):603–14.

13. Hansmann G. Pulmonary hypertension in infants, children, and young adults. *J Am Coll Cardiol* 2017; 69(20):2551–69.

14. Morrell NW, Adnot S, Archer SL, Dupuis J, Jones PL, MacLean MR, McMurtry IF, Stenmark KR, Thistlethwaite PA, Weissmann N, Yuan JX, Weir EK. Cellular and molecular basis of pulmonary arterial hypertension. *J Am Coll Cardiol* 2009; 54(1 Suppl):S20–31.

15. Schermuly RT, Ghofrani HA, Wilkins MR, Grimminger F. Mechanisms of disease: pulmonary arterial hypertension. *Nat Rev Cardiol* 2011; 8(8):443–55.

16. Barst RJ, Gibbs JS, Ghofrani HA, Hoeper MM, McLaughlin VV, Rubin LJ, Sitbon O, Tapson VF, Galie N. Updated evidence-based treatment algorithm in pulmonary arterial hypertension. *J Am Coll Cardiol* 2009; 54(1 Suppl):S78–84.

17. McLaughlin VV, Archer SL, Badesch DB, Barst RJ, Farber HW, Lindner JR, Mathier MA, McGoon MD, Park MH, Rosenson RS, Rubin LJ, Tapson VF, et al. ACCF/AHA 2009 expert consensus document on pulmonary hypertension: a report of the American College of Cardiology Foundation Task Force on Expert Consensus Documents and the American Heart Association: developed in collaboration with the American College of Chest Physicians, American Thoracic Society, Inc., and the Pulmonary Hypertension Association. *Circulation* 2009; 119(16):2250–94.

18. Galie N, Corris PA, Frost A, Girgis RE, Granton J, Jing ZC, Klepetko W, McGoon MD, McLaughlin VV, Preston IR, Rubin LJ, Sandoval J, et al. Updated treatment algorithm of pulmonary arterial hypertension. *J Am Coll Cardiol* 2013; 62(25 Suppl):D60–72.

19. McLaughlin VV, Gaine SP, Howard LS, Leuchte HH, Mathier MA, Mehta S, Palazzini M, Park MH, Tapson VF, Sitbon O. Treatment goals of pulmonary hypertension. *J Am Coll Cardiol* 2013; 62(25 Suppl):D73–81.

20. McLaughlin VV, Archer SL, Badesch DB, Barst RJ, Farber HW, Lindner JR, Mathier MA, McGoon MD, Park MH, Rosenson RS, Rubin LJ, Tapson VF, et al. ACCF/AHA 2009 expert consensus document on pulmonary hypertension: a report of the American College of Cardiology Foundation Task Force on Expert Consensus Documents and the American Heart Association developed in collaboration with the American College of Chest Physicians; American Thoracic Society, Inc.; and the Pulmonary Hypertension Association. *J Am Coll Cardiol* 2009; 53(17):1573–619.

21. Taichman DB, Ornelas J, Chung L, Klinger JR, Lewis S, Mandel J, Palevsky HI, Rich S, Sood N, Rosenzweig EB, Trow TK, Yung R, et al. Pharmacologic therapy for pulmonary arterial hypertension in adults: CHEST guideline and expert panel report. *Chest* 2014; 146(2):449–75.

22. Abman SH, Hansmann G, Archer SL, Ivy DD, Adatia I, Chung WK, Hanna BD, Rosenzweig EB, Raj JU, Cornfield D, Stenmark KR, Steinhorn R, et al. Pediatric pulmonary hypertension: guidelines from the American Heart Association and American Thoracic Society. *Circulation* 2015; 132(21):2037–99.

23. Vachiery JL, Adir Y, Barbera JA, Champion H, Coghlan JG, Cottin V, De Marco T, Galie N, Ghio S, Gibbs JS, Martinez F, Semigran M, et al. Pulmonary hypertension due to left heart diseases. *J Am Coll Cardiol* 2013; 62(25 Suppl):D100–8.

24. Hoeper MM, Madani MM, Nakanishi N, Meyer B, Cebotari S, Rubin LJ. Chronic thromboembolic pulmonary hypertension. *Lancet Respir Med* 2014; 2(7):573–82.

CHAPTER 7

New Drugs for Pulmonary Hypertension

CHAPTER HIGHLIGHTS

- Recent advancements in developing novel drugs targeting specific pathophysiological processes have changed the paradigm of the clinical management of pulmonary hypertension, especially pulmonary arterial hypertension (PAH).
- Over the past five years, the United States Food and Drug Administration (US FDA) has approved three new drugs for treating pulmonary hypertension. They are macitentan, riociguat, and selexipag.
- While macitentan is the newest third member of the endothelin receptor antagonist drug class, both riociguat and selexipag are first-in-class members, belonging to the soluble guanylate cyclase stimulator drug class and the prostacyclin IP receptor agonist drug class, respectively.
- All three new drugs are indicated for treating PAH, and riociguat is also approved for treating chronic thromboembolic pulmonary hypertension (CTEPH).

KEYWORDS | Chronic thromboembolic pulmonary hypertension; Endothelin receptor antagonist; Macitentan; Prostacyclin IP receptor agonist; Pulmonary arterial hypertension; Pulmonary hypertension; Riociguat; Selexipag; Soluble guanylate cyclase stimulator

CITATION | *Li YR. Cardiovascular Medicine: New Therapeutic Drugs Approved by the US FDA (2013–2017). Cell Med Press, Raleigh, NC, USA. 2018. http://dx.doi.org/10.20455/ndcvd.2018.07*

ABBREVIATIONS | ABCG2, ATP binding cassette protein G2; cAMP, cyclic adenosine monophosphate; cGMP, cyclic guanosine monophosphate; CTEPH, chronic thromboembolic pulmonary hypertension; CYP, cytochrome P450; ET, Endothelin; ET_A, endothelin receptor type A; ET_B, endothelin receptor type B; HRQoL, health-related quality of life; NT-proBNP, N-terminal proB-type natriuretic peptide; PAH, pulmonary arterial hypertension; PAH-CTD, pulmonary arterial hypertension associated with connective tissue disease; PDE, phosphodiesterase; sGC, soluble guanylate cyclase; UGT, UDP-glucuronosyltransferase; US FDA, the United States Food and Drug Administration; WHO, the World Health Organization

CHAPTER AT A GLANCE

1. INTRODUCTION

Drug treatment of pulmonary hypertension, especially pulmonary arterial hypertension (PAH) has been evolving progressively over the past two decades. This is due primarily to the advancements in the understanding of the molecular pathophysiology of the disease and the availability of new drugs with efficacy demonstrated in randomized controlled trials [1–3]. As noted in Chapter 6, several classes of specific drugs are now available for treating pulmonary hypertension, which include endothelin receptor antagonists, phosphodiesterase type 5 inhibitors, soluble guanylate cyclase stimulators, prostacyclin analogues, and prostacyclin IP receptor agonists [4–6]. This chapter covers the new drugs approved by the United States Food and Drug Administration (US FDA) over the past five years (2013–2017). These include the endothelin receptor antagonist macitentan (approved in October 2013), the soluble guanylate cyclase stimulator riociguat (approved in October 2013), and the prostacyclin IP receptor agonist selexipag (approved in December 2015).

2. THE ENDOTHELIN RECEPTOR ANTAGONIST: MACITENTAN (OPSUMIT)

2.1. Overview

Endothelin (ET) is an important factor involved in the regulation of vascular tone as well as other vascular processes. Three endothelins, namely, ET-1, ET-2, and ET-3, are expressed in humans. They are all 21-amino acid peptides. ET-1 is the main endothelin secreted by endothelial cells. It is also the endothelin that has been shown to play an important role in cardiovascular physiology and pathophysiology. ET-2 is produced mainly by the kidney and the intestine, whereas ET-3 is primarily localized in the brain, the intestine, and kidney tubular cells. ET-1 acts in an autocrine/paracrine manner to activate G protein-coupled receptors—endothelin type A (ET_A) and type B (ET_B)—to produce its physiological effects on vessels. Endothelin receptors are expressed in endothelial cells and vascular smooth muscle cells with both ET_A and ET_B being expressed in vascular smooth muscle cells and ET_B in endothelial cells. Binding of ET-1 to ET_A and ET_B receptors in smooth muscle causes vasoconstriction, as well as inflammatory responses in the vascular wall. The vasoconstriction results from inositol triphosphate-induced release of calcium ions from sarcoplasmic reticulum. Both vasoconstriction and vascular inflammation are involved in the detrimental actions of ET-1 on blood vessels in hypertension and other vascular disorders [7, 8]. Evidence suggests that binding of ET-1 to ET_B receptors in endothelial cells may lead to vasodilation via a nitric oxide-dependent mechanism. ET_B receptors are also involved in the clearance of circulating ET-1 which has a half-life of ~1 min.

Over the past two decades, the US FDA has approved three endothelin receptor antagonists. Bosentan (Tracleer) is the first member approved in November 2001. The second member, ambrisentan (Letairis) was approved in June 2007. As noted earlier, macitentan is the newest member of the drug class, which was approved on October 18, 2013. Ambrisentan has a high selectivity for the ET_A receptor versus the ET_B receptor, whereas bosentan and macitentan block both receptors. The clinical significance of high selectivity for the ET_A receptor is not known. All 3 drugs are approved by the US FDA for the treatment of PAH.

The approval of macitentan (Actelion Pharmaceuticals, Allschwil, Switzerland) by the US FDA was based on a randomized controlled trial (SERAPHIN) involving 742 subjects with symptomatic PAH. Treatment with macitentan at 10 mg once daily significantly reduced the morbidity and mortality among patients with PAH in this event-driven study [9]. This section primarily focuses on macitentan, and comparisons with ambrisentan and bosentan are also made.

2.2. Chemistry and Pharmacokinetics

The structures of macitentan and the other two members of the endothelin receptor antagonist class are shown in **Figure 7.1**. Ambrisentan is a propionic acid derivative, whereas bosentan belongs to a class of highly substituted pyrimidine derivatives. The newly approved macitentan is a bosentan-derivative. **Table 7.1** summarizes the major pharmacokinetic properties of macitentan as well as ambrisentan and bosentan.

2.3. Molecular Mechanisms and Pharmacological/Clinical Effects

2.3.1. Molecular Mechanisms

As noted earlier, ET-1 is a potent autocrine and paracrine peptide. Two receptor subtypes, namely, ET_A and ET_B, mediate the biological effects of ET-1 in the vascular smooth muscle and endothelium. The primary consequences of ET_A and ET_B activation in smooth muscle

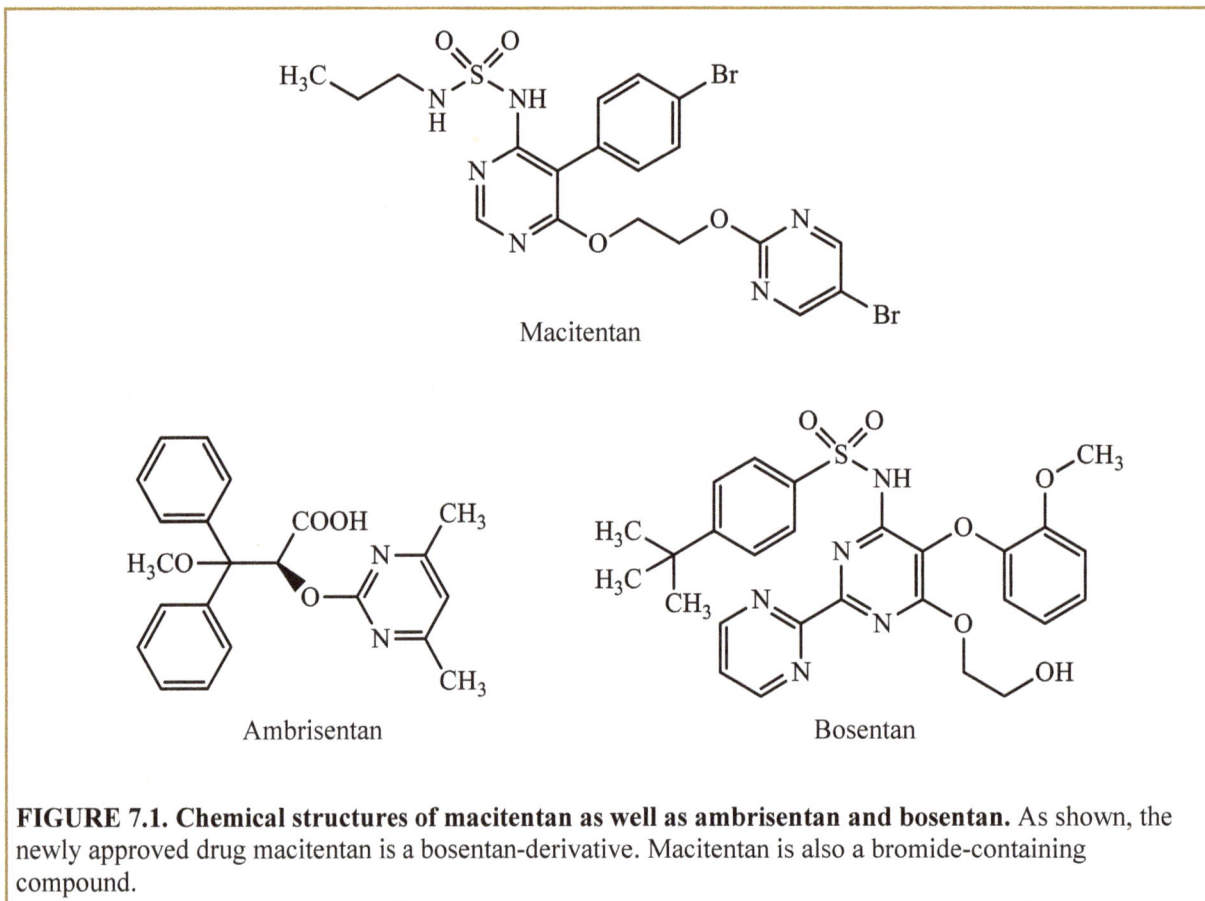

FIGURE 7.1. Chemical structures of macitentan as well as ambrisentan and bosentan. As shown, the newly approved drug macitentan is a bosentan-derivative. Macitentan is also a bromide-containing compound.

cells are vasoconstriction, cell proliferation, and vascular inflammation, while the predominant actions of ET_B activation in endothelial cells are vasodilation, antiproliferation, and ET-1 clearance. In patients with PAH, plasma ET-1 levels are elevated as much as 10-fold and correlate with increased mean right atrial pressure and disease severity. Notably, both protein and mRNA expression of ET-1 are increased as much as 9-fold in the lung tissue of patients with PAH, primarily in the endothelium of pulmonary arteries [10]. These findings suggest that dysregulation of ET-1 may play a critical role in the pathogenesis and progression of PAH. Indeed, endothelin receptor antagonists via blocking ET-1-mediated receptor activation are effective therapy of PAH (**Figure 7.2**).

Ambrisentan is a high-affinity ET_A receptor antagonist with a high selectivity for the ET_A versus ET_B receptors (>4,000-fold). Bosentan is a specific and competitive antagonist at ET_A and ET_B receptors, and has a slightly higher affinity for ET_A receptors than for ET_B receptors. Macitentan displays high affinity and sustained occupancy of both ET_A and ET_B receptors in human pulmonary arterial smooth muscle cells. Although ET_B activation in endothelial cells appears to be vascular protective, the clinical impact of selective ET_A inhibition or dual receptor (ET_A/ET_B) blockage is currently unknown. In other words, there is currently no evidence suggesting a better clinical efficacy for the ET_A-selective inhibitor (i.e., ambrisentan) as compared with the ET_A/ET_B-dual receptor antagonists (i.e., macitentan and bosentan; also see **Figure 7.2**).

2.3.2. Pharmacological/Clinical Effects

Treatment with macitentan 10 mg once daily results in a 45% reduction in the occurrence of the primary endpoint up to the end (36 months) of double-blind treatment compared to placebo [9]. The primary endpoint includes the time from the initiation of treatment to the first occurrence of a composite endpoint of death, atrial septostomy, lung transplantation, initiation of treatment with intravenous or subcutaneous prostacyclin analogues, or worsening of PAH. Macitentan is noted for its ability to reduce mortality in patients with PAH. Like macitentan, both ambrisentan and bosentan are able to reduce clinical worsening in patients with PAH. Clinical worsening refers to decreased 6-min walk distance, worsened PAH symptoms, and need for additional PAH treatment. However, neither ambrisentan nor bosentan has been shown to reduce the mortality in PAH patients.

TABLE 7.1. Major pharmacokinetic properties of endothelin receptor antagonists

Drug	Oral bioavailability	Half-life	Metabolism and excretion
Macitentan	Unknown	16 h	Hepatic CYP3A4; hepatic CYP2C19 (minor); urinary and biliary excretion
Ambrisentan	Unknown	9 h	Hepatic CYP3A4 and CYP2C19; glucuronidation; biliary excretion
Bosentan	50%	5 h	Hepatic CYP2C9 and CYP3A4; also an inducer of CYP2C9 and CYP3A4; biliary excretion

2.4. Clinical Uses

Macitentan is indicated for treating PAH to delay disease progression. Disease progression includes death, initiation of intravenous or subcutaneous prostacyclin analogues, or clinical worsening of PAH (decreased 6-min walk distance, worsened PAH symptoms, and need for additional PAH treatment). Macitentan also reduces hospitalization for PAH [11]. Notably, macitentan reduces mortality due to PAH [9], which represents a significant advantage over the other two members (i.e., ambrisentan and bosentan), for which, as mentioned above, the mortality benefit has not been established.

Ambrisentan and bosentan are approved for treating PAH to improve exercise ability and delay clinical worsening. Ambrisentan is also approved to be used in combination with tadalafil, a phosphodiesterase type 5 (PDE5) inhibitor (also see Table 6.5 of Chapter 6), to reduce the risks of disease progression and hospitalization for worsening PAH, and to improve exercise ability. Approval of this new indication for ambrisentan was based on the efficacy demonstrated in a randomized controlled trial [12].

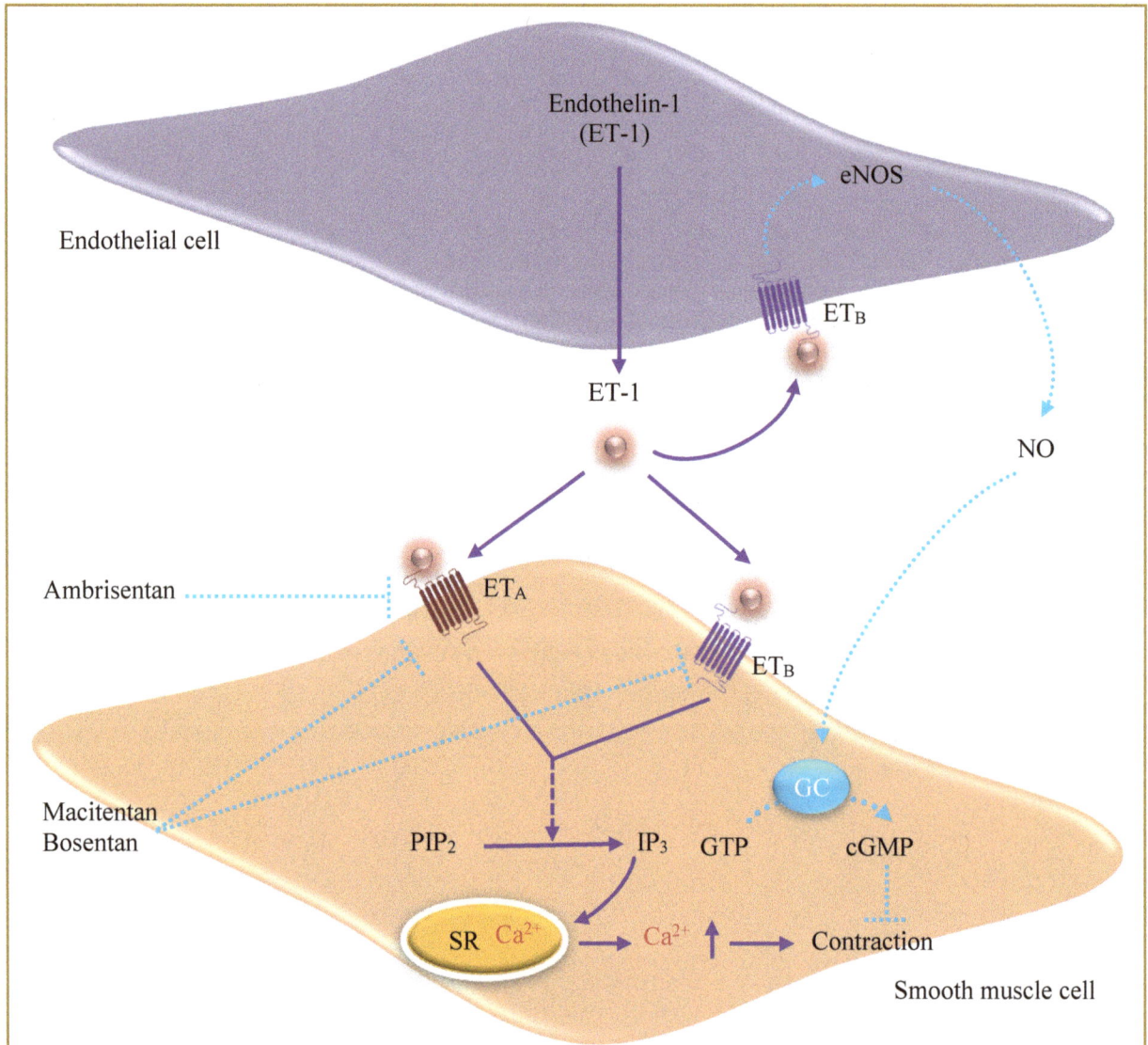

FIGURE 7.2. Molecular mechanisms of action of endothelin receptor antagonists (ERAs). Endothelial cell-derived ET-1 activates type A and type B receptors (ET_A and ET_B) on smooth muscle cells (SMCs), leading to the formation of inositol 1,4,5-triphosphate (IP_3) through phospholipase C-catalyzed hydrolysis of phosphatidylinositol 4,5-bisphosphate (PIP_2). IP_3 then causes Ca^{2+} release from sarcoplasmic reticulum (SR), inducing SMC contraction. Abnormal activation of ET_A and ET_B on SMCs may also cause cell proliferation and vascular inflammation (not shown). Blocking ET_A and ET_B on SMCs by ERAs thus inhibits the above detrimental effects of ET-1. Notably, activation of ET_B receptors by ET-1 on endothelial cells results in increased production of nitric oxide (NO), which activates guanylate cyclase (GC), leading to increased formation of cGMP, and the subsequent SMC relaxation. However, the clinical significance of this vasodilating effect of activation of ET_B receptors on endothelial cells remains to be elucidated.

2.5. Therapeutic Dosages

The dosage forms and strengths of macitentan as well as ambrisentan and bosentan are listed below, and the dosage regimens of these drugs in treating PAH are summarized in **Table 7.2**. As noted, all the three endothelial receptor antagonists are administered orally, and macitentan has only one dosage strength (10 mg).

- Macitentan: oral, 10 mg tablets
- Ambrisentan: oral, 5, 10 mg tablets
- Bosentan: oral, 62.5, 125 mg tablets

TABLE 7.2. Dosage regimens of macitentan as well as ambrisentan and bosentan

Drug	Indication	Dosage regimen
Macitentan	PAH	10 mg once daily; doses higher than 10 mg once daily have not been studied in patients with PAH and are not recommended
Ambrisentan	PAH	Initial dose: 5 mg once daily; the dose may be increased to 10 mg once daily if 5 mg once daily is tolerated
Bosentan	PAH	Initial dose: 62.5 mg twice daily for 4 weeks; the dose may then be increased to maintenance dose of 125 mg twice daily

2.6. Adverse Effects and Drug Interactions

2.6.1. Adverse Effects

The most common adverse effects of macitentan as well as ambrisentan and bosentan are upper respiratory infections, peripheral edema, and anemia. Use of macitentan and bosentan is also associated with liver toxicity. In contrast, risk of liver injury in patients treated with ambrisentan is low. Among the above adverse effects, peripheral edema is the most common one that requires attention. Mild cases can be managed with diuretics, but more severe cases warrant discontinuation of the medication. Macitentan as well as ambrisentan and bosentan are potent teratogens, requiring meticulous contraception if used by women who have childbearing potential, and are contraindicated during pregnancy (also see Section 2.6.3).

2.6.2. Drug Interactions

2.6.2.1. MACITENTAN

Macitentan is primarily metabolized by cytochrome P450 (CYP) 3A4, and as such, drugs that affect CYP3A4 may significantly alter the metabolism of macitentan. Strong inducers of CYP3A4 such as rifampin significantly reduce macitentan levels in the plasma. Hence, the concomitant use of macitentan with strong CYP3A4 inducers should be avoided. On the other hand, concomitant use of strong CYP3A4 inhibitors (such as ketoconazole and many anti-human immunodeficiency virus drugs) may markedly increase the plasma concentrations of macitentan.

2.6.2.2. AMBRISENTAN

Drug interactions for ambrisentan at therapeutic doses are less dramatic than macitentan and bosentan. This is because ambrisentan does not significantly affect drug metabolism enzymes at therapeutic doses. The only clinically significant drug interaction is that co-treatment with ambrisentan and cyclosporine results in a 2-fold increase in ambrisentan exposure, and as such, the dose of ambrisentan should be reduced when co-administered with cyclosporine.

2.6.2.3. BOSENTAN

Bosentan may cause significant drug interactions due to its ability to alter CYP enzymes (also see **Table 7.1**). Bosentan is metabolized by CYP2C9 and CYP3A4. Inhibition of these enzymes may increase the plasma concentrations of bosentan. Concomitant administration of both a CYP2C9 inhibitor (e.g., fluconazole or amiodarone) and a strong CYP3A4 inhibitor (e.g., ketoconazole or itraconazole) or a moderate CYP3A4 inhibitor (e.g., amprenavir, erythromycin, fluconazole, or diltiazem) with bosentan can lead to large increases in plasma concentrations of bosentan. As such, co-administration of such combinations of a CYP2C9 inhibitor plus a strong or moderate CYP3A4 inhibitor with bosentan is not recommended. Bosentan is also an inducer of CYP3A4 and CYP2C9. Consequently, plasma concentrations of drugs metabolized by these two isozymes will be decreased when bosentan is co-administered. In this regard, combination use of bosentan decreases the bioavailability of simvastatin and other CYP3A4-metabolized statins, resulting in decreased efficacy of the statin therapy in treating dyslipidemia and atherosclerotic cardiovascular diseases (see Chapter 4 for statin drugs).

Notably, initial concomitant administration of cyclosporine may increase the plasma concentrations of bosentan by ~30-fold. The mechanism of this interaction is most likely related to the inhibition of transport protein-mediated uptake of bosentan into hepatocytes by cyclosporine. Steady-state bosentan plasma concentrations are 3–4-fold higher than those in the absence of cyclosporine. As such, concomitant administration of bosentan and cyclosporine is contraindicated. Bosentan also decreases the plasma concentrations of cyclosporine (a CYP3A4 substrate) by ~50% upon co-administration.

2.6.3. Contraindications and FDA Pregnancy Category

As noted above, all the three endothelin receptor antagonists are contraindicated in pregnancy (FDA pregnancy category: X) because of their potential to cause fetal harm. While pregnancy is the only contraindication for macitentan therapy, as described below, ambrisentan and bosentan also have other contraindications.

2.6.3.1. AMBRISENTAN

Ambrisentan is also contraindicated in patients with idiopathic pulmonary fibrosis (IPF), including IPF patients with pulmonary hypertension (WHO Group 3; see Chapter 6 for classification of pulmonary hypertension). A randomized controlled study in IPF patients with or without pulmonary hypertension (WHO Group 3) comparing ambrisentan (n = 329) to placebo (n = 163) was terminated after 34 weeks for lack of efficacy and a greater risk of disease progression or death on ambrisentan [13].

2.6.3.2. BOSENTAN

Bosentan is also contraindicated for the following conditions.

- *Concomitant use with cyclosporine*: As noted earlier, co-administration of cyclosporine and bosentan results in markedly increased plasma concentrations of bosentan. As such, concomitant use of bosentan and cyclosporine is contraindicated.
- *Concomitant use with glyburide*: An increased risk of liver enzyme elevations has been observed in patients receiving glyburide (an anti-diabetic drug) concomitantly with bosentan. Therefore, co-administration of glyburide and bosentan is contraindicated.
- *Hypersensitivity*: Bosentan is contraindicated in patients who are hypersensitive to bosentan or any component of the product. Observed hypersensitivity reactions include rash and angioedema. Angioedema refers to pronounced swelling of the deep dermis, subcutaneous or submucosal tissue, or mucous membranes as a result of vascular leakage.

2.7. Comparison with Existing Members and New Development since the US FDA Approval

The biggest advantage with macitentan therapy is its ability to reduce mortality in patients with PAH. On the other hand, the mortality-reducing capacity of ambrisentan and bosentan has not been established. In this context, a recent randomized controlled trial involving 500 subjects reported that among participants with PAH who had not received previous treatment, initial combination therapy with ambrisentan and tadalafil (a PDE5 inhibitor; see Table 6.4 of Chapter 6) resulted in a 50% lower risk of clinical-failure events than with ambrisentan or tadalafil monotherapy. The clinical-failure event was defined as a composite of death, hospitalization for worsening PAH, disease progression, or unsatisfactory long-term clinical response in the trial [12]. The results of the above trial suggested a potential mortality-reducing efficacy of ambrisentan when combined with a PDE5 inhibitor. Likewise, combination of macitentan and a PDE5 inhibitor has also been suggested to be effective and well-tolerated in the management of PAH [14].

The safety profile of macitentan is favorable with respect to edema/fluid retention and other effects, and may be better than that of bosentan and ambrisentan. Unlike bosentan, macitentan has limited interactions with other drugs. Because of these characteristics, macitentan has become an important new addition to the treatment of PAH [15]. Indeed, a recent study demonstrated that macitentan therapy also improved the health-related quality of life (HRQoL) for patients with PAH and reduced the risk of HRQoL deterioration, likely leading to improved long-term outcomes [16].

> **HRQoL**
> Health-related quality of life (HRQoL) is a multi-dimensional concept that includes domains related to physical, mental, emotional, and social functioning. It goes beyond direct measures of population health, life expectancy, and causes of death, and focuses on the impact health status has on quality of life. A related concept of HRQoL is well-being, which assesses the positive aspects of a person's life, such as positive emotions and life satisfaction (https://www.healthypeople.gov)

In addition to its proven efficacy in treating PAH, macitentan may also be effective in treating other forms of pulmonary hypertension. In this regard, a recent phase 2 double-blind, randomized, placebo-controlled trial (MERIT-1) involving 80 patients with inoperable chronic thromboembolic pulmonary hypertension (CTEPH; also see Table 6.1 of Chapter 6) reported that, as compared with the placebo, macitentan treatment (10 mg once daily for 10 weeks) significantly decreased the pulmonary vascular resistance by 16% and that the macitentan treatment was well tolerated [17]. The efficacy of macitentan therapy in improving the clinical outcomes of CTEPH patients as well as patients with other groups of pulmonary hypertension (e.g., pulmonary hypertension owing to left heart disease) warrants further investigation through large clinical trials.

3. THE SOLUBLE GUANYLATE CYCLASE STIMULATOR: RIOCIGUAT (ADEMPAS)

3.1. Overview

Soluble guanylate cyclase (sGC) is activated by nitric oxide and catalyzes the formation of cyclic guanosine monophosphate (cGMP) from guanosine triphosphate (GTP). It plays an important role in a wide variety of physiological and pathophysiological processes, particularly in the cardiovascular system. As such, sGC has become a potential therapeutic target in cardiovascular disorders, including myocardial infarction, stroke, and pulmonary hypertension. Multiple drug compounds have been developed to stimulate sGC to treat pulmonary hypertension. Among them, riociguat has recently been approved by the US FDA (initial approval date: October 8, 2013), and is the first-in-class member for treating pulmonary hypertension, including both PAH and CTEPH.

   The approval of riociguat (Bayer, Leverkusen, Germany) by the US FDA was based on two randomized controlled trials, namely, PATENT-1 and CHEST-1. The PATENT-1 trial involving 443 patients with symptomatic PAH demonstrated that riociguat treatment resulted in significant improvements in pulmonary vascular resistance, N-terminal proB-type natriuretic peptide (NT-proBNP) levels, the WHO functional class, time to clinical worsening, and Borg dyspnea score [18]. On the other hand, the CHEST-1 trial involved 261 patients with inoperable CTEPH or persistent or recurrent pulmonary hypertension after pulmonary endarterectomy (see Section 3.2.3 of Chapter 6 for pulmonary endarterectomy). This trial demonstrated that riociguat treatment led to significant improvements in pulmonary vascular resistance, exercise capacity, NT-proBNP levels, and the WHO functional class [19].

3.2. Chemistry and Pharmacokinetics

Riociguat is chemically known as methyl 4,6-diamino-2-[1-(2-fluorobenzyl)-1H-pyrazolo[3,4-b]pyridin-3-yl]-5-pyrimidinyl(methyl)carbamate, and its structure is shown in **Figure 7.3**. Riociguat is readily absorbed through the gut and its oral bioavailability is about

BNP and NT-proBNP
The 32-amino acid polypeptide, namely, brain-natriuretic peptide (BNP) is secreted attached to a 76-amino acid N-terminal fragment in the prohormone called NT-proBNP, which is biologically inactive. Cleavage of this 76-amino acid N-terminal fragment releases BNP. BNP and NT-proBNP are synthesized in the cardiomyocytes in response to ventricular stretch and ischemic injury. It is called brain natriuretic peptide because the peptide was originally identified in extracts of pig brain. Measurement of the concentrations of BNP and NT-proBNP, especially the latter, in the blood has been used as a biomarker for diagnosis and management of heart failure as well as other cardiovascular conditions, including pulmonary hypertension.

Borg dyspnea score
Dyspnea is a subjective experience of breathing discomfort that consists of qualitatively distinct sensations that vary in intensity. Gunnar Borg in the 1970s elaborated a categorical scale, known as the Rating of Perceived Exertion (RPE), and the subsequent modified version of the so called 10 Category-Ratio (CR 10), both used to assess the sensation of exertional dyspnea and fatigue perceived during physical activity. The CR 10 is a categorical scale with a score from 0 to 10, where 0 (as a measure of dyspnea) corresponds to the sensation of normal breathing (absence of dyspnea) and 10 corresponds to the subject's maximum possible sensation of dyspnea.

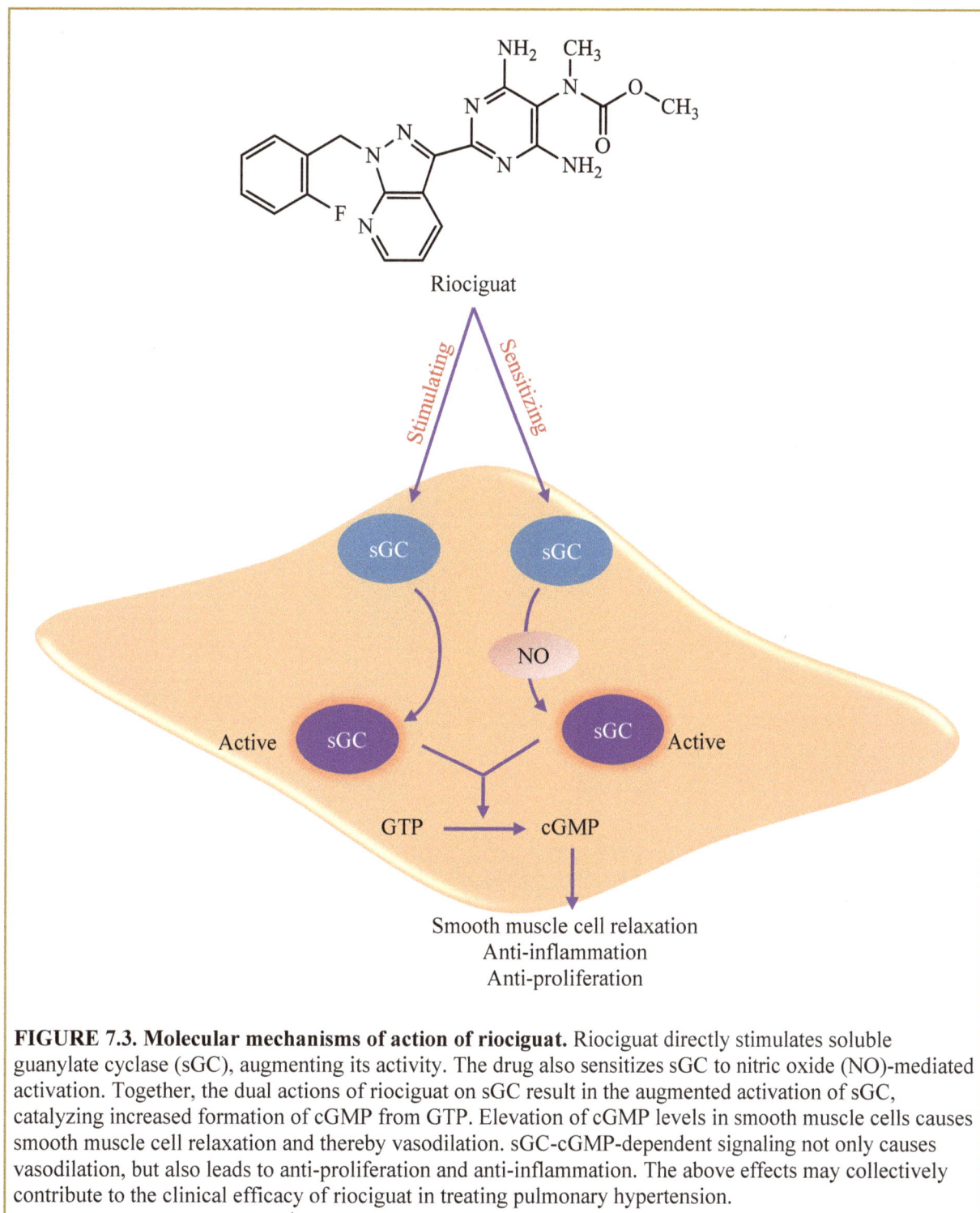

FIGURE 7.3. Molecular mechanisms of action of riociguat. Riociguat directly stimulates soluble guanylate cyclase (sGC), augmenting its activity. The drug also sensitizes sGC to nitric oxide (NO)-mediated activation. Together, the dual actions of riociguat on sGC result in the augmented activation of sGC, catalyzing increased formation of cGMP from GTP. Elevation of cGMP levels in smooth muscle cells causes smooth muscle cell relaxation and thereby vasodilation. sGC-cGMP-dependent signaling not only causes vasodilation, but also leads to anti-proliferation and anti-inflammation. The above effects may collectively contribute to the clinical efficacy of riociguat in treating pulmonary hypertension.

94%. It is also a substrate of P-glycoprotein and ATP binding cassette protein G2 (ABCG2). Riociguat is metabolized by CYP1A1, CYP3A, CYP2C8, and CYP2J2, and eliminated via both urinary and biliary excretion. Its emanation half-life is 7–12 h.

3.3. Molecular Mechanisms and Pharmacological Effects

3.3.1. Molecular Mechanisms

When nitric oxide binds to sGC, the enzyme catalyzes the synthesis of the signaling molecule cGMP. Intracellular cGMP plays an important role in regulating processes that influence vascular tone, proliferation, fibrosis, and inflammation. Pulmonary hypertension is associated with endothelial dysfunction, impaired synthesis of nitric oxide, and insufficient stimulation of the nitric oxide-sGC-cGMP pathway. Riociguat stimulates the nitric oxide-sGC-cGMP pathway and leads to increased generation of intracellular cGMP with subsequent smooth muscle relaxation and vasodilation. Riociguat has a dual mode of action. It sensitizes sGC to endogenous nitric oxide by stabilizing the nitric oxide-sGC binding. Riociguat also directly stimulates sGC via a different binding site, independently of nitric oxide (**Figure 7.3**). It should be noted that the sGC-cGMP-dependent signaling has been shown to not only cause vasodilation, but also lead to anti-proliferation and anti-inflammation [20, 21].

3.3.2. Pharmacological Effects

Riociguat treatment results in decreases in systemic vascular resistance, systolic blood pressure, pulmonary vascular resistance, and pulmonary arterial pressure [22]. Riociguat therapy also significantly reduces NT-proBNP levels, a biomarker for pulmonary hypertension. Riociguat treatment resulted in a reduction of 432 pg/ml of NT-proBNP in the PATENT-1 study [18], and a reduction of 444 pg/ml of NT-proBNP in the CHEST-1 study [19].

3.4. Clinical Uses

Riociguat is currently the only drug approved by the US FDA for treating two different forms of pulmonary hypertension, namely, CTEPH and PAH.

- CTEPH: riociguat is indicated for the treatment of adult patients with persistent/recurrent CTEPH (WHO Group 4) after surgical treatment, or inoperable CTEPH, to improve exercise capacity and the WHO functional class.
- PAH: riociguat is indicated for the treatment of adult patients with PAH (WHO Group 1), to improve exercise capacity, the WHO functional class, and to delay clinical worsening.

3.5. Therapeutic Dosages

The dosage forms and strengths of riociguat are listed below.

- Oral: 0.5, 1, 1.5, 2, 2.5 mg tablets

The recommended starting dosage is 1 mg taken 3 times a day. For patients who may not tolerate the hypotensive effect of riociguat (see Section 3.6 below for adverse effects), a starting dose of 0.5 mg taken three times a day may be considered. If systolic blood pressure remains greater than 95 mm Hg and the patient has no signs or symptoms of hypotension, the dose can be up-titrated by 0.5 mg taken three times a day. Dose increases should be no sooner than 2 weeks apart. The dose can be increased to the highest tolerated dosage, up to a maximum of 2.5 mg taken three times a day. If at any time, the patient has symptoms of hypotension, decrease the dosage by 0.5 mg taken three times a day.

3.6. Adverse Effects and Drug Interactions

3.6.1. Adverse Effects

Adverse effects of riociguat may include headache, dyspepsia/gastritis, dizziness, nausea, diarrhea, hypotension, vomiting, anemia, gastroesophageal reflux, and constipation. Riociguat may also cause bleeding, pulmonary edema in patients with pulmonary veno-occlusive disease, and fetal harm. Like the endothelin receptor antagonists, riociguat is contraindicated in pregnancy (also see Section 3.6.3).

3.6.2. Drug Interactions

Due to the involvement of multiple pathways in the metabolism of riociguat, drug interactions can be significant. For example, cigarette smoking (an inducer of CYP1A1) augments metabolism of riociguat, and the plasma concentrations of the drug in smokers can thus be reduced by 50–60% compared to nonsmokers. Concomitant use of riociguat with strong cytochrome CYP inhibitors and P-glycoprotein/ABCG2 inhibitors such as azole antimycotics (e.g., ketoconazole, itraconazole) or human immunodeficiency virus protease inhibitors (e.g., ritonavir) increases riociguat exposure and may result in hypotension. Strong inducers of CYP3A (e.g., rifampin, phenytoin, carbamazepine, phenobarbital, or St. John's Wort) may significantly reduce riociguat exposure. Finally, antacids, such as aluminum hydroxide/magnesium hydroxide, decrease riociguat absorption and should not be taken within one hour of taking riociguat.

3.6.3. Contraindications and FDA Pregnancy Category

- Co-administration of riociguat with nitrates or nitric oxide donors in any form is contraindicated because of additive blood pressure-lowering effects.
- Concomitant administration of riociguat with specific PDE5 inhibitors (e.g., sildenafil, tadalafil, or vardenafil) or nonspecific PDE inhibitors (e.g., dipyridamole or theophylline) is contraindicated due to additive blood pressure-lowering effects.
- FDA pregnancy category: X

3.7. Comparison with Existing Members and New Development since the US FDA Approval

Riociguat is the first-in-class and the only member of the sGC stimulator drug class. Comparative studies on riociguat versus other drugs in patients with pulmonary hypertension are currently lacking. Recently, follow-up studies of the patients enrolled in the PATENT-1 and CHEST-1 trials further demonstrated the long-term benefits and safety profile of riociguat therapy in patients with either PAH or CTEPH [23–26].

4. THE PROSTACYCLIN IP RECEPTOR AGONIST: SELEXIPAG (UPTRAVI)

4.1. Overview

Prostacyclin (also called prostaglandin I_2 or PGI_2) is produced in vascular endothelial cells and acts via the prostacyclin IP receptors to cause vasodilation and inhibit smooth muscle cell proliferation and platelet aggregation. Prostacyclin production is reduced in PAH, and drugs targeting the prostacyclin pathway are one of the pharmacotherapeutic options for PAH [27, 28]. Indeed, administration of prostanoids (i.e., prostacyclin analogues; also see Table 6.4 of Chapter 6) has been a mainstay of PAH therapy for more than a decade. There are currently three US FDA-approved prostacyclin analogues for treating PAH: epoprostenol, iloprost, and treprostinil. In addition to supplementing prostacyclin analogues, another effective way of reducing pulmonary vascular resistance is to potently stimulate the prostacyclin IP receptors via the use of novel non-prostanoid agonists. In this context, on December 21, 2015, the US FDA approved selexipag, the first-in-class and currently the only member of the prostacyclin IP receptor agonist drug class.

Approval of selexipag (Actelion Pharmaceuticals, Allschwil, Switzerland) by the US FDA was based on a randomized controlled trial (GRIPHON) involving 1,156 patients with symptomatic PAH. Treatment with selexipag resulted in a significant delay of disease progression and reduction of the risk of hospitalization for PAH. However, there was no significant difference in mortality between the treated and placebo groups [29].

4.2. Chemistry and Pharmacokinetics

Selexipag is a selective non-prostanoid IP prostacyclin receptor agonist (structure shown in **Figure 7.4**). The major pharmacokinetic properties of selexipag are summarized in **Table 7.3**.

4.3. Molecular Mechanisms and Pharmacological Effects

4.3.1. Molecular Mechanisms

Selexipag is an oral prostacyclin IP receptor agonist that is structurally distinct from prostacyclin. Selexipag is hydrolyzed by carboxylesterase 1 in the liver and intestine to yield its active metabolite, which is approximately 37-fold as potent as selexipag. Selexipag and its active metabolite are selective for the IP receptors versus other prostanoid receptors (EP1–4, DP, FP, and TP). Activation of prostacyclin IP receptors by selexipag causes vasodilation and inhibits

---

Prostacyclin and prostanoid receptors

Prostacyclin IP receptor belongs to the family of prostanoid receptors. Prostanoid receptors are activated by the endogenous ligands prostaglandins PGD_2, PGE_1, PGE_2, $PGF_{2\alpha}$, PGH_2, and prostacyclin (PGI_2), as well as thromboxane A_2 (TxA_2). As prostacyclin is also known as PGI_2, the receptor for prostacyclin is thus called IP receptor meaning the receptor for the I_2 type of the prostaglandin. To signify the ligand (i.e., prostacyclin), IP receptor is commonly called prostacyclin IP receptor or IP prostacyclin receptor. The major prostaglandins PGD_2, PGE_2, $PGF_{2\alpha}$, PGI_2, and TxA_2 preferentially interact with dedicated receptors designated as DP, EP, FP, IP, and TP, respectively (TP is also activated by PGH_2). Four subtypes of EP receptors (EP_1, EP_2, EP_3, and EP_4) have been described. Although two subtypes of DP receptors (DP_1 and DP_2) have been described, the DP_2 receptor has little structural resemblance to DP_1 and other receptors. DP_2 receptors are more closely related to chemoattractant receptors (based primarily on Woodward DF, Jones RL, Narumiya S. International Union of Basic and Clinical Pharmacology. LXXXIII: classification of prostanoid receptors, updating 15 years of progress. *Pharmacol Rev* 2011; 63(3):471–538).

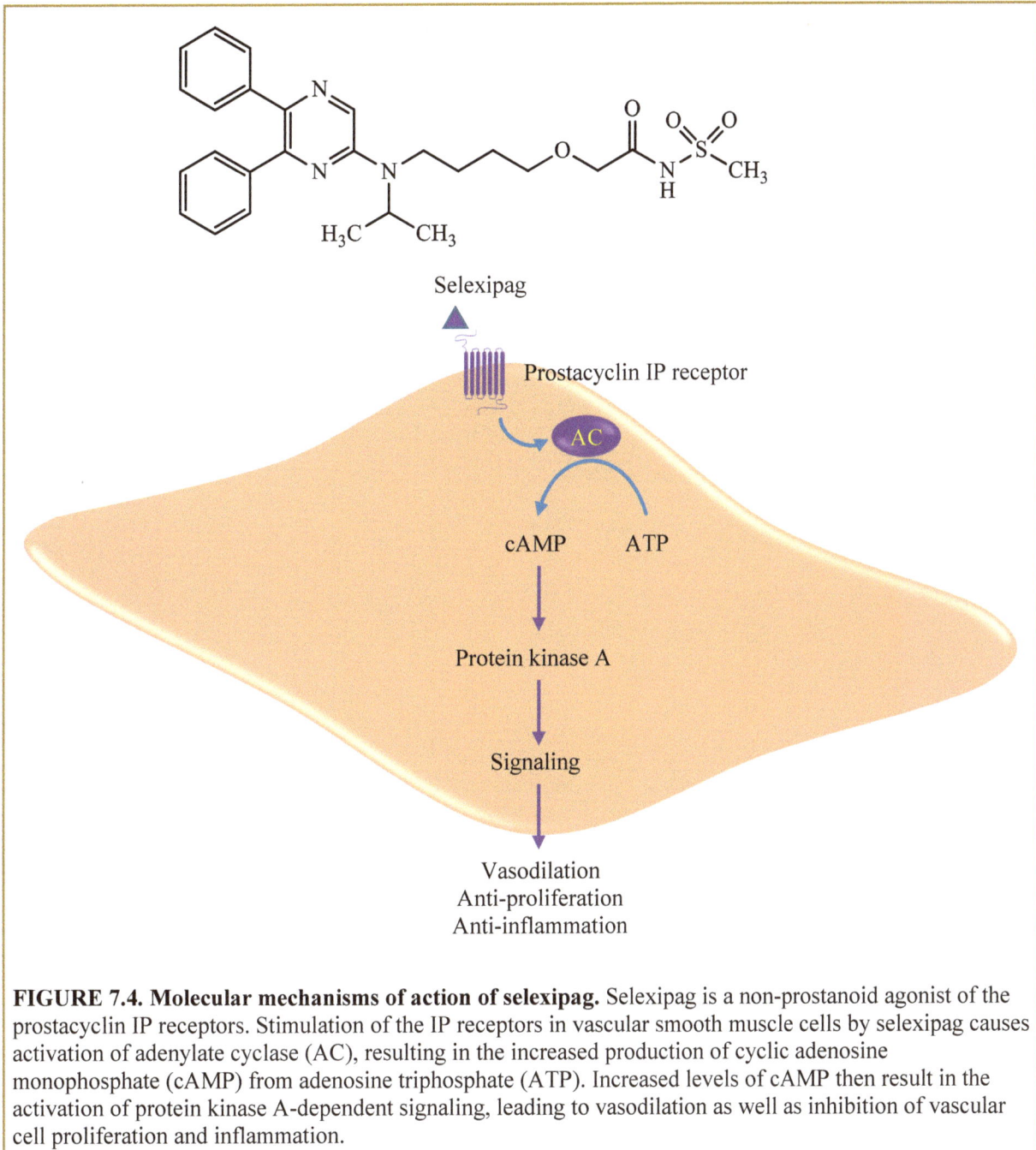

FIGURE 7.4. Molecular mechanisms of action of selexipag. Selexipag is a non-prostanoid agonist of the prostacyclin IP receptors. Stimulation of the IP receptors in vascular smooth muscle cells by selexipag causes activation of adenylate cyclase (AC), resulting in the increased production of cyclic adenosine monophosphate (cAMP) from adenosine triphosphate (ATP). Increased levels of cAMP then result in the activation of protein kinase A-dependent signaling, leading to vasodilation as well as inhibition of vascular cell proliferation and inflammation.

smooth muscle cell proliferation and vascular inflammation via adenylate cyclase-cyclic adenosine monophosphate (cAMP)-dependent signaling (**Figure 7.4**).

4.3.2. Pharmacological Effects

Selexipag treatment reduces pulmonary vascular resistance by ~30% in patients with PAH. Selexipag treatment of PAH patients also results in an increase in cardiac index (median treatment effect) of 0.41

L/min/m^2. Cardiac index is an assessment of the cardiac output value based on the patient's size. Cardiac index = [cardiac output (L/min)] ÷ [body surface area (m^2)].

TABLE 7.3. Major pharmacokinetic properties of selexipag

Oral bioavailability	49%
t_{max}	1–3 h (selexipag); 3–4 h (active metabolite)
Vd	11.7 L per 70 kg body weight
Metabolism	Hydrolysis to its active metabolite (a free carboxylic acid) in the liver and intestine by carboxylesterase 1; oxidation by CYP2C8 and CYP3A4; glucuronidation of the active metabolite by UGT1A3 and UGT2B7
Elimination route	~90% via feces; ~10% via urine
Clearance	17.9 L/h
$t_{1/2}$	0.8–2.5 h (selexipag); 6.2–13.5 h (active metabolite)

Note: $t_{1/2}$, elimination half-life; t_{max}, the time when the maximum plasma concentration is reached; Vd, volume of distribution; UGT, UDP-glucuronosyltransferase.

4.4. Clinical Uses

Selexipag is indicated for the treatment of PAH (WHO Group I) to delay disease progression and reduce the risk of hospitalization for PAH.

4.5. Therapeutic Dosages

The dosage forms and strengths of selexipag are listed below.

- Oral: 200, 400, 600, 800, 1000, 1200, 1400, 1600 µg (mcg) tablets

The recommended starting dose of selexipag is 200 µg (mcg) given twice daily. The dose can be increased by 200 µg (mcg) twice daily at weekly intervals to the highest tolerated dose of up to 1600 µg (mcg) twice daily. Tolerability may be improved when taken with food. For patients with moderate hepatic impairment, the recommended starting dose is 200 µg (mcg) once daily, and the dose can be increased by 200 µg (mcg) once daily at weekly intervals, as tolerated.

4.6. Adverse Effects and Drug Interactions

4.6.1. Adverse Effects

Selexipag is generally well tolerated. Common adverse effects include headache, diarrhea, jaw pain, nausea, myalgia, vomiting, pain in extremity, and flushing.

4.6.2. Drug Interactions

Oxidation of selexipag is primarily catalyzed by CYP2C8. As such, concomitant use of a strong CYP2C8 inhibitor (e.g., gemfibrozil) can double the exposure to selexipag and increase exposure to the active metabolite by over 10-fold [30]. Because of this, concomitant administration of selexipag with strong inhibitors of CYP2C8 is contraindicated. Concomitant use of a moderate CYP2C8 inhibitor (e.g., deferasirox or teriflunomide) also increases the exposure to selexipag, but to a much less extent, compared to strong inhibitors. A such, the dose of selexipag should be reduced when a moderate CYP2C8 inhibitor is initiated. On the other hand, CYP2C8 inducers (e.g., rifampin) decrease exposure to the active metabolite. Accordingly, the standard dose of selexipag needs to be doubled when used concomitantly with rifampin.

4.6.3. Contraindications and FDA Pregnancy Category

- Concomitant use of selexipag and strong inhibitors of CYP2C8 (e.g., gemfibrozil) is contraindicated.
- FDA pregnancy category: not assigned. No data available on use of selexipag in pregnant women to inform a drug-related risk.

4.7. Comparison with Existing Members and New Development since the US FDA Approval

Selexipag is the first-in-class and presently the only member of the prostacyclin IP receptor agonist dug class. Studies directly comparing the efficacy and safety of selexipag with those of other PAH drugs are currently not available. The results of the ongoing phase 3 studies (TRITON and TRANSIT-1) are expected to throw more light on the safety and efficacy of this novel drug across various treatment scenarios [31]. Meanwhile, a recent post-hoc analysis of the subpopulation of patients with connective tissue disease-associated pulmonary arterial hypertension (PAH-CTD; n = 334) enrolled in the GRIPHON trial demonstrated that selexipag treatment was well tolerated and delayed the progression of PAH irrespective of CTD subtype (e.g., systemic sclerosis and systemic lupus erythematosus) and baseline PAH therapy [32]. This finding is encouraging as patients with PAH-CTD have a poor prognosis compared with other etiologies and have been considered difficult to treat.

> **Connective tissue disease**
> The term connective tissue disease (CTD) refers to a heterogeneous group of diseases including systemic sclerosis and systemic lupus erythematosus. PAH is a serious complication of CTD, and historically, patients with PAH associated with CTD (PAH-CTD) have had worse outcomes compared with those with idiopathic PAH (IPAH).

5. SELF-ASSESSMENT QUESTIONS

5.1. A 38-year-old man is diagnosed with chronic thromboembolic pulmonary hypertension (CTEPH), which is also judged to be inoperable. A decision is made to treat the patient pharmacologically. Which of the following drugs is most appropriate for treating the patient's condition?

A. Ambrisentan
B. Bosentan

C. Riociguat
D. Selexipag
E. Tadalafil

5.2. A 41-year-old woman with heritable pulmonary arterial hypertension (PAH) is prescribed a recently approved drug for treating her condition. This new drug is a non-prostanoid compound and acts via stimulating the prostacyclin IP receptors in vascular smooth muscle cells to reduce pulmonary vascular resistance. Which of the following drugs is mostly likely prescribed?

A. Bosentan
B. Macitentan
C. Riociguat
D. Selexipag
E. Sildenafil

5.3. A 37-year-old man is diagnosed with idiopathic pulmonary arterial hypertension (IPAH). The patient is treated with an endothelin receptor antagonist, but he continues to experience significant symptoms. A decision is made to add to the regimen another drug which acts via directly inhibiting the hydrolysis of cyclic guanosine monophosphate (cGMP) in pulmonary vascular cells. Which of the following drugs is most likely added?

A. Ambrisentan
B. Iloprost
C. Riociguat
D. Selexipag
E. Tadalafil

5.4. Treatment with which of the following drugs is most likely capable of reducing the mortality in patients with pulmonary arterial hypertension?

A. Ambrisentan
B. Bosentan
C. Macitentan
D. Riociguat
E. Sildenafil

5.5. A 50-year-old man is diagnosed with pulmonary arterial hypertension associated with connective tissue disease (PAH-CTD) and hyperlipidemia. A decision is made to treat both of his conditions simultaneously with drugs. If the patient is to be treated with selexipag for his PAH-CTD, which of the following lipid-lowering drugs should be avoided?

A. Atorvastatin
B. Ezetimibe
C. Gemfibrozil
D. Simvastatin
E. Vascepa

ANSWERS AND EXPLANATIONS

5.1. The correct answer is C. Among the drugs listed, only riociguat is approved by the US FDA for treating chronic thromboembolic pulmonary hypertension to improve exercise capacity and the WHO functional class. Riociguat is also indicated for treating pulmonary arterial hypertension.

5.2. The correct answer is D. Among the drugs listed, only selexipag acts via stimulating prostacyclin IP receptors. It is the first-in-class and currently only member of the prostacyclin IP receptor agonist drug class.

5.3. The correct answer is E. Although both riociguat and tadalafil are able to increase the cGMP levels in pulmonary vascular cells, leading to decreased pulmonary vascular pressure, only tadalafil is able to directly inhibit the hydrolysis of cGMP by phosphodiesterase type 5. Riociguat, on the other hand, increases cGMP levels via stimulating soluble guanylate cyclase, thereby leading to increased synthesis of cGMP. The prostacyclin analogue iloprost increases cyclic adenosine monophosphate (cAMP) levels in vascular smooth muscle.

5.4. The correct answer is C. Among the drugs listed, only macitentan has been demonstrated to decrease mortality in patients with pulmonary arterial hypertension. At the present time, the mortality-reducing ability of the other drugs listed (ambrisentan, bosentan, riociguat, sildenafil) has not been established.

5.5. The correct answer is C. Oxidation of selexipag is primarily catalyzed by cytochrome P450 (CYP) 2C8. Concomitant use of a strong CYP2C8 inhibitor, such as the lipid-lowering drug gemfibrozil, can double the exposure to selexipag and increase exposure to the active metabolite by over 10-fold, potentially leading to serious adverse reactions. As such, concomitant administration of selexipag with gemfibrozil is contraindicated.

REFERENCES

1. McLaughlin VV, Archer SL, Badesch DB, Barst RJ, Farber HW, Lindner JR, Mathier MA, McGoon MD, Park MH, Rosenson RS, Rubin LJ, Tapson VF, et al. ACCF/AHA 2009 expert consensus document on pulmonary hypertension: a report of the American College of Cardiology Foundation Task Force on Expert Consensus Documents and the American Heart Association: developed in collaboration with the American College of Chest Physicians, American Thoracic Society, Inc., and the Pulmonary Hypertension Association. *Circulation* 2009; 119(16):2250–94.
2. Taichman DB, Ornelas J, Chung L, Klinger JR, Lewis S, Mandel J, Palevsky HI, Rich S, Sood N, Rosenzweig EB, Trow TK, Yung R, et al. Pharmacologic therapy for pulmonary arterial hypertension in adults: CHEST guideline and expert panel report. *Chest* 2014; 146(2):449–75.
3. Galie N, Humbert M, Vachiery JL, Gibbs S, Lang I, Torbicki A, Simonneau G, Peacock A, Vonk Noordegraaf A, Beghetti M, Ghofrani A, Gomez Sanchez MA, et al. 2015 ESC/ERS guidelines for the diagnosis and treatment of pulmonary hypertension: the Joint Task Force for the Diagnosis and Treatment of Pulmonary Hypertension of the European Society of Cardiology (ESC) and the European Respiratory Society (ERS): endorsed by: Association for European Paediatric and Congenital Cardiology

(AEPC), International Society for Heart and Lung Transplantation (ISHLT). *Eur Heart J* 2016; 37(1):67–119.

4. Hoeper MM, McLaughlin VV, Dalaan AM, Satoh T, Galie N. Treatment of pulmonary hypertension. *Lancet Respir Med* 2016; 4(4):323–36.

5. Maron BA, Galie N. Diagnosis, treatment, and clinical management of pulmonary arterial hypertension in the contemporary era: a review. *JAMA Cardiol* 2016; 1(9):1056–65.

6. Hansmann G. Pulmonary hypertension in infants, children, and young adults. *J Am Coll Cardiol* 2017; 69(20):2551–69.

7. Jandeleit-Dahm KA, Watson AM. The endothelin system and endothelin receptor antagonists. *Curr Opin Nephrol Hypertens* 2012; 21(1):66–71.

8. Rautureau Y, Schiffrin EL. Endothelin in hypertension: an update. *Curr Opin Nephrol Hypertens* 2012; 21(2):128–36.

9. Pulido T, Adzerikho I, Channick RN, Delcroix M, Galie N, Ghofrani HA, Jansa P, Jing ZC, Le Brun FO, Mehta S, Mittelholzer CM, Perchenet L, et al. Macitentan and morbidity and mortality in pulmonary arterial hypertension. *N Engl J Med* 2013; 369(9):809–18.

10. Giaid A, Yanagisawa M, Langleben D, Michel RP, Levy R, Shennib H, Kimura S, Masaki T, Duguid WP, Stewart DJ. Expression of endothelin-1 in the lungs of patients with pulmonary hypertension. *N Engl J Med* 1993; 328(24):1732–9.

11. Channick RN, Delcroix M, Ghofrani HA, Hunsche E, Jansa P, Le Brun FO, Mehta S, Pulido T, Rubin LJ, Sastry BK, Simonneau G, Sitbon O, et al. Effect of macitentan on hospitalizations: results from the SERAPHIN trial. *JACC Heart Fail* 2015; 3(1):1–8.

12. Galie N, Barbera JA, Frost AE, Ghofrani HA, Hoeper MM, McLaughlin VV, Peacock AJ, Simonneau G, Vachiery JL, Grunig E, Oudiz RJ, Vonk-Noordegraaf A, et al. Initial use of ambrisentan plus tadalafil in pulmonary arterial hypertension. *N Engl J Med* 2015; 373(9):834–44.

13. Raghu G, Behr J, Brown KK, Egan JJ, Kawut SM, Flaherty KR, Martinez FJ, Nathan SD, Wells AU, Collard HR, Costabel U, Richeldi L, et al. Treatment of idiopathic pulmonary fibrosis with ambrisentan: a parallel, randomized trial. *Ann Intern Med* 2013; 158(9):641–9.

14. Jansa P, Pulido T. Macitentan in pulmonary arterial hypertension: a focus on combination therapy in the SERAPHIN trial. *Am J Cardiovasc Drugs* 2017.

15. Dingemanse J, Sidharta PN, Maddrey WC, Rubin LJ, Mickail H. Efficacy, safety and clinical pharmacology of macitentan in comparison to other endothelin receptor antagonists in the treatment of pulmonary arterial hypertension. *Expert Opin Drug Saf* 2014; 13(3):391–405.

16. Mehta S, Sastry BK, Souza R, Torbicki A, Ghofrani HA, Channick RN, Delcroix M, Pulido T, Simonneau G, Wlodarczyk J, Rubin LJ, Jansa P, et al. Macitentan improves health-related quality of life for patients with pulmonary arterial hypertension: results from the randomized controlled SERAPHIN trial. *Chest* 2017; 151(1):106–18.

17. Ghofrani HA, Simonneau G, D'Armini AM, Fedullo P, Howard LS, Jais X, Jenkins DP, Jing ZC, Madani MM, Martin N, Mayer E, Papadakis K, et al. Macitentan for the treatment of inoperable chronic thromboembolic pulmonary hypertension (MERIT-1): results from the multicentre, phase 2, randomised, double-blind, placebo-controlled study. *Lancet Respir Med* 2017; 5(10):785–94.

18. Ghofrani HA, Galie N, Grimminger F, Grunig E, Humbert M, Jing ZC, Keogh AM, Langleben D, Kilama MO, Fritsch A, Neuser D, Rubin LJ, et al. Riociguat for the treatment of pulmonary arterial hypertension. *N Engl J Med* 2013; 369(4):330–40.

19. Ghofrani HA, D'Armini AM, Grimminger F, Hoeper MM, Jansa P, Kim NH, Mayer E, Simonneau G, Wilkins MR, Fritsch A, Neuser D, Weimann G, et al. Riociguat for the treatment of chronic thromboembolic pulmonary hypertension. *N Engl J Med* 2013; 369(4):319–29.

20. Ahluwalia A, Foster P, Scotland RS, McLean PG, Mathur A, Perretti M, Moncada S, Hobbs AJ. Antiinflammatory activity of soluble guanylate cyclase: cGMP-dependent down-regulation of P-selectin expression and leukocyte recruitment. *Proc Natl Acad Sci USA* 2004; 101(5):1386–91.

21. Stasch JP, Pacher P, Evgenov OV. Soluble guanylate cyclase as an emerging therapeutic target in cardiopulmonary disease. *Circulation* 2011; 123(20):2263–73.

22. Ghofrani HA, Humbert M, Langleben D, Schermuly R, Stasch JP, Wilkins MR, Klinger

JR. Riociguat: mode of action and clinical development in pulmonary hypertension. *Chest* 2017; 151(2):468–80.

23. Simonneau G, D'Armini AM, Ghofrani HA, Grimminger F, Hoeper MM, Jansa P, Kim NH, Wang C, Wilkins MR, Fritsch A, Davie N, Colorado P, et al. Riociguat for the treatment of chronic thromboembolic pulmonary hypertension: a long-term extension study (CHEST-2). *Eur Respir J* 2015; 45(5):1293–302.

24. Rubin LJ, Galie N, Grimminger F, Grunig E, Humbert M, Jing ZC, Keogh A, Langleben D, Fritsch A, Menezes F, Davie N, Ghofrani HA. Riociguat for the treatment of pulmonary arterial hypertension: a long-term extension study (PATENT-2). *Eur Respir J* 2015; 45(5):1303–13.

25. Simonneau G, D'Armini AM, Ghofrani HA, Grimminger F, Jansa P, Kim NH, Mayer E, Pulido T, Wang C, Colorado P, Fritsch A, Meier C, et al. Predictors of long-term outcomes in patients treated with riociguat for chronic thromboembolic pulmonary hypertension: data from the CHEST-2 open-label, randomised, long-term extension trial. *Lancet Respir Med* 2016; 4(5):372–80.

26. Ghofrani HA, Grimminger F, Grunig E, Huang Y, Jansa P, Jing ZC, Kilpatrick D, Langleben D, Rosenkranz S, Menezes F, Fritsch A, Nikkho S, et al. Predictors of long-term outcomes in patients treated with riociguat for pulmonary arterial hypertension: data from the PATENT-2 open-label, randomised, long-term extension

trial. *Lancet Respir Med* 2016; 4(5):361–71.

27. Humbert M, Sitbon O, Simonneau G. Treatment of pulmonary arterial hypertension. *N Engl J Med* 2004; 351(14):1425–36.

28. Lau EMT, Giannoulatou E, Celermajer DS, Humbert M. Epidemiology and treatment of pulmonary arterial hypertension. *Nat Rev Cardiol* 2017.

29. Sitbon O, Channick R, Chin KM, Frey A, Gaine S, Galie N, Ghofrani HA, Hoeper MM, Lang IM, Preiss R, Rubin LJ, Di Scala L, et al. Selexipag for the treatment of pulmonary arterial hypertension. *N Engl J Med* 2015; 373(26):2522–33.

30. Bruderer S, Petersen-Sylla M, Boehler M, Remenova T, Halabi A, Dingemanse J. Effect of gemfibrozil and rifampicin on the pharmacokinetics of selexipag and its active metabolite in healthy subjects. *Br J Clin Pharmacol* 2017; 83(12):2778–88.

31. Ghosh RK, Ball S, Das A, Bandyopadhyay D, Mondal S, Saha D, Gupta A. Selexipag in pulmonary arterial hypertension: most updated evidence from recent preclinical and clinical studies. *J Clin Pharmacol* 2017; 57(5):547–57.

32. Gaine S, Chin K, Coghlan G, Channick R, Di Scala L, Galie N, Ghofrani HA, Lang IM, McLaughlin V, Preiss R, Rubin LJ, Simonneau G, et al. Selexipag for the treatment of connective tissue disease-associated pulmonary arterial hypertension. *Eur Respir J* 2017; 50(2):1602493.

UNIT IV

ACUTE CORONARY SYNDROMES AND OTHER THROMBOTIC DISORDERS

CHAPTER 8

Overview of Acute Coronary Syndromes and Drug Therapy

CHAPTER HIGHLIGHTS

- Acute coronary syndromes (ACS) include unstable angina (UA), non-ST elevation myocardial infarction (NSTEMI), and ST elevation myocardial infarction (STEMI). UA and NSTEMI are also called non-ST elevation ACS (NSTE-ACS).
- Acute myocardial infarction (MI) is predominantly caused by rupture (or erosion) of an atherosclerotic plaque and partial or complete thrombotic occlusion of the inflicted coronary artery. Acute MI in the absence of critical coronary artery disease accounts for ~10% of cases.
- Drug targeting for ACS includes thrombus- and inflammation-based targeting. Thrombus-based drug therapies involve the use of platelet inhibitors and anticoagulants, as well as fibrinolytic agents (for STEMI). Inflammation-based drug therapies are currently investigational.
- Management of ACS involves the use of both drugs and non-pharmacological approaches (e.g., percutaneous coronary intervention). Drugs used in the acute management of ACS include oxygen, nitrates, β-blockers, calcium channel blockers, morphine, statins, platelet inhibitors, anticoagulants, and fibrinolytic agents (for STEMI only).
- Long-term management of ACS involves the use of dual-antiplatelet therapy (DAPT) and drugs to treat risk factors and comorbidities (e.g., lipid-lowering drugs, anti-diabetic drugs), as well as lifestyle modifications, cardiac rehabilitation, and patient/family education.

KEYWORDS | Acute coronary syndromes; Acute myocardial infarction; Anticoagulants; Fibrinolytic agents; Non-ST elevation myocardial infarction; Percutaneous coronary intervention; Platelet inhibitors; ST-elevation myocardial infarction; Unstable angina

CITATION | *Li YR. Cardiovascular Medicine: New Therapeutic Drugs Approved by the US FDA (2013–2017). Cell Med Press, Raleigh, NC, USA. 2018. http://dx.doi.org/10.20455/ndcvd.2018.08*

ABBREVIATIONS | ACE, angiotensin-converting enzyme; ACS, acute coronary syndromes; ASCVD, atherosclerotic cardiovascular disease; CABG, coronary artery bypass grafting; CAD, coronary artery disease; CCB, calcium channel blocker; CHD, coronary heart disease; CI, confidence interval; DAPT, dual-antiplatelet therapy; DVT, deep vein thrombosis; ECG, electrocardiography; HIT, heparin-induced thrombocytopenia; hsCRP, high-sensitivity C-reactive protein; IHD, ischemic heart disease; IL, interleukin; Lp-PLA$_2$, lipoprotein-associated phospholipase A$_2$; MAPK, mitogen-activated protein kinase; MI, myocardial infarction; MMP, matrix metalloproteinase; NSTE-ACS, non-ST elevation acute coronary syndromes; NSTEMI, non-ST elevation myocardial infarction; NVAF, nonvalvular atrial fibrillation; PCI, percutaneous coronary intervention; PE, pulmonary embolism; SMC, smooth muscle cell; sPLA$_2$, secretory lipoprotein-associated phospholipase A$_2$; STEMI, ST elevation myocardial infarction; VTE, venous thromboembolism

CHAPTER AT A GLANCE

1. INTRODUCTION

Unstable angina (UA), acute non-ST elevation myocardial infarction (NSTEMI), and acute ST elevation myocardial infarction (STEMI) are the three presentations of acute coronary syndromes (ACS). This chapter provides an overview of the definitions and epidemiology of ACS. It also surveys the current understanding of the molecular pathophysiology of ACS and the principles of mechanistically based drug therapy. This sets a stage for the subsequent discussion of the new drugs for ACS in Chapter 9.

2. MOLECULAR MEDICINE OF ACS

2.1. Definitions and General Considerations

2.1.1. Definitions of Ischemic Heart Disease

The term ischemic heart disease (IHD) refers to a spectrum of diseases of the heart caused by decreased oxygen supply to the myocardium. The International Statistical Classification of Diseases and Related Health Problems 10th Revision (ICD-10) classifies IHD into the following six categories, with each category consisting of multiple disease entities.

(1) Angina pectoris
(2) Acute myocardial infarction
(3) Certain current complications following acute myocardial infarction
(4) Subsequent myocardial infarction
(5) Other acute ischemic heart diseases
(6) Chronic ischemic heart disease including coronary artery disease among others

The above ICD-10 classification of IHD is comprehensive and authoritative; however, it is complicated and often times causes confusion. Hence, a simplified classification scheme is frequently used to divide IHD into two general categories (**Figure 8.1**): (1) stable IHD

ICD-10
The International Statistical Classification of Diseases and Related Health Problems, more commonly known as the International Classification of Diseases (ICD), is the standard diagnostic tool for epidemiology, health management, and clinical purposes. The ICD is revised periodically and is currently in its tenth revision, namely, ICD-10 (http://apps.who.int/classifications/icd10/browse/2016/en). ICD-10 is used by more than 100 countries around the world. (ICD-11 is expected to be released in 2018.) ICD-10 defines the universe of diseases, disorders, injuries, and other related health conditions, listed in a comprehensive, hierarchical fashion that allows for: (1) easy storage, retrieval, and analysis of health information for evidenced-based decision-making; (2) sharing and comparing health information between hospitals, regions, settings, and countries; and (3) data comparisons in the same location across different time.

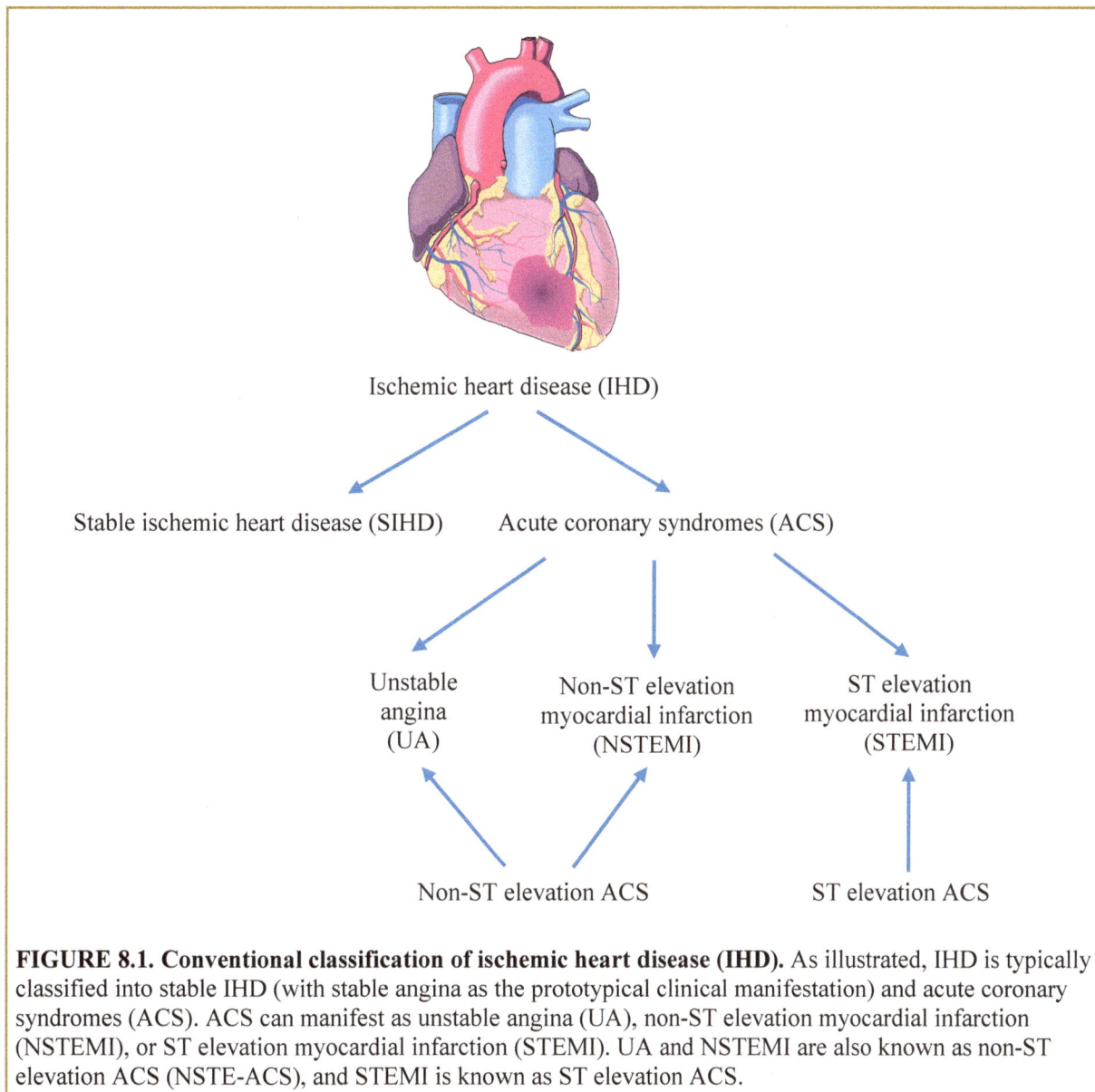

FIGURE 8.1. Conventional classification of ischemic heart disease (IHD). As illustrated, IHD is typically classified into stable IHD (with stable angina as the prototypical clinical manifestation) and acute coronary syndromes (ACS). ACS can manifest as unstable angina (UA), non-ST elevation myocardial infarction (NSTEMI), or ST elevation myocardial infarction (STEMI). UA and NSTEMI are also known as non-ST elevation ACS (NSTE-ACS), and STEMI is known as ST elevation ACS.

with stable angina as the prototypical manifestation, and (2) ACS, which, as noted earlier, include UA, NSTEMI, and STEMI (see Section 2.1.3 below). Stable IHD is frequently also known as stable coronary artery disease or chronic coronary artery disease. Regardless of the nomenclature, stable angina is the chief manifestation of stable IHD [1].

2.1.2. Definitions of Coronary Artery Disease and Coronary Heart Disease

Coronary artery disease (CAD) and coronary heart disease (CHD) are frequently used synonymously by health care professionals. However, strictly speaking there are differences between these two terms. CAD is generally used to refer to the pathological process affecting the coronary arteries (usually atherosclerosis). On the other hand, CHD is actually a result of CAD. With CAD, plaque first develops in the coronary arteries until the blood flow to the myocardium is limited. This is also known as myocardial ischemia. It may be chronic, caused by narrowing of the coronary artery and limitation of the blood supply to part of the myocardium. Or it can be acute, resulting from a sudden plaque rupture with subsequent thrombosis. Hence, CHD includes the diagnoses of angina pectoris, myocardial infarction, silent myocardial ischemia, and CHD mortality that results from CAD [1]. Nevertheless, the terms CAD and CHD are frequently used interchangeably in the medical literature and in clinical practice.

2.1.3. Definition of ACS

As mentioned above, the term ACS refers to a spectrum of clinical presentations ranging from those for STEMI to presentations found in NSTEMI or in UA. In terms of pathogenesis, ACS are predominantly associated with rupture (or erosion) of an atherosclerotic plaque and partial or complete thrombotic occlusion of the inflicted coronary artery. While UA and NSTEMI are caused by incomplete coronary blockage, STEMI typically results from complete coronary occlusion. UA and NSTEMI are also known as non-ST elevation ACS (NSTE-ACS), and STEMI as ST elevation ACS.

2.1.4. Historical Overview of ACS

The condition commonly referred to as ACS, today, has a long and storied history in the annals of medicine. The dreaded symptoms were eloquently described by the esteemed English physician, William Heberden (1710–1801) in 1772 as "a most disagreeable sensation in the breast, which seems as if it would take their life away, if it were to increase or continue". Sir William Osler (1849–1919) formalized the definition of ACS and highlighted its profound implications for the patient in his famous Lumleian Lecture on "Angina Pectoris" delivered before the Royal College of Physicians in London in 1910: "There are two primary features of the disease, pain and sudden death: pain, paroxysmal, intense, peculiar, usually pectoral, and with well-known lines of radiation; death in a higher percentage than any known disorder, and usually sudden." With the advent of diagnostic tools, such as the electrocardiography (ECG) and laboratory tests for myocardial damage, the term ACS has evolved as an umbrella diagnosis to capture the full spectrum of disease severity and protean clinical manifestations of critical coronary atherosclerosis from UA to NSTEMI and STEMI [2].

2.1.5. Diagnostic Criteria for UA and NSTEMI

UA and NSTEMI differ primarily in whether the ischemia is severe enough to cause sufficient myocardial damage to release detectable quantities of a marker of myocardial injury (e.g., cardiac troponins) (**Figure 8.2**). The key diagnostic criteria for UA and NSTEMI are outlined below.

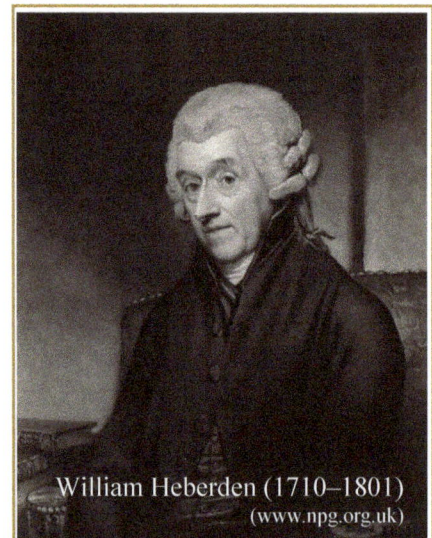

William Heberden (1710–1801)
(www.npg.org.uk)

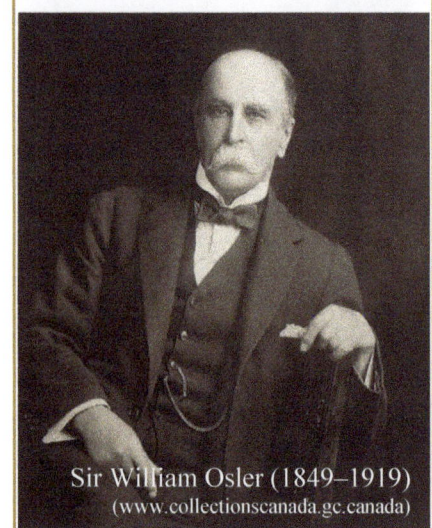

Sir William Osler (1849–1919)
(www.collectionscanada.gc.canada)

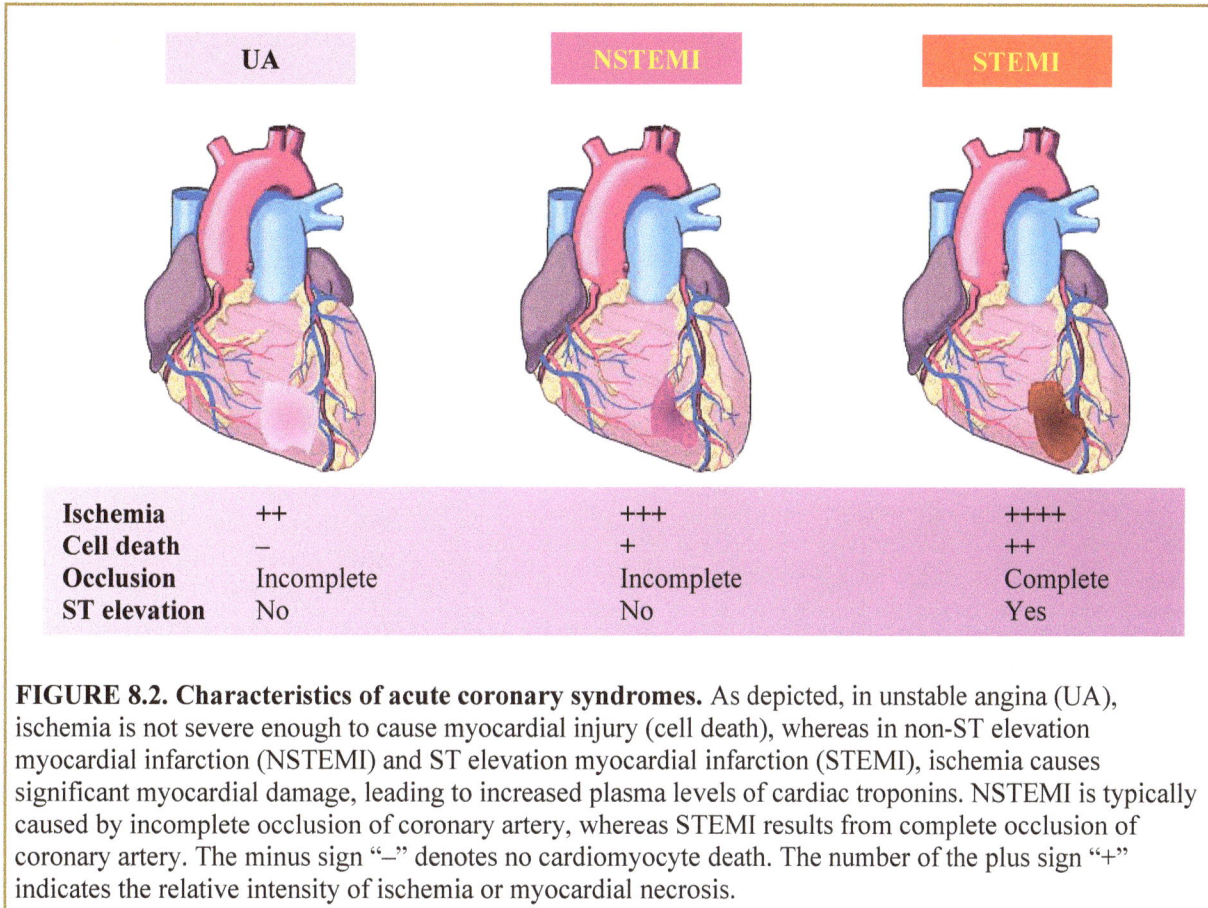

	UA	NSTEMI	STEMI
Ischemia	++	+++	++++
Cell death	–	+	++
Occlusion	Incomplete	Incomplete	Complete
ST elevation	No	No	Yes

FIGURE 8.2. Characteristics of acute coronary syndromes. As depicted, in unstable angina (UA), ischemia is not severe enough to cause myocardial injury (cell death), whereas in non-ST elevation myocardial infarction (NSTEMI) and ST elevation myocardial infarction (STEMI), ischemia causes significant myocardial damage, leading to increased plasma levels of cardiac troponins. NSTEMI is typically caused by incomplete occlusion of coronary artery, whereas STEMI results from complete occlusion of coronary artery. The minus sign "–" denotes no cardiomyocyte death. The number of the plus sign "+" indicates the relative intensity of ischemia or myocardial necrosis.

- UA is considered to be present in patients with ischemic symptoms suggestive of an ACS and no elevation in troponins, with or without ECG changes indicative of ischemia (e.g., ST segment depression or transient elevation or new T wave inversion).
- NSTEMI is considered to be present in patients having the same manifestations as those in UA, but in whom an elevation in troponins is present.

Since an elevation in cardiac troponins may not be detectable for hours after presentation, UA and NSTEMI are frequently indistinguishable at initial evaluation. As such, the initial management is the same for these two syndromes. For this reason, and because the pathophysiological mechanisms of the two conditions are similar, UA and NSTEMI are often considered together.

2.1.6. The Third Universal Definition of Acute Myocardial Infarction

When discussing ACS, an important term cannot be ignored: it is acute myocardial infarction (MI) [3]. Both NSTEMI and STEMI under the ACS umbrella belong to the acute MI category. The term refers to a condition when there is evidence of myocardial necrosis in a clinical setting consistent with acute myocardial ischemia [4]. This definition emphasizes that the myocardial necrosis is caused by ischemia as opposed to other etiologies such as myocarditis or trauma. According to the Third Universal Definition of Myocardial Infarction [4], MI is classified into six types, as outlined below.

Type 1 (spontaneous MI): It is related to atherosclerotic plaque rupture, ulceration, assuring, erosion, or dissection with resulting intraluminal thrombus in one or more of the coronary arteries leading to decreased myocardial blood flow or distal platelet emboli with ensuing myocyte necrosis. Type 1 MI is the predominant form of MI, accounting for ~90% of cases of acute MI. On the other hand, the occurrence of acute MI in the absence of critical coronary artery disease is increasingly recognized and accounting for ~10% of cases [3].

Type 2 (MI secondary to an ischemic imbalance): It is caused by an imbalance between myocardial oxygen supply and demand that is not the result of acute atherothrombosis and that is due to factors, such as coronary endothelial dysfunction, coronary artery spasm, coronary embolism, cardiac arrhythmias, anemia, respiratory failure, hypotension, and hypertension with or without left ventricular hypertrophy.

Type 3 (MI resulting in death when biomarker values are unavailable): It refers to cardiac death with symptoms suggestive of myocardial ischemia and presumed new ischemic ECG changes or new left bundle branch block, but death occurring before blood samples could be obtained, before cardiac biomarker could rise, or in rare cases cardiac biomarkers were not collected.

Type 4a (MI related to percutaneous coronary intervention [PCI]): It refers to MI that occurs as a result of the various insults introduced during the mechanical revascularization via PCI. MI associated with PCI is arbitrarily defined by elevation of cardiac troponin values greater than 5 times of the 99th percentile upper reference limit in patients with normal baseline values (<99th percentile upper reference limit) or a rise of cardiac troponin values >20% if the baseline values are elevated and are stable or falling. In addition, one of the following also occurs: (1) symptoms suggestive of myocardial ischemia; (2) new ischemic ECG changes or new left bundle branch block; (3) angiographic loss of patency of a major coronary artery or a side branch or persistent slow- or no-flow or embolization; or (4) imaging demonstration of new loss of viable myocardium or new regional wall motion abnormality.

Type 4b (MI related to stent thrombosis): It refers to MI that occurs as a result of stent thrombosis and restenosis following a primary PCI. MI associated with stent thrombosis is detected by coronary angiography or autopsy in the setting of myocardial ischemia and with a rise and/or fall of the values of cardiac biomarkers with at least one value above the 99th percentile upper reference limit.

Type 5 (MI related to coronary artery bypass grafting [CABG]): It refers to MI that occurs as a result of the various insults introduced

Universal definition of myocardial infarction (MI)
In 2000, the First Global MI Task Force presented a new definition of MI, which implied that any necrosis in the setting of myocardial ischemia should be labelled as MI. This may be considered the "first" international consensus on MI definition. The principles in the "first definition" were further refined by the Second Global MI Task Force, leading to the publication of the so called "universal definition of MI" consensus document in 2007, which emphasized the different conditions that might lead to an MI and provided a universal definition of MI (types 1 through 5). This may be considered as the "second" international consensus on MI definition. Given the development of more sensitive assays for markers of myocardial necrosis, revision of the definitions for myocardial necrosis, particularly in the setting of critical illness and after revascularization, prompted the publication of the third universal definition of MI in 2012 [4]. The "third" definition is also the most current one (see Section 2.1.6).

Percutaneous coronary intervention (PCI)
PCI, also known as angioplasty, is a medical procedure in which a balloon is used to open narrowed or blocked coronary arteries. With a PCI, a catheter with a deflated balloon on its tip is passed into the narrowed artery segment, and the balloon is inflated and the narrowed segment widened. Then the balloon is deflated and the catheter is removed. Coronary stents are now used in nearly all PCI procedures helping keep the artery from narrowing or closing again.

during the mechanical revascularization via CABG. MI associated with CABG is arbitrarily defined by elevation of cardiac biomarker values greater than 10 times of the 99th percentile upper reference limit in patients with normal baseline cardiac troponin values (<99th percentile upper reference limit). In addition, one of the following also occurs: (1) new pathological Q waves or new left bundle branch block; (2) angiographic documented new graft or new native coronary artery occlusion; or (3) imaging evidence of new loss of viable myocardium or new regional wall motion abnormality.

2.2. Epidemiology

2.2.1. IHD/ACS and Global Burden of Diseases

The epidemic of IHD is truly global, with more than 80% of the burden of this disease carried by the developing nations. IHD (with its manifestation as ACS) carries enormous personal, societal, and economic burdens, and is a major determinant of morbidity and mortality among all races, ethnic groups, and cultures [2, 5, 6]. Indeed, the Global Burden of Disease Study 2016 reported that for non-communicable diseases in 2016, the largest number of deaths were caused by cardiovascular diseases (17.6 million deaths) followed by neoplasms (8.93 million deaths) and chronic respiratory diseases (3.54 million deaths). Globally, deaths from cardiovascular diseases increased by 14.5% between 2006 and 2016. Notably, IHD and cerebrovascular disease (stroke) combined accounted for more than 85% of all cardiovascular disease deaths in 2016. Total deaths from IHD rose by 19%, increasing from 7.96 million deaths in 2006 to 9.48 million deaths in 2016, which largely accounts for the overall increase in total deaths from cardiovascular diseases [7].

2.2.2. IHD/ACS in the United States

According to the American Heart Association Heart Disease and Stroke Statistics—2017 Update [8], an estimated 16.5 million Americans ≥20 years of age have coronary heart disease, accounting for 6.3% of the US adults ≥20 years of age. The overall prevalence for MI is 3.0% in US adults ≥20 years of age. Thus, nearly 50% of coronary heart disease patients have MI. The estimated annual incidence of MI is 580,000 new attacks and 210,000 recurrent attacks. Currently, coronary heart disease is responsible for approximately one in every 7 deaths in the United States, accounting for more than 360,000 deaths each year. MI is responsible for over 110,000 deaths annually. A recent estimate for the number of inpatient hospital discharges with ACS in the United States was 1,141,000, and of the total, 813,000 were for MI alone, 322,000 were for UA alone, and 6,000 hospitalizations received both diagnoses [8].

2.2.3. Trends of STEMI

While the prevalence of ACS has reached a pandemic level as a consequence of modernization of the developing world, the demographics of ACS have also evolved, with a precipitous decline in

> **Coronary artery bypass grafting (CABG)**
> CABG is a type of surgery that improves blood flow to the heart and used to treat people with severe coronary artery disease. During CABG, a healthy artery or vein from the patient's body is connected, or grafted, to the blocked coronary artery. The grafted artery or vein bypasses the blocked portion of the coronary artery. This creates a new path for oxygen-rich blood to flow to the myocardium (www.nhlbi.nih.gov).

the incidence of STEMI and a progressive rise in the incidence of NSTEMI [2]. In an analysis of 46,086 hospitalizations for ACS in the Kaiser Permanente Northern California study, the percentage of STEMI cases decreased from 47.0% to 22.9% between 1999 and 2008 [8, 9].

2.3. Pathophysiology

2.3.1. Historical Overview

The causative link between arterial thrombosis and ACS has a controversial history [10, 11]. The initial link between coronary thrombosis and acute MI was recognized in the late 1800s and gained widespread acceptance within the medical community throughout the early 1900s. But after a series of pathological studies that cast doubt on this association, alternative mechanisms were sought. It was not until the use of coronary angiography in people with an acute MI in the late 1970s, in combination with the success of thrombolytic therapies in the 1980s, that the causative role for thrombosis in precipitating UA and acute MI was unequivocally established. Since then, there has been dramatic improvement in the understanding and treatment options for ACS, with antithrombotic therapy taking center stage in the disease management [1].

2.3.2. Molecular Pathophysiology

ACS represent life-threatening manifestations of atherosclerosis. Atherosclerosis alone may obstruct coronary blood flow and cause stable angina, but this is rarely fatal in the absence of scarring of the myocardium, which can elicit an arrhythmia presenting as sudden cardiac arrest [12, 13]. ACS are predominantly precipitated by acute thrombosis induced by a ruptured or eroded atherosclerotic coronary plaque with or without concomitant vasospasm, causing a sudden and critical reduction in blood flow [13, 14].

2.3.2.1. PLAQUE RUPTURE

In the complex process of plaque disruption, inflammation has been revealed as a key pathophysiological element [12, 13, 15]. Plaque rupture occurs where the cap is thinnest and most infiltrated by foam cells (macrophages). In eccentric plaques, the weakest spot is often the cap margin or shoulder region, and only extremely thin fibrous caps are at risk of rupturing. Thinning of the fibrous cap probably involves two concurrent mechanisms. One is the gradual loss of vascular smooth muscle cells (SMCs) from the fibrous cap. Indeed, ruptured caps contain fewer SMCs and less collagen than do intact caps, and SMCs are usually absent at the actual site of rupture. Concurrently, infiltrating macrophages in the plaque degrade the collagen-rich cap matrix via releasing matrix metalloproteinases (MMPs), especially MMP-1, -8, and -13 [12, 15]. With plaque rupture, cap collagen and the highly thrombogenic lipid core, enriched in tissue factor-expressing apoptotic microparticles, are exposed to the thrombogenic factors of the blood, leading to thrombogenesis [12, 15].

2.3.2.2. PLAQUE EROSION

In addition to plaque rupture, superficial plaque erosion also causes thrombus formation responsible for 20–25% of the cases of fatal MI [13, 16, 17]. This anatomical substrate for coronary thrombosis occurs more frequently in women than in men and in persons with certain risk factors, such as hypertriglyceridemia. Many lesions, that cause coronary thrombosis because of superficial erosion, lack prominent inflammatory infiltrates, and such plaques typically exhibit proteoglycan accumulation. The exact molecular mechanisms of superficial erosion are less clear than those involved in the rupture of the fibrous cap. The surface endothelium under the thrombus is usually absent, but no distinct morphological features of the underlying plaque have been identified.

Eroded and thrombosed plaques causing sudden cardiac death are often scarcely calcified, often associated with negative remodeling, and contain fewer macrophages than ruptured plaques. Apoptosis of endothelial cells could contribute to their desquamation. Reactive oxygen species and oxidative stress may play an important role in endothelial apoptosis. As endothelial cells undergo apoptosis, they produce the procoagulant tissue factor, resulting in local thrombosis in coronary arteries. Endothelial cells also express proteinases that may sever their tethers to the underlying basement membrane. In this context, modified low-density lipoprotein induces the expression of the enzyme MMP-14 by human endothelial cells. MMP-14 can activate MMP-2, an enzyme that degrades basement-membrane forms of nonfibrillar collagen (i.e., type IV collagen). These events may collectively contribute to the superficial erosion of the atheroma, thereby promoting thrombogenesis and the eventual formation of a thrombus that severely restricts the blood flow of the inflicted coronary artery, leading to myocardial injury [12, 13, 15].

2.3.2.3. SECONDARY MECHANISMS

In up to 10% cases, ACS may have a nonatherosclerotic etiology, such as arteritis, dissection, coronary artery spasm, thromboembolism, congenital anomalies, cocaine abuse, or complications of cardiac catheterization. These are collectively known as secondary mechanisms of ACS. Hence, the key pathophysiological mechanisms, including plaque rupture and plaque erosion, as well as the secondary mechanisms of ACS, need to be understood for the correct use of the available therapeutic strategies.

3. OVERVIEW OF MECHANISTICALLY BASED DRUG THERAPY

This section introduces the big picture of mechanistically based drug therapy of ACS, including NSTE-ACS and STEMI. It first examines the overall drug targeting strategies and introduces current guideline-directed treatment strategies for ACS. The section then provides an overview of the drugs commonly used in the management of ACS as well as the United States Food and Drug Administration (US FDA)-

approved antithrombotic drugs for ACS, which include anticoagulants, platelet inhibitors, and fibrinolytic agents. This will lay a basis for the subsequent discussion of the newly approved drugs for ACS in Chapter 9.

3.1. Overview of Mechanistically Based Drug Targeting for ACS

3.1.1. Thrombus-Based Targeting

In STEMI, because of the complete occlusion, prompt reopening of the occluded artery via either mechanical (e.g., percutaneous coronary intervention [PCI]) or pharmacological (i.e., fibrinolysis) approach is the therapeutic priority that limits the extent of myocardial injury and saves lives. On the other hand, the therapeutic goals in NSTE-ACS management are to prevent progression of the thrombus to total occlusion, plaque thromboembolization, and recurrent infarction. In-hospital mortality rates in STEMI patients remain 50% higher than those for NSTEMI patients. However, the high rates of recurrent ischemic events in NSTE-ACS patients result in similar one-year mortality rates in the two conditions, emphasizing the need for selecting appropriate early management strategies and secondary prevention measures for NSTE-ACS as well. In this context, mechanical revascularization via PCI has been becoming an important approach in the management of NSTE-ACS. Regardless of the modalities used to restore coronary blood flow in ACS patients, additional drugs are necessary to inhibit or prevent thrombogenesis.

Drugs targeting the thrombus, also known as antithrombotic drugs, include three groups of agents, namely anticoagulants, platelet inhibitors, and fibrinolytics (also known as thrombolytics). While anticoagulants and platelet inhibitors prevent or inhibit thrombus formation (thrombogenesis), fibrinolytic agents degrade the already formed thrombus. While all three groups of antithrombotic drugs are indicated in the management of STEMI, fibrinolytic drugs are not recommended for treating NSTE-ACS due to their potential harm and lack of benefit in this setting [18, 19].

3.1.2. Inflammation-Based Targeting

Given the critical role of inflammation in the pathophysiological aspects of plaque rupture and thrombogenesis, multiple studies have been carried out over the past few years to assess the safety and efficacy of various anti-inflammatory agents other than statins in reducing the risk of cardiovascular events and mortality in patients with MI. This subsection introduces some of the recent trials on anti-inflammatory therapies in ACS and discusses the potential implications of such emerging modalities.

3.1.2.1. COLCHICINE

The presence of activated neutrophils in culprit atherosclerotic plaques of patients with unstable coronary disease raises the possibility that inhibition of neutrophil function with colchicine may reduce the risk of plaque instability and thereby improve clinical outcomes in patients with stable coronary heart disease. In this regard, in a recent randomized controlled trial, 532 patients with stable coronary heart disease receiving aspirin and/or clopidogrel (93%) and statins (95%) were randomly assigned to receive colchicine 0.5 mg/day or no colchicine and followed for a median of 3 years. The primary outcome was the composite incidence of ACS, out-of-hospital cardiac arrest, or noncardioembolic ischemic stroke. The primary outcome occurred in 15 of 282 patients (5.3%) who received colchicine and 40 of 250 patients (16.0%) assigned to no colchicine (hazard ratio: 0.33; 95% confidence interval [CI] 0.18 to 0.59; p <0.001; number needed to treat: 11). In a pre-specified secondary on-treatment analysis that excluded 32 patients (11%) assigned to colchicine who withdrew within 30 days due to intestinal intolerance and a further 7 patients (2%) who did not start treatment, the primary outcome occurred in 4.5% versus 16.0% (hazard ratio: 0.29; 95% CI: 0.15 to 0.56; p <0.001). The study concluded that colchicine, 0.5 mg/day administered in addition to statins and other standard secondary prevention therapies, appeared effective for the prevention of cardiovascular events in patients with stable coronary heart disease [20].

The above colchicine trial was relatively small (532 patients, with a total of 55 events), and the investigators did not use a double-blind design and did not report levels of inflammatory biomarkers, which might have provided a glimpse into the possible mechanisms underlying the effects of colchicine [15, 21]. Nevertheless, the above encouraging results have prompted additional studies, including mechanistic studies and large-scale, randomized controlled trials of this inexpensive agent, which has a long history of clinical use and a well-known and acceptable risk profile [15, 22]. In this context, a recent study with 40 ACS patients demonstrated that ACS patients exhibited increased local cardiac production of inflammatory cytokines, including interleukin (IL)-1β, IL-6, and IL-18, and short-term colchicine administration rapidly and significantly reduced the levels of these cytokines by 40–88% [23]. A more recent study involving 80 patients with recent ACS (<1 month) reported that low-dose colchicine therapy favorably modified coronary plaque, independent of high-dose statin intensification therapy and substantial low-density lipoprotein reduction. The study also suggested that improvement in plaque morphology was likely driven by the anti-inflammatory properties of colchicine, as evidenced by reductions in high-sensitivity C-reactive protein (hsCRP), rather than changes in lipoproteins [24]. A much larger randomized controlled trial, known as Colchicine Cardiovascular Outcomes Trial (COLCOT), involving >4,000 participants, is currently underway to evaluate whether long-term treatment with colchicine reduces rates of cardiovascular events in patients after MI. This trial is expected to be completed in September 2019 (https://clinicaltrials.gov/ct2/show/NCT02551094).

3.1.2.2. N-3 FATTY ACIDS

As noted in Chapter 3, n-3 fatty acids (also known as omega-3 fatty acids) possess anti-inflammatory activities, possibly via interacting with G protein-coupled receptor 120 [25–27]. The anti-inflammatory properties of n-3 fatty acids may also underlie the protective effects of these fatty acids in diverse cardiovascular conditions, including ACS [28–31] (also see Chapter 3). Notably, a recent randomized controlled trial involving 241 patients with ACS in Japan reported that initiation of a combination therapy of pitavastatin (2 mg/day) and eicosapentaenoic acid (EPA; a major form of n-3 fatty acids) (1.8 g/day) within 24 hours after PCI in patients with acute MI not only suppressed inflammation and ventricular arrhythmia, but also reduced cardiovascular events by 58% compared with statin monotherapy during a 12-month follow-up [32]. The cardiovascular events included death from a cardiovascular cause, nonfatal stroke, nonfatal MI, and revascularization.

In another recent trial, 285 subjects with stable coronary heart disease on statins were randomized to omega-3 ethyl-ester (1.86 g of eicosapentaenoic acid and 1.5 g of docosahexaenoic acid daily) or no omega-3 (control) for 30 months. The trial demonstrated that the co-treatment with the high dose n-3 fatty acids prevented the progression of fibrous coronary plaque in subjects on low-intensity statin therapy, but not in subjects on high-intensity statin therapy [33]. The results of the trial implicate that n-3 fatty acid therapy may provide additional benefits to those coronary heart disease patients who can only receive low-intensity statin therapy due to intolerability to high-intensity statin treatment.

3.1.2.3. IL-1β INHIBITORS

In line with the inflammatory stress mechanism of cardiovascular degeneration, substantial evidence from studies in experimental animal models as well as human subjects supports a critical causal role for IL-1β signaling cascade (i.e., IL-1β to IL-6 cascade) in the development of atherosclerotic cardiovascular diseases (ASCVDs) [34–38]. Identification of IL-1β as a critical pathophysiological factor in ASCVDs has prompted clinical trials on the efficacy of canakinumab, a therapeutic antibody targeting IL-1β, in treating ASCVDs. In this regard, a major randomized controlled trial, known as CANTOS (Canakinumab Anti-inflammatory Thrombosis Outcomes Study), has recently been completed with encouraging results.

The CANTOS trial and cardiovascular events: CANTOS is a randomized, double-blind, controlled trial involving 10,061 patients with previous MI and a hsCRP level of ≥2 mg/L. The trial compared three doses of canakinumab (50 mg, 150 mg, and 300 mg, administered subcutaneously once every 3 months) with placebo. The primary efficacy endpoint was nonfatal MI, nonfatal stroke, or cardiovascular death [39]. As expected, canakinumab as compared with placebo significantly reduced hsCRP (a downstream clinical biomarker of inflammation) and IL-6 (a likely causal effector in the critical IL-1 to IL-6 cascade). When compared with placebo, the lowest dose of canakinumab (50 mg) reduced hsCRP and IL-6 by 20–25%, whereas the two higher doses (150 and 300 mg) each reduced hsCRP and IL-6 by 35–40%. In contrast, canakinumab had virtually no effect on either lower-density lipoprotein cholesterol or high-density lipoprotein cholesterol. At a median follow-up period of 3.7 years, treatment with 150 mg or 300 mg dose of canakinumab caused a ~15% reduction in the trial primary endpoint inclusive of nonfatal MI, nonfatal stroke, and cardiovascular death. Moreover, for the pre-specified secondary cardiovascular endpoint additionally inclusive of hospitalization for unstable angina requiring urgent revascularization, the two higher doses both reduced the event rates by 17% [39]. It should be mentioned that the CANTOS trial also revealed that canakinumab treatment was associated with a higher incidence of fatal infection than placebo, affirming a critical role of IL-1β in innate immunity against infections.

The CANTOS trial and residual inflammation: Further analysis of the data from the CANTOS trial revealed that among CANTOS participants treated with any dose of canakinumab who achieved hsCRP levels below 2 mg/L after drug initiation, a 26% reduction in the risk of major adverse cardiovascular events was observed. Furthermore, among these robust responders, both cardiovascular mortality and all-cause mortality were reduced by 31%. On the other hand, for those treated with canakinumab who had a less pronounced anti-inflammatory response, the effects on these endpoints were smaller and no longer significant. These data suggest that suppression of the residual inflammatory stress by canakinumab is a viable approach to further reducing cardiovascular events and mortality [40, 41].

The CANTOS trial and lung cancer: While IL-1β is an important player in innate immunity against infections, IL-1β-mediated inflammation in tumor microenvironment also has a major role in cancer invasiveness, progression, and metastasis, and as such, may be a promising target for cancer therapy [42]. Indeed, analysis of the CANTOS participants showed that treatment with canakinumab was associated with a dose-dependent reduction of total cancer mortality (with a >50% reduction in total cancer mortality at the 300 mg dosage). The 300 mg dosage was also associated with a >75% reduction in lung cancer mortality. Notably, the incident lung cancer rate was also reduced dose-dependently, with a 67% reduction at 300 mg dosage [43]. These provocative data point to that despite an increased risk of fatal infections, the anti-inflammatory therapy with canakinumab targeting the IL-1β innate immunity pathway could drastically reduce incident lung cancer rate and lung cancer mortality. Confirmation of such an anticancer efficacy of canakinumab in additional clinical trials with formal settings of cancer screening and treatment would obviously be a major breakthrough in the field of cancer therapeutics.

The CANTOS trial and the inflammatory stress mechanism of ASCVDs: Dysregulated inflammation or inflammatory stress has been proposed to be a major pathophysiological mechanism underlying the development of ASCVDs [44, 45]. Indeed, measurement of the CRP level, a gauge of the overall inflammatory state, has been used as a biomarker for predicting cardiovascular events [46–48]. Furthermore, the cardiovascular benefits of statin therapy appear to result partially from the suppression of inflammation [49–51]. The promising results of the CANTOS trial provide one of the strongest and cleanest lines of evidence supporting the inflammatory stress mechanism of ASCVDs. The CANTOS trial has also convincingly demonstrated the feasibility of ASCVD intervention via a monoclonal antibody-mediated precise targeting of IL-1β. This will certainly prompt additional studies to develop novel drugs targeting critical inflammatory pathways for the more effective management of ASCVDs, including ACS [41, 52]. The firm establishment of the efficacy of the anti-IL-1β-based therapy in ASCVDs/ACS will also have a major impact on the paradigm of precise and individualized treatment of patients with heightened inflammatory state and thereby at high risk of developing adverse cardiovascular events.

3.1.2.4. OTHER ANTI-INFLAMMATORY MODALITIES

Despite the encouraging findings on the efficacy of the anti-IL-1β therapy, clinical trials on several other anti-inflammatory modalities have yielded inconsistent and/or null results. These include phospholipase A2 inhibitors, p38 mitogen-activated protein kinase (MAPK) inhibitors, cyclosporine A, and methotrexate, among others.

Phospholipase A2 inhibitors: Elevated lipoprotein-associated phospholipase A_2 (Lp-PLA$_2$) activity promotes the development of vulnerable atherosclerotic plaques, and elevated plasma levels of this enzyme are associated with an increased risk of coronary events. Hence, inhibition of Lp-PLA$_2$ activity may be an effective strategy for ACS intervention. In this regard, darapladib has been developed as a selective oral inhibitor of Lp-PLA$_2$. In a randomized controlled trial of 15,828 patients with stable coronary heart disease, darapladib (160 mg, once daily) did not significantly reduce the risk of the primary composite endpoint of cardiovascular death, MI, or stroke; however, it significantly reduced the rate of major coronary events and total coronary events, each by ~10% compared to placebo [53]. On the other hand, the SOLID-TIMI 52 study, a multi-national randomized controlled trial, involving 13,026 participants, concluded that in patients who experienced an ACS event, direct inhibition of Lp-PLA$_2$ with darapladib added to optimal medical therapy and initiated within 30 days of hospitalization did not reduce the risk of major coronary events [54]. Likewise, a randomized, multicenter trial of 5145 patients with recent ACS (VISTA-16) showed that varespladib, an inhibitor of secretory PLA$_2$ (sPLA$_2$), did not reduce the risk of recurrent cardiovascular events, and instead significantly increased the risk of MI. Hence, the sPLA$_2$ inhibition with varespladib may be harmful and is not a useful strategy to reduce adverse cardiovascular outcomes after ACS [55]. Although one cannot state with certainty whether the observed harmful effects in the VISTA-16 trial were a direct consequence of sPLA$_2$ inhibition, this specific enzyme target is unlikely to be investigated further. Nonetheless, these findings do not argue against a central role for inflammation in atherogenesis, but rather highlight that much still needs to be learned regarding the complexity of inflammatory pathways in ACS and effective targeting of the pathways with novel agents [56–58].

p38 MAPK inhibitors: The p38 MAPK-mediated inflammation is implicated in atherogenesis, plaque destabilization, and maladaptive processes in MI [59]. A randomized phase 2 trial involving 526 NSTEMI patients suggested that p38 MAPK inhibition with oral losmapimod was well tolerated and might improve outcomes after ACS [60]. Subsequently, a larger multi-national trial involving 3,503 patients hospitalized with acute MI concluded that among patients with acute MI, use of losmapimod compared with placebo did not reduce the risk of major ischemic cardiovascular events [61].

Cyclosporine A and methotrexate: Both cyclosporine A and methotrexate are immunosuppressive agents that have been demonstrated to attenuate myocardial ischemia-reperfusion injury in certain animal models [62]. A recent multicenter, randomized controlled trial involving 970 patients with STEMI who were undergoing PCI within 12 hours after symptom onset, demonstrated that intravenous cyclosporine A (2.5 mg/kg) before PCI did not result in better clinical outcomes than those with placebo and did not prevent adverse left ventricular remodeling at one year [63]. Similarly, in the CYCLE (CYCLosporinE A in Reperfused Acute Myocardial Infarction) trial, a single intravenous cyclosporine A (2.5 mg/kg) bolus just before primary PCI had no effect on ST-segment resolution or high-sensitivity cardiac troponin T, and did not improve clinical outcomes or left ventricular remodeling up to 6 months [64]. A pilot study involving 84 patients with STEMI reported that methotrexate did not reduce infarction size and instead worsened left ventricular dysfunction at 3 months [65]. The ongoing Cardiovascular Inflammation Reduction Trial (CIRT) is designed to determine the effect of low-dose methotrexate (10 to 20 mg/week) on cardiovascular events in 7,000 patients with prior acute MI, elevated C-reactive protein levels, and diabetes (https://clinicaltrials.gov/ct2/show/NCT01594333). This trial is expected to be completed in December 2019, and the results would shed more light on the role of methotrexate in the long-term management of patients with ACS.

3.2. Overview of Guideline-Directed Treatment Strategies for ACS

3.2.1. General Considerations

All patients with suspected ACS must be admitted to an emergency department and evaluated rapidly, because the benefits of therapy are greatest when performed soon after hospital presentation. For patients presenting to the emergency department with chest pain or other atypical symptoms suspicious of an ACS, the diagnosis of MI (NSTEMI and STEMI) can be confirmed by the ECG changes and elevation of serum cardiac biomarkers (e.g., cardiac troponins). On the other hand, the diagnosis of UA is relied heavily on the history (e.g., a pressure-type chest pain occurring at rest or with minimal exertion lasting ≥10 minutes). Over the past decade, a number of guidelines have been released by various professional organizations to provide evidence-based recommendations on the management of patients with ACS. Among them, the most notable ones are recent guidelines from the American Heart Association (AHA)/the American College of Cardiology (ACC) [66, 67] and from the European

Society of Cardiology (ESC) [68, 69]. In view of the critical role of antiplatelet therapy in ACS, the AHA/ACC and ESC have also provided evidence-based recommendations on dual antiplatelet therapy (DAPT) in patients with ACS as well as in patients with stable coronary heart disease [70, 71].

3.2.2. NSTE-ACS

Once the diagnosis of either UA or an acute NSTEMI is made, the management of the patient involves the simultaneous achievement of several goals, which are outlined below [66, 68].

(1) Relief of ischemic pain
(2) Assessment of the patient's hemodynamic status and correction of abnormalities
(3) Estimation of the level of risk of death and nonfatal cardiac ischemic events
(4) Initiation of a treatment strategy to minimize myocardial injury and reduce mortality, i.e., an early invasive strategy (with angiography and intent for revascularization with PCI or coronary artery bypass grafting [CABG]) versus a conservative strategy with drug therapy (e.g., anticoagulants and platelet inhibitors)
(5) Long-term care to prolong survival, including lifestyle modifications and drug therapy

As mentioned earlier (Section 3.1.1), thrombolytic drugs are not recommended for treating NSTE-ACS due to their potential harm and lack of benefit. Hence, the mechanical approach (e.g., PCI or CABG) is the only option for revascularization, if needed, in patients with NSTE-ACS. On the other hand (see below), reperfusion therapy with thrombolytic drugs is indicated in patients with STEMI.

3.2.3. STEMI

Once the diagnosis of an acute STEMI is made, the early management of the patient involves the simultaneous achievement of several goals (similar, in principle, to those for NSTE-ACS, except for the indication of thrombolytic drugs), including: (1) relief of ischemic pain; (2) assessment of the hemodynamic state and correction of abnormalities that are present; (3) initiation of reperfusion therapy with primary PCI or fibrinolysis by thrombolytic agents; and (4) initiation of antithrombotic therapy. The above acute management is then followed by the initiation of short- and long-term interventions aimed at improving in-hospital and long-term outcomes. This non-acute management in the hours and days following the very early decision-making period includes use of various types of cardiovascular drugs as well as risk assessment and post-hospitalization plan of care [67, 69].

3.3. Overview of Drugs Commonly Used in the Management of ACS

As outlined below and summarized in **Table 8.1**, drugs used in the management of ACS are generally classified into two groups.

(1) *Drugs used in the acute management of ACS*: The major drugs include oxygen, anti-ischemic drugs (e.g., nitrates, β-blockers, or calcium channel blockers) and analgesics (e.g., morphine), statins, anticoagulants and platelet inhibitors, and thrombolytic drugs (thrombolytic agents are indicated only for STEMI).

(2) *Drugs used in the long-term management of ACS*: These include platelet inhibitors, statins, as well as other drugs for secondary prevention (e.g., drugs for dyslipidemias and diabetes).

3.4. Overview of the US FDA-Approved Antithrombotic Drugs for Treating ACS

Considering the essential role of antithrombotic drugs in the management of ACS as well as other thrombotic disorders, substantial efforts have been devoted to the development of new and more effective antithrombotics, especially novel anticoagulants and platelet inhibitors. Indeed, as listed in **Tables 8.2–8.4**, a number of antithrombotic drugs have been approved by the US FDA over the past two decades.

TABLE 8.1. Drugs used in the management of ACS

Drug treatment	Pharmacological/clinical effects and/or other comments
Drugs used in the acute management of ACS	
Oxygen	Oxygen therapy is indicated for clinically significant hypoxemia (oxygen saturation <90%)
Nitrates (e.g., nitroglycerin)	Nitroglycerin decreases myocardial ischemia and improves chest pain; nitrates are contraindicated with recent use of a phosphodiesterase inhibitor (e.g., sildenafil) due to hypotension
β-Blockers (e.g., metoprolol succinate, carvedilol, bisoprolol)	β-Blockers decrease myocardial ischemia, inhibit ventricular arrhythmias, and increase long-term survival. β-Blockers are contraindicated in hemodynamically unstable patients
Calcium channel blockers (CCBs) (e.g., diltiazem, verapamil)	CCBs decrease myocardial ischemia and are used when β-blockers are ineffective or contraindicated. CCBs do not prolong survival. The use of the immediate-release nifedipine is contraindicated in patients with STEMI because of hypotension and reflex sympathetic activation with tachycardia
Analgesics (morphine sulfate)	Morphine is a potent analgesic with favorable anxiolytic and hemodynamic actions. Non-steroid anti-inflammatory drugs (except aspirin) should not be used due to their detrimental effects
Statins (e.g., atorvastatin)	Statins reduce cardiovascular events and death due, at least partially, to its anti-inflammatory/other pluripotent actions
Inhibitors of renin-angiotensin-aldosterone system (e.g., lisinopril, captopril, ramipril, trandolapril, valsartan)	Angiotensin-converting enzyme (ACE) inhibitors reduce mortality in MI patients with left ventricular dysfunction. The angiotensin receptor blocker valsartan is used if ACE inhibitors cannot be tolerated

TABLE 8.1. (*continued*)

Drug treatment	Pharmacological/clinical effects and/or other comments
Platelet inhibitors (e.g., aspirin, P2Y$_{12}$ inhibitors, glycoprotein IIb/IIIa inhibitors)	Antiplatelet drugs inhibit thrombogenesis and are the mainstay of medical therapy of ACS. These drugs are used with primary PCI (for both NSTE-ACS and STEMI) and fibrinolytic agents (only for STEMI). Some (such as aspirin and P2Y$_{12}$ inhibitors) are used also for long-term management (see below)
Anticoagulants (e.g., heparins, selective Xa inhibitors, direct thrombin inhibitors)	Anticoagulants inhibit thrombogenesis and are important agents for medical therapy of ACS. These drugs are used with primary PCI (for both NSTE-ACS and STEMI) and fibrinolytic agents (only for STEMI)
Fibrinolytic drugs (e.g., alteplase, reteplase, tenecteplase)	Fibrinolytic drugs are used for reperfusion therapy in patients with STEMI when performing primary PCI is impossible or there is an anticipated delay for doing it. Fibrinolytic drugs are contraindicated in NSTE-ACS

Drugs used in the long-term management of ACS

Antiplatelet drugs (e.g., aspirin, clopidogrel, prasugrel, ticagrelor)	Dual antiplatelet therapy (i.e., aspirin plus a P2Y$_{12}$ inhibitor) reduces cardiovascular events and mortality. Aspirin should be taken indefinitely unless contraindicated, and the P2Y$_{12}$ inhibitor for 12 months
Drugs for treating risk factors and secondary prevention (e.g., lipid-lowering drugs, drugs for hypertension, drugs for diabetes, drugs for other comorbidities)	Drug therapy is only a part of the comprehensive post-hospitalization plan of care of ACS patients. The non-pharmacological components include lifestyle modifications, cardiac rehabilitation, and patient/family education, among others

TABLE 8.2. The US FDA-approved platelet inhibitors for treating ACS and other thrombotic disorders

Drug	FDA approval date	Major indication
Cyclooxygenase inhibitors		
Aspirin	Prior to January 1, 1982	The US FDA-approved use of aspirin is for pain relief. The cardiovascular indication is off-label use. Aspirin at low doses (81–325 mg/day) is indicated in patients with ACS and should be given as soon as possible after presentation and continued indefinitely unless contraindicated
Aspirin (Durlaza), extended release	September 2015	(1) Reduction of the risk of death and MI in patients with chronic coronary artery disease; (2) reduction of the risk of death and recurrent stroke in patients who have had an ischemic stroke or transient ischemic attack. Use immediate-release aspirin, not Durlaza in situations where a rapid onset of action is required, such as ACS

TABLE 8.2. (*continued*)

Drug	FDA approval date	Major indication
P2Y$_{12}$ inhibitors		
Cangrelor (Kengreal)	June 2015	As an adjunct to PCI for reducing the risk of periprocedural MI, repeat coronary revascularization, and stent thrombosis in patients who have not been treated with a P2Y$_{12}$ inhibitor and are not being given a GP IIb/IIIa inhibitor
Clopidogrel (Plavix)	November 1997	(1) ACS to reduce the rate of MI and stroke; (2) recent MI, recent stroke, or established peripheral arterial disease to reduce the rate of MI and stroke
Prasugrel (Effient)	July 2009	Reduction of thrombotic cardiovascular events (including stent thrombosis) in patients with ACS who are to be managed with PCI
Ticagrelor (Brilinta)	July 2011	Reduction of the rate of cardiovascular death, MI, and stroke in patients with ACS or a history of MI
Glycoprotein (GP) IIb/IIIa inhibitors		
Abciximab (ReoPro)	November 1997	As an adjunct to PCI for the prevention of cardiac ischemic complications in patients undergoing PCI or in patients with UA not responding to conventional medical therapy when PCI is planned within 24 h
Eptifibatide (Integrilin)	May 1998	(1) Treatment of ACS managed medically or with PCI; (2) treatment of patients undergoing PCI (including intracoronary stenting)
Tirofiban (Aggrastat)	May 1998	Reduction of the rate of thrombotic cardiovascular events in patients with NSTE-ACS
Phosphodiesterase (PDE) inhibitors		
Cilostazol (Pletal)	January 1999	Cilostazol is a platelet inhibitor and vasodilator, and it is predominantly used for reduction of symptoms of intermittent claudication (see Note below)
Dipyridamole (Persantine)	December 1986	As an adjunct to warfarin in the prevention of postoperative thromboembolic complications of cardiac valve replacement
Thrombin receptor inhibitors		
Vorapaxar (Zontivity)	May 2014	Reduction of thrombotic cardiovascular events in patients with a history of MI or with peripheral arterial disease
Combination of two platelet inhibitors		
Aspirin-dipyridamole (Aggrenox)	November 1999	Reduction of the risk of stroke in patients who have had transient ischemia of the brain or completed ischemic stroke due to thrombosis

Note: Cilostazol is a cyclic adenosine monophosphate (cAMP) phosphodiesterase III inhibitor that has vasodilatory and antiplatelet effects. While cilostazol is predominantly used for the management of intermittent claudication associated with peripheral artery disease, the drug may provide benefits when added to dual antiplatelet therapy (e.g., aspirin + clopidogrel) in ACS patients.

TABLE 8.3. The US FDA-approved anticoagulants for ACS and other thrombotic disorders

Drug	FDA approval date	Major indication
Vitamin K antagonists		
Warfarin (Coumadin)	Prior to January 1, 1982	(1) Prophylaxis and treatment of venous thrombosis and pulmonary embolism (PE), and thromboembolic complications associated with atrial fibrillation and/or cardiac valve replacement; (2) reduction in the risk of death, recurrent MI, and thromboembolic events such as stroke or systemic embolization after MI
Heparins (unfractionated heparin and low-molecular-weight heparins)		
Unfractionated heparin	Prior to January 1, 1982	(1) Prophylaxis and treatment of venous thrombosis, PE, and peripheral arterial embolism; (2) atrial fibrillation with embolization
Dalteparin (Fragmin)	December 1994	(1) Prophylaxis of ischemic complications in NSTE-ACS, when concurrently administered with aspirin therapy; (2) prophylaxis of deep vein thrombosis (DVT) and PE; (3) the extended treatment of symptomatic venous thromboembolism (VTE) in cancer patients
Enoxaparin (Lovenox)	March 1993	(1) Prophylaxis and treatment of DVT and PE; (2) prophylaxis of ischemic complications of NSTE-ACS; (3) treatment of acute STEMI
Tinzaparin (Innohep)	July 2000	Treatment of acute symptomatic DVT with or without PE when administered in conjunction with warfarin.
Selective Xa inhibitors		
Apixaban (Eliquis)	December 2012	(1) Reduction of the risk of stroke and systemic embolism in nonvalvular atrial fibrillation (NVAF); (2) prophylaxis and treatment of DVT and PE
Betrixaban (Bevyxxa)	June 2017	Prophylaxis of VTE in adult patients hospitalized for an acute medical illness who are at risk for thromboembolic complications
Edoxaban (Savaysa)	January 2015	(1) Reduction of the risk of stroke and systemic embolism in NVAF; (2) treatment of DVT and PE
Fondaparinux (Arixtra)	December 2001	Prophylaxis and treatment of DVT and PE
Rivaroxaban (Xarelto)	July 2011	(1) Reduction of the risk of stroke and systemic embolism in NVAF; (2) treatment and prophylaxis of DVT and PE
Direct thrombin inhibitors (hirudin analogues and small-molecule inhibitors)		
Bivalirudin (Angiomax)	December 2000	For patients (1) with UA undergoing percutaneous transluminal coronary angioplasty; (2) undergoing PCI with provisional use of a GP IIb/IIIa inhibitor; (3) with, or at risk of, heparin-induced thrombocytopenia (HIT) or heparin-induced thrombocytopenia and thrombosis syndrome undergoing PCI

TABLE 8.3. (*continued*)

Drug	FDA approval date	Major indication
Desirudin (Iprivask)	April 2003	Prophylaxis of DVT and PE in patients undergoing elective hip replacement surgery
Lepirudin (Refludan)	March 1998	Treatment of HIT
Argatroban (Acova)	June 2000	(1) Prophylaxis or treatment of thrombosis in adult patients with HIT; (2) as an anticoagulant in patients with or at risk for HIT undergoing PCI
Dabigatran (Pradaxa)	October 2010	Reduction of the risk of stroke and systemic embolism in patients with NVAF

TABLE 8.4. The US FDA-approved fibrinolytic drugs for ACS and other thrombotic disorders

Drug	FDA approval date	Major indication
Recombinant human tissue plasminogen activators (tPA)		
Alteplase (Activase)	November 13, 1987	Treatment of (1) acute ischemic stroke; (2) acute STEMI; (3) acute massive PE.
Reteplase (Retavase)	October 30, 1996	Treatment of acute STEMI
Tenecteplase (TNKase)	June 2, 2000	Treatment of acute STEMI
Non-tPA fibrinolytic agents		
Anistreplase (streptokinase + plasminogen) (Eminase)	November 28, 1989	Treatment of (1) STEMI; (2) PE
Streptokinase (Streptase)	November 5, 1987	Treatment of (1) acute STEMI; (2) PE, DVT, arterial thrombosis or embolism
Urokinase (Kinlytic)	Prior to January 1, 1982	Treatment of (1) acute massive PE; (2) pulmonary emboli accompanied by unstable hemodynamics

4. SELF-ASSESSMENT QUESTIONS

4.1. A 43-year-old man is brought to the emergency department because of severe chest pain immediately after his dinner. ECG shows ST-segment depression and T wave inversion. Blood chemistry reveals elevated levels of cardiac troponins. Which of the following is most likely responsible for the patient's condition?

A. Coronary arteritis
B. Coronary artery rupture
C. Coronary embolism

D. Coronary plaque rupture
E. Coronary vasospasm

4.2. A 55-year-old woman is diagnosed with acute myocardial infarction. History and cardiac tests exclude critical coronary artery disease. Which of the following types of myocardial infarction does the patient mostly likely have?

A. Type 1
B. Type 2
C. Type 3
D. Type 4a
E. Type 5

4.3. A 65-year-old obese patient is brought to the emergency room because of a pressure-type chest pain following climbing the stairs. Serum chemistry shows that cardiac troponins are significantly elevated. Which of the following is the most likely diagnosis?

A. Acute decompensated heart failure
B. Microvascular angina
C. Non-ST elevation myocardial infarction
D. Stable ischemic heart disease
E. Unstable angina

4.4. A 48-year-old man is brought to the emergency department because he feels like "an elephant is sitting on his chest". ECG shows ST-segment elevation. Serum chemistry reveals marked elevations of cardiac troponins and creatine phosphokinase activity. Which of the following is most likely responsible for the patient's condition?

A. Complete coronary occlusion
B. Coronary arteritis
C. Coronary artery rupture
D. Coronary congenital abnormalities
E. Partial coronary occlusion

4.5. A 57-year-old man, brought to the emergency department of a rural hospital due to crushing chest pain, is put on thrombolytic therapy to reopen his occluded coronary artery. Which of the following conditions is the patient most likely having?

A. Acute heart failure
B. Acute non-ST elevation myocardial infarction
C. Acute ST elevation myocardial infarction
D. Stable angina
E. Unstable angina

ANSWERS AND EXPLANATIONS

4.1. The correct answer is D. Coronary atherosclerotic plaque rupture and the subsequent thrombogenesis are the predominant cause of acute myocardial infarction. The occurrence of acute myocardial infarction in the absence of critical coronary artery disease is increasingly recognized and accounting for ~10% of cases of acute MI. The possible causes include coronary spasm, coronary arteritis, and coronary embolism.

4.2. The correct answer is B. Type 2 myocardial infarction is caused by an imbalance between myocardial oxygen supply and demand that is not the result of acute atherothrombosis and that is due to factors, such as coronary endothelial dysfunction, coronary artery spasm, or coronary embolism.

4.3. The correct answer is C. Cardiomyocyte death occurs in non-ST elevation myocardial infarction, but not in unstable angina and the other conditions listed.

4.4. The correct answer is A. The patient is having ST-elevation myocardial infarction, which typically results from complete coronary occlusion. Non-ST elevation myocardial infarction, on the other hand, is typically caused by partial coronary occlusion.

4.5. The correct answer is C. Reperfusion therapy with fibrinolytic agents is indicated for treating patients with acute ST-elevation myocardial infarction. Due to harm and lack of efficacy, fibrinolytic therapy is not recommended for treating patients with non-ST elevation acute coronary syndromes (i.e., unstable angina and non-ST elevation myocardial infarction).

REFERENCES

1. Li YR. *Cardiovascular Diseases: From Molecular Pharmacology to Evidence-Based Therapeutics*. John Wiley & Sons, New Jersey, USA. 2015.
2. Ruff CT, Braunwald E. The evolving epidemiology of acute coronary syndromes. *Nat Rev Cardiol* 2011; 8(3):140–7.
3. Anderson JL, Morrow DA. Acute myocardial infarction. *N Engl J Med* 2017; 376(21):2053–64.
4. Thygesen K, Alpert JS, Jaffe AS, Simoons ML, Chaitman BR, White HD, Joint ESC/ACCF/AHA/WHF Task Force for Universal Definition of Myocardial Infarction, Authors/Task Force Members Chairpersons, Thygesen K, Alpert JS, White HD, Biomarker Subcommittee, et al. Third universal definition of myocardial infarction. *J Am Coll Cardiol* 2012; 60(16):1581–98.
5. Moran AE, Forouzanfar MH, Roth GA, Mensah GA, Ezzati M, Flaxman A, Murray CJ, Naghavi M. The global burden of ischemic heart disease in 1990 and 2010: the global burden of disease 2010 study. *Circulation* 2014; 129(14):1493–501.
6. Moran AE, Forouzanfar MH, Roth GA, Mensah GA, Ezzati M, Murray CJ, Naghavi M. Temporal trends in ischemic heart disease mortality in 21 world regions, 1980 to 2010: the global burden of disease 2010 study. *Circulation* 2014; 129(14):1483–92.
7. GBD 2016 Causes of Death Collaborators. Global, regional, and national age-sex specific mortality for 264 causes of death, 1980–2016: a systematic analysis for the Global Burden of Disease Study 2016. *Lancet* 2017; 390(10100):1151–210.
8. Benjamin EJ, Blaha MJ, Chiuve SE, Cushman M, Das SR, Deo R, de Ferranti SD, Floyd J, Fornage M, Gillespie C, Isasi CR, Jimenez MC, et al. Heart Disease and Stroke Statistics–2017 Update: a report from the American Heart Association. *Circulation* 2017; 135(10):e146–e603.
9. Yeh RW, Sidney S, Chandra M, Sorel M, Selby JV, Go AS. Population trends in the incidence

and outcomes of acute myocardial infarction. *N Engl J Med* 2010; 362(23):2155–65.

10. Muller JE. Coronary artery thrombosis: historical aspects. *J Am Coll Cardiol* 1983; 1(3):893–6.

11. Jackson SP. Arterial thrombosis: insidious, unpredictable and deadly. *Nat Med* 2011; 17(11):1423–36.

12. Bentzon JF, Otsuka F, Virmani R, Falk E. Mechanisms of plaque formation and rupture. *Circ Res* 2014; 114(12):1852–66.

13. Crea F, Libby P. Acute coronary syndromes: the way forward from mechanisms to precision treatment. *Circulation* 2017; 136(12):1155–66.

14. Hamm CW, Bassand JP, Agewall S, Bax J, Boersma E, Bueno H, Caso P, Dudek D, Gielen S, Huber K, Ohman M, Petrie MC, et al. ESC guidelines for the management of acute coronary syndromes in patients presenting without persistent ST-segment elevation: the Task Force for the management of acute coronary syndromes (ACS) in patients presenting without persistent ST-segment elevation of the European Society of Cardiology (ESC). *Eur Heart J* 2011; 32(23):2999–3054.

15. Libby P. Mechanisms of acute coronary syndromes and their implications for therapy. *N Engl J Med* 2013; 368(21):2004–13.

16. Arbab-Zadeh A, Nakano M, Virmani R, Fuster V. Acute coronary events. *Circulation* 2012; 125(9):1147–56.

17. Falk E, Nakano M, Bentzon JF, Finn AV, Virmani R. Update on acute coronary syndromes: the pathologists' view. *Eur Heart J* 2013; 34(10):719–28.

18. TIMI IIIB Investigators. Effects of tissue plasminogen activator and a comparison of early invasive and conservative strategies in unstable angina and non-Q-wave myocardial infarction. Results of the TIMI IIIB Trial. Thrombolysis in Myocardial Ischemia. *Circulation* 1994; 89(4):1545–56.

19. Anderson HV, Cannon CP, Stone PH, Williams DO, McCabe CH, Knatterud GL, Thompson B, Willerson JT, Braunwald E. One-year results of the Thrombolysis in Myocardial Infarction (TIMI) IIIB clinical trial: a randomized comparison of tissue-type plasminogen activator versus placebo and early invasive versus early conservative strategies in unstable angina and non-Q wave myocardial infarction. *J Am Coll Cardiol* 1995; 26(7):1643–50.

20. Nidorf SM, Eikelboom JW, Budgeon CA, Thompson PL. Low-dose colchicine for secondary prevention of cardiovascular disease. *J Am Coll Cardiol* 2013; 61(4):404–10.

21. Vogel RA, Forrester JS. Cooling off hot hearts: a specific therapy for vulnerable plaque? *J Am Coll Cardiol* 2013; 61(4):411–2.

22. Hemkens LG, Ewald H, Gloy VL, Arpagaus A, Olu KK, Nidorf M, Glinz D, Nordmann AJ, Briel M. Colchicine for prevention of cardiovascular events. *Cochrane Database Syst Rev* 2016; (1):CD011047.

23. Martinez GJ, Robertson S, Barraclough J, Xia Q, Mallat Z, Bursill C, Celermajer DS, Patel S. Colchicine acutely suppresses local cardiac production of inflammatory cytokines in patients with an acute coronary syndrome. *J Am Heart Assoc* 2015; 4(8):e002128.

24. Vaidya K, Arnott C, Martinez GJ, Ng B, McCormack S, Sullivan DR, Celermajer DS, Patel S. Colchicine therapy and plaque stabilization in patients with acute coronary syndrome: a CT coronary angiography study. *JACC Cardiovasc Imaging* 2017; 11(2 Pt 2):305–16.

25. Oh DY, Talukdar S, Bae EJ, Imamura T, Morinaga H, Fan W, Li P, Lu WJ, Watkins SM, Olefsky JM. GPR120 is an omega-3 fatty acid receptor mediating potent anti-inflammatory and insulin-sensitizing effects. *Cell* 2010; 142(5):687–98.

26. Oh DY, Olefsky JM. Omega 3 fatty acids and GPR120. *Cell Metab* 2012; 15(5):564–5.

27. Oh DY, Walenta E, Akiyama TE, Lagakos WS, Lackey D, Pessentheiner AR, Sasik R, Hah N, Chi TJ, Cox JM, Powels MA, Di Salvo J, et al. A Gpr120-selective agonist improves insulin resistance and chronic inflammation in obese mice. *Nat Med* 2014; 20(8):942–7.

28. Tavazzi L, Maggioni AP, Marchioli R, Barlera S, Franzosi MG, Latini R, Lucci D, Nicolosi GL, Porcu M, Tognoni G, GISSI-HF Investigators. Effect of n-3 polyunsaturated fatty acids in patients with chronic heart failure (the GISSI-HF trial): a randomised, double-blind, placebo-controlled trial. *Lancet* 2008; 372(9645):1223–30.

29. Joensen AM, Overvad K, Dethlefsen C, Johnsen SP, Tjonneland A, Rasmussen LH, Schmidt EB. Marine n-3 polyunsaturated fatty acids in adipose tissue and the risk of acute coronary syndrome. *Circulation* 2011; 124(11):1232–8.

30. Del Gobbo LC, Imamura F, Aslibekyan S, Marklund M, Virtanen JK, Wennberg M,

Yakoob MY, Chiuve SE, Dela Cruz L, Frazier-Wood AC, Fretts AM, Guallar E, et al. Omega-3 polyunsaturated fatty acid biomarkers and coronary heart disease: pooling project of 19 cohort studies. *JAMA Intern Med* 2016; 176(8):1155–66.

31. Heydari B, Abdullah S, Pottala JV, Shah R, Abbasi S, Mandry D, Francis SA, Lumish H, Ghoshhajra BB, Hoffmann U, Appelbaum E, Feng JH, et al. Effect of omega-3 acid ethyl esters on left ventricular remodeling after acute myocardial infarction: the OMEGA-REMODEL randomized clinical trial. *Circulation* 2016; 134(5):378–91.

32. Nosaka K, Miyoshi T, Iwamoto M, Kajiya M, Okawa K, Tsukuda S, Yokohama F, Sogo M, Nishibe T, Matsuo N, Hirohata S, Ito H, et al. Early initiation of eicosapentaenoic acid and statin treatment is associated with better clinical outcomes than statin alone in patients with acute coronary syndromes: 1-year outcomes of a randomized controlled study. *Int J Cardiol* 2017; 228:173–9.

33. Alfaddagh A, Elajami TK, Ashfaque H, Saleh M, Bistrian BR, Welty FK. Effect of eicosapentaenoic and docosahexaenoic acids added to statin therapy on coronary artery plaque in patients with coronary artery disease: a randomized clinical trial. *J Am Heart Assoc* 2017; 6(12):e006981.

34. Suzuki K, Murtuza B, Smolenski RT, Sammut IA, Suzuki N, Kaneda Y, Yacoub MH. Overexpression of interleukin-1 receptor antagonist provides cardioprotection against ischemia-reperfusion injury associated with reduction in apoptosis. *Circulation* 2001; 104(12 Suppl 1):I308–I3.

35. Ikonomidis I, Lekakis JP, Nikolaou M, Paraskevaidis I, Andreadou I, Kaplanoglou T, Katsimbri P, Skarantavos G, Soucacos PN, Kremastinos DT. Inhibition of interleukin-1 by anakinra improves vascular and left ventricular function in patients with rheumatoid arthritis. *Circulation* 2008; 117(20):2662–9.

36. Ridker PM, Howard CP, Walter V, Everett B, Libby P, Hensen J, Thuren T, CANTOS Pilot Investigative Group. Effects of interleukin-1beta inhibition with canakinumab on hemoglobin A1c, lipids, C-reactive protein, interleukin-6, and fibrinogen: a phase IIb randomized, placebo-controlled trial. *Circulation* 2012; 126(23):2739–48.

37. Sager HB, Heidt T, Hulsmans M, Dutta P, Courties G, Sebas M, Wojtkiewicz GR, Tricot B, Iwamoto Y, Sun Y, Weissleder R, Libby P, et al. Targeting interleukin-1beta reduces leukocyte production after acute myocardial infarction. *Circulation* 2015; 132(20):1880–90.

38. Ridker PM. From C-reactive protein to interleukin-6 to interleukin-1: moving upstream to identify novel targets for atheroprotection. *Circ Res* 2016; 118(1):145–56.

39. Ridker PM, Everett BM, Thuren T, MacFadyen JG, Chang WH, Ballantyne C, Fonseca F, Nicolau J, Koenig W, Anker SD, Kastelein JJP, Cornel JH, et al. Antiinflammatory therapy with canakinumab for atherosclerotic disease. *N Engl J Med* 2017; 377(12):1119–31.

40. Ridker PM, MacFadyen JG, Everett BM, Libby P, Thuren T, Glynn RJ, Group CT. Relationship of C-reactive protein reduction to cardiovascular event reduction following treatment with canakinumab: a secondary analysis from the CANTOS randomised controlled trial. *Lancet* 2018; 391(10118):319–28.

41. Ridker PM. Canakinumab for residual inflammatory risk. *Eur Heart J* 2017; 38(48):3545–8.

42. Mantovani A, Barajon I, Garlanda C. IL-1 and IL-1 regulatory pathways in cancer progression and therapy. *Immunol Rev* 2018; 281(1):57–61.

43. Ridker PM, MacFadyen JG, Thuren T, Everett BM, Libby P, Glynn RJ, CANTOS Trial Group. Effect of interleukin-1beta inhibition with canakinumab on incident lung cancer in patients with atherosclerosis: exploratory results from a randomised, double-blind, placebo-controlled trial. *Lancet* 2017; 390(10105):1833–42.

44. Ross R. Atherosclerosis: an inflammatory disease. *N Engl J Med* 1999; 340(2):115–26.

45. Hansson GK. Inflammation, atherosclerosis, and coronary artery disease. *N Engl J Med* 2005; 352(16):1685–95.

46. Ridker PM, Hennekens CH, Buring JE, Rifai N. C-reactive protein and other markers of inflammation in the prediction of cardiovascular disease in women. *N Engl J Med* 2000; 342(12):836–43.

47. Ridker PM, Rifai N, Rose L, Buring JE, Cook NR. Comparison of C-reactive protein and low-density lipoprotein cholesterol levels in the prediction of first cardiovascular events. *N Engl J Med* 2002; 347(20):1557–65.

48. Emerging Risk Factors C, Kaptoge S, Di Angelantonio E, Pennells L, Wood AM, White IR, Gao P, Walker M, Thompson A, Sarwar N,

Caslake M, Butterworth AS, et al. C-reactive protein, fibrinogen, and cardiovascular disease prediction. *N Engl J Med* 2012; 367(14):1310–20.

49. Ridker PM, Danielson E, Fonseca FA, Genest J, Gotto AM, Jr., Kastelein JJ, Koenig W, Libby P, Lorenzatti AJ, MacFadyen JG, Nordestgaard BG, Shepherd J, et al. Rosuvastatin to prevent vascular events in men and women with elevated C-reactive protein. *N Engl J Med* 2008; 359(21):2195–207.

50. Oesterle A, Laufs U, Liao JK. Pleiotropic effects of statins on the cardiovascular system. *Circ Res* 2017; 120(1):229–43.

51. Bohula EA, Giugliano RP, Cannon CP, Zhou J, Murphy SA, White JA, Tershakovec AM, Blazing MA, Braunwald E. Achievement of dual low-density lipoprotein cholesterol and high-sensitivity C-reactive protein targets more frequent with the addition of ezetimibe to simvastatin and associated with better outcomes in IMPROVE-IT. *Circulation* 2015; 132(13):1224–33.

52. Libby P. Interleukin-1 beta as a target for atherosclerosis therapy: biological basis of CANTOS and beyond. *J Am Coll Cardiol* 2017; 70(18):2278–89.

53. STABILITY Investigators, White HD, Held C, Stewart R, Tarka E, Brown R, Davies RY, Budaj A, Harrington RA, Steg PG, Ardissino D, Armstrong PW, et al. Darapladib for preventing ischemic events in stable coronary heart disease. *N Engl J Med* 2014; 370(18):1702–11.

54. O'Donoghue ML, Braunwald E, White HD, Lukas MA, Tarka E, Steg PG, Hochman JS, Bode C, Maggioni AP, Im K, Shannon JB, Davies RY, et al. Effect of darapladib on major coronary events after an acute coronary syndrome: the SOLID-TIMI 52 randomized clinical trial. *JAMA* 2014; 312(10):1006–15.

55. Nicholls SJ, Kastelein JJ, Schwartz GG, Bash D, Rosenson RS, Cavender MA, Brennan DM, Koenig W, Jukema JW, Nambi V, Wright RS, Menon V, et al. Varespladib and cardiovascular events in patients with an acute coronary syndrome: the VISTA-16 randomized clinical trial. *JAMA* 2014; 311(3):252–62.

56. O'Donoghue ML. Acute coronary syndromes: targeting inflammation-what has the VISTA-16 trial taught us? *Nat Rev Cardiol* 2014; 11(3):130–2.

57. Held C, White HD, Stewart RAH, Budaj A, Cannon CP, Hochman JS, Koenig W, Siegbahn A, Steg PG, Soffer J, Weaver WD, Ostlund O, et al. Inflammatory biomarkers interleukin-6 and C-reactive protein and outcomes in stable coronary heart disease: experiences from the STABILITY (Stabilization of Atherosclerotic Plaque by Initiation of Darapladib Therapy) trial. *J Am Heart Assoc* 2017; 6(10):e005077.

58. Fanola CL, Morrow DA, Cannon CP, Jarolim P, Lukas MA, Bode C, Hochman JS, Goodrich EL, Braunwald E, O'Donoghue ML. Interleukin-6 and the risk of adverse outcomes in patients after an acute coronary syndrome: observations from the SOLID-TIMI 52 (Stabilization of Plaque Using Darapladib-Thrombolysis in Myocardial Infarction 52) trial. *J Am Heart Assoc* 2017; 6(10):e005637.

59. Denise Martin E, De Nicola GF, Marber MS. New therapeutic targets in cardiology: p38 alpha mitogen-activated protein kinase for ischemic heart disease. *Circulation* 2012; 126(3):357–68.

60. Newby LK, Marber MS, Melloni C, Sarov-Blat L, Aberle LH, Aylward PE, Cai G, de Winter RJ, Hamm CW, Heitner JF, Kim R, Lerman A, et al. Losmapimod, a novel p38 mitogen-activated protein kinase inhibitor, in non-ST-segment elevation myocardial infarction: a randomised phase 2 trial. *Lancet* 2014; 384(9949):1187–95.

61. O'Donoghue ML, Glaser R, Cavender MA, Aylward PE, Bonaca MP, Budaj A, Davies RY, Dellborg M, Fox KA, Gutierrez JA, Hamm C, Kiss RG, et al. Effect of losmapimod on cardiovascular outcomes in patients hospitalized with acute myocardial infarction: a randomized clinical trial. *JAMA* 2016; 315(15):1591–9.

62. Lim WY, Messow CM, Berry C. Cyclosporin variably and inconsistently reduces infarct size in experimental models of reperfused myocardial infarction: a systematic review and meta-analysis. *Br J Pharmacol* 2012; 165(7):2034–43.

63. Cung TT, Morel O, Cayla G, Rioufol G, Garcia-Dorado D, Angoulvant D, Bonnefoy-Cudraz E, Guerin P, Elbaz M, Delarche N, Coste P, Vanzetto G, et al. Cyclosporine before PCI in patients with acute myocardial infarction. *N Engl J Med* 2015; 373(11):1021–31.

64. Ottani F, Latini R, Staszewsky L, La Vecchia L, Locuratolo N, Sicuro M, Masson S, Barlera S, Milani V, Lombardi M, Costalunga A, Mollichelli N, et al. Cyclosporine A in reperfused myocardial infarction: the multicenter, controlled, open-label CYCLE trial. *J Am Coll Cardiol* 2016; 67(4):365–74.

65. Moreira DM, Lueneberg ME, da Silva RL, Fattah T, Gottschall CAM. Methotrexate therapy in ST-segment elevation myocardial infarctions: a randomized double-blind, placebo-controlled trial (TETHYS Trial). *J Cardiovasc Pharmacol Ther* 2017; 22(6):538–45.

66. Amsterdam EA, Wenger NK, Brindis RG, Casey DE, Jr., Ganiats TG, Holmes DR, Jr., Jaffe AS, Jneid H, Kelly RF, Kontos MC, Levine GN, Liebson PR, et al. 2014 AHA/ACC guideline for the management of patients with non-ST-elevation acute coronary syndromes: a report of the American College of Cardiology/American Heart Association Task Force on Practice Guidelines. *J Am Coll Cardiol* 2014; 64(24):e139–e228.

67. O'Gara PT, Kushner FG, Ascheim DD, Casey DE, Jr., Chung MK, de Lemos JA, Ettinger SM, Fang JC, Fesmire FM, Franklin BA, Granger CB, Krumholz HM, et al. 2013 ACCF/AHA guideline for the management of ST-elevation myocardial infarction: a report of the American College of Cardiology Foundation/American Heart Association Task Force on Practice Guidelines. *Circulation* 2013; 127(4):e362–425.

68. Roffi M, Patrono C, Collet JP, Mueller C, Valgimigli M, Andreotti F, Bax JJ, Borger MA, Brotons C, Chew DP, Gencer B, Hasenfuss G, et al. 2015 ESC guidelines for the management of acute coronary syndromes in patients presenting without persistent ST-segment elevation: Task Force for the management of acute coronary syndromes in patients presenting without persistent ST-segment elevation of the European Society of Cardiology (ESC). *Eur Heart J* 2016; 37(3):267–315.

69. Ibanez B, James S, Agewall S, Antunes MJ, Bucciarelli-Ducci C, Bueno H, Caforio ALP, Crea F, Goudevenos JA, Halvorsen S, Hindricks G, Kastrati A, et al. 2017 ESC guidelines for the management of acute myocardial infarction in patients presenting with ST-segment elevation: the Task Force for the management of acute myocardial infarction in patients presenting with ST-segment elevation of the European Society of Cardiology (ESC). *Eur Heart J* 2018; 39(2):119-77.

70. Levine GN, Bates ER, Bittl JA, Brindis RG, Fihn SD, Fleisher LA, Granger CB, Lange RA, Mack MJ, Mauri L, Mehran R, Mukherjee D, et al. 2016 ACC/AHA guideline focused update on duration of dual antiplatelet therapy in patients with coronary artery disease: a report of the American College of Cardiology/American Heart Association Task Force on Clinical Practice Guidelines: an update of the 2011 ACCF/AHA/SCAI guideline for percutaneous coronary intervention, 2011 ACCF/AHA guideline for coronary artery bypass graft surgery, 2012 ACC/AHA/ACP/AATS/PCNA/SCAI/STS guideline for the diagnosis and management of patients with stable ischemic heart disease, 2013 ACCF/AHA guideline for the management of ST-elevation myocardial infarction, 2014 AHA/ACC guideline for the management of patients with non-ST-elevation acute coronary syndromes, and 2014 ACC/AHA guideline on perioperative cardiovascular evaluation and management of patients undergoing noncardiac surgery. *Circulation* 2016; 134(10):e123–55.

71. Valgimigli M, Bueno H, Byrne RA, Collet JP, Costa F, Jeppsson A, Juni P, Kastrati A, Kolh P, Mauri L, Montalescot G, Neumann FJ, et al. 2017 ESC focused update on dual antiplatelet therapy in coronary artery disease developed in collaboration with EACTS: the Task Force for dual antiplatelet therapy in coronary artery disease of the European Society of Cardiology (ESC) and of the European Association for Cardio-Thoracic Surgery (EACTS). *Eur Heart J* 2018; 39(3):213–60.

CHAPTER 9

New Drugs for Acute Coronary Syndromes

CHAPTER HIGHLIGHTS

- Advancement in developing novel antiplatelet therapies has greatly contributed to the improved management of acute coronary syndromes. Over the past five years, the United States Food and Drug Administration (US FDA) has approved two new antiplatelet drugs: cangrelor and vorapaxar.
- Cangrelor is the newest member of the platelet $P2Y_{12}$ receptor-inhibiting drug class that also includes clopidogrel, prasugrel, and ticagrelor. All four drugs selectively block ADP-mediated $P2Y_{12}$ receptor activation, thereby inhibiting platelet aggregation, a critical event in thrombogenesis.
- Cangrelor is the only $P2Y_{12}$ receptor inhibitor administered intravenously to achieve a rapid and reversible platelet inhibition. It is indicated as an adjunct to percutaneous coronary intervention to reduce the risk of periprocedural myocardial infarction, repeat coronary revascularization, and stent thrombosis.
- Vorapaxar is the first-in-class and presently the only member of the thrombin receptor antagonist drug class approved for clinical use. It is a selective inhibitor of platelet protease-activated receptor-1 (PAR-1) and inhibits thrombin-mediated activation of PAR-1 and the subsequent platelet aggregation.
- Vorapaxar is indicated for reducing thrombotic cardiovascular events in patients with a history of myocardial infarction or with peripheral arterial disease.

KEYWORDS | Acute coronary syndromes; Cangrelor; Clopidogrel; Myocardial infarction; Non-ST elevation myocardial infarction; $P2Y_{12}$ receptor inhibitor; PAR-1 inhibitor; Peripheral arterial disease; Prasugrel; Protease-activated receptor; ST elevation myocardial infarction; Ticagrelor; Unstable angina; Vorapaxar

CITATION | Li YR. *Cardiovascular Medicine: New Therapeutic Drugs Approved by the US FDA (2013–2017). Cell Med Press, Raleigh, NC, USA. 2018. http://dx.doi.org/10.20455/ndcvd.2018.09*

ABBREVIATIONS | ACS, acute coronary syndromes; ADP, adenosine diphosphate; COX-1, cyclooxygenase-1; CYP, cytochrome P450; EPAD, established peripheral arterial disease; GPI, glycoprotein IIb/IIIa inhibitor; IV, intravenous; MI, myocardial infarction; NSAID, nonsteroidal anti-inflammatory drug; NSTEMI, non-ST elevation myocardial infarction; PAD, peripheral arterial disease; PAR-1, protease-activated receptor-1; PCI, percutaneous coronary intervention; STEMI, ST elevation myocardial infarction; TRAP, thrombin receptor agonist peptide; TxA_2, thromboxane A_2; UA, unstable angina; US FDA, the United States Food and Drug Administration

CHAPTER AT A GLANCE

1. INTRODUCTION

The advancement in the development of novel platelet inhibitors (also known as antiplatelet drugs) has greatly contributed to the effective management of thrombotic disorders, especially acute coronary syndromes (ACS) [1–4]. Over the past five years, the United States Food and Drug Administration (US FDA) has approved two new members of drugs that belong to the antiplatelet drug family. They are the $P2Y_{12}$ receptor inhibitor cangrelor (approved in June 2015) and the thrombin receptor antagonist vorapaxar (approved in May 2014).

2. $P2Y_{12}$ RECEPTOR ANTAGONIST: CANGRELOR (KENGREAL)

Cangrelor is the newest member of the $P2Y_{12}$ receptor antagonist drug class which currently consists of four members. This section focuses on cangrelor, and comparisons with the other three members are also made.

2.1. Overview

$P2Y_{12}$ receptor antagonists are also known as $P2Y_{12}$ ADP receptor antagonists, $P2Y_{12}$ receptor inhibitors, or simply as $P2Y_{12}$ inhibitors. Adenosine diphosphate (ADP) binding to the platelet $P2Y_{12}$ receptors plays an important role in platelet activation and aggregation, amplifying the initial platelet response to vascular damage. As such, the antagonism of the $P2Y_{12}$ receptors is a major therapeutic strategy in the management of ACS as well as certain other thrombotic disorders. The $P2Y_{12}$ inhibitor class currently includes 3 thienopyridine drugs, namely clopidogrel (Plavix), prasugrel (Effient), and ticlopidine (ticlopidine is not commonly used due to its significant adverse effects, and as such, is not covered here), and two cyclopentyltriazolopyrimidine drugs, namely, ticagrelor (Brilinta) and cangrelor. Cangrelor is the newest member of the drug class, approved by the US FDA on June 22, 2015.

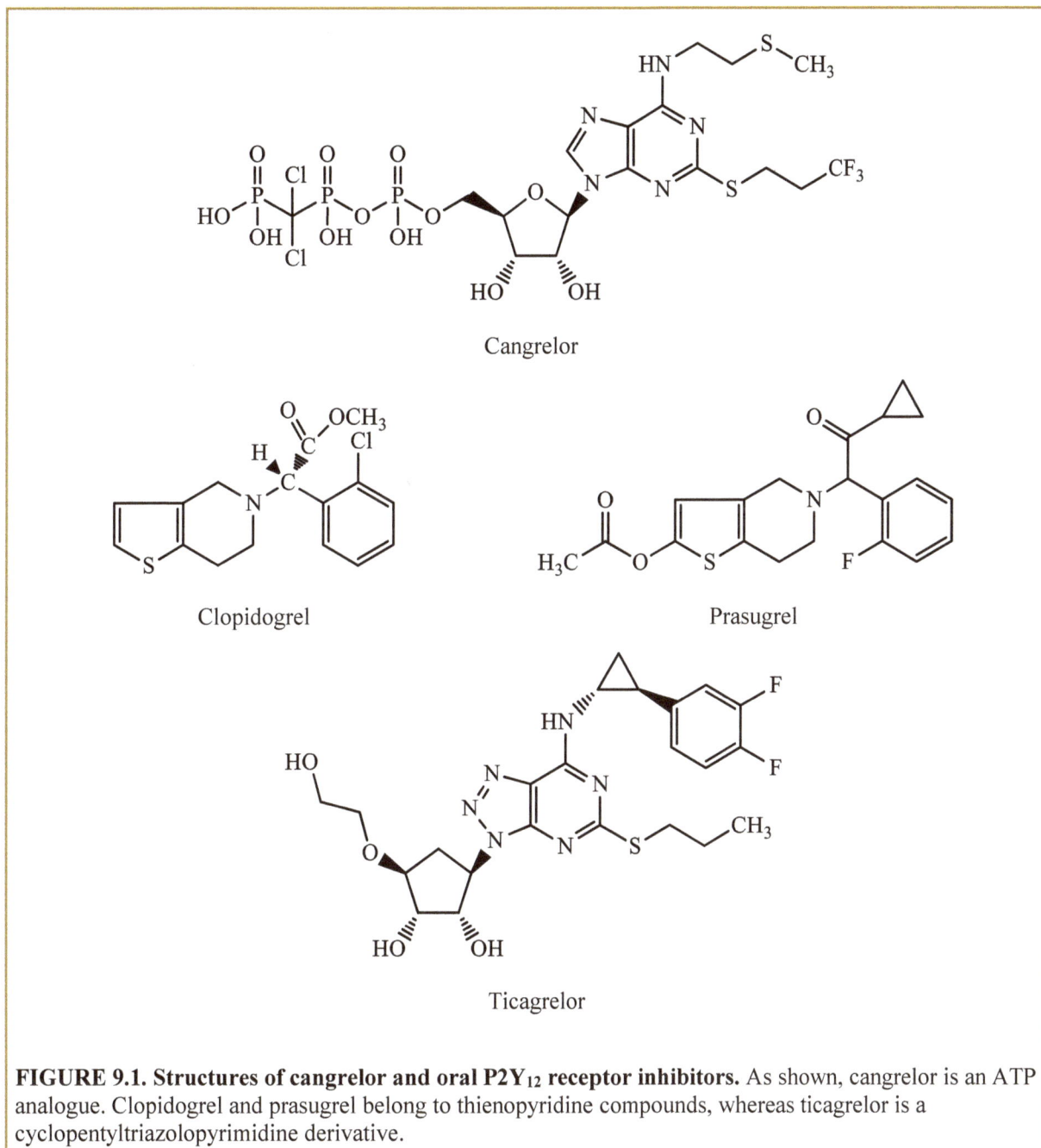

FIGURE 9.1. Structures of cangrelor and oral P2Y$_{12}$ receptor inhibitors. As shown, cangrelor is an ATP analogue. Clopidogrel and prasugrel belong to thienopyridine compounds, whereas ticagrelor is a cyclopentyltriazolopyrimidine derivative.

The approval of cangrelor (Chiesi Farmaceutici S.p.A., Parma, Italy) by the US FDA was based on a randomized controlled trial (CHAMPION PHOENIX) involving 11,145 patients who were undergoing either urgent or elective percutaneous coronary intervention (PCI) and were receiving guideline-recommended therapy [5]. The CHAMPION PHOENIX trial was intended to test whether faster platelet inhibition with cangrelor at the time of PCI would reduce the rate of periprocedural thrombotic events compared to a drug with a slower antiplatelet effect, clopidogrel, given at about the time of PCI.

Cangrelor significantly reduced the occurrence of primary composite endpoint events compared to clopidogrel (with a relative risk reduction of 22%). Most of the effect was a reduction in post-procedural myocardial infarction (MI) detected solely by elevations in creatine kinase-MB (type 4a MI; see Chapter 8 for definition of type 4a MI). The mortality and the risk of severe bleeding were not different between cangrelor and clopidogrel [5].

2.2. Chemistry and Pharmacokinetics

Cangrelor is a direct-acting $P2Y_{12}$ inhibitor that blocks ADP-induced platelet activation and aggregation. The chemical structure of cangrelor is similar to that of adenosine triphosphate (ATP), and can be considered as an ATP analogue. As noted above, clopidogrel and prasugrel belong to thienopyridine compounds, whereas ticagrelor is a cyclopentyltriazolopyrimidine derivative (structures shown in **Figure 9.1**). Clopidogrel and prasugrel are prodrugs that undergo biotransformation to form the active metabolites that bind irreversibly to $P2Y_{12}$ receptors. On the other hand, cangrelor and ticagrelor are reversible inhibitors. The major pharmacokinetic properties of the $P2Y_{12}$ receptor antagonists are summarized in **Table 9.1**.

TABLE 9.1. Major pharmacokinetic properties of cangrelor and the other $P2Y_{12}$ receptor inhibitors

Drug	Oral BA	t_{max}	Vd	Metabolism and excretion	$t_{1/2}$
Cangrelor	Injection only	<2 min	3.9 L	Dephosphorylated in the circulation to become inactive; metabolism independent of the liver function; eliminated in urine and feces	3–6 min
Clopidogrel	50%	30–60 min	Not available	Hydrolyzed by esterases to form an inactive derivative; metabolized by CYP2C19 (major), CYP3A4, CYP2B6, and CYP1A2 to form the active metabolite; eliminated in urine and feces	6 h (0.5 h for the active metabolite)
Prasugrel	80%	30 min	44–68 L	Rapidly hydrolyzed in the intestine to a thioactone, which is then converted to the active metabolite primarily by CYP3A4 and CYP2B6 and, to a lesser extent, by CYP2C9 and CYP2C19; eliminated in urine (major) and feces	7 h for the active metabolite
Ticagrelor	36%	1–4 h (1–5 h for the active metabolite)	88 L	Metabolized by CYP3A4 and the major metabolite is also pharmacologically active; eliminated in feces (major) and urine	7 h (9 h for the active metabolite)

Note: Both ticagrelor and its major metabolite inhibit $P2Y_{12}$ receptors. Ticagrelor and its major active metabolite are also weak P-glycoprotein substrates and inhibitors. BA, bioavailability; CYP, cytochrome P450; $t_{1/2}$, elimination half-life; t_{max}, the time when the maximum plasma concentration is reached; Vd, volume of distribution per 70 kg body weight.

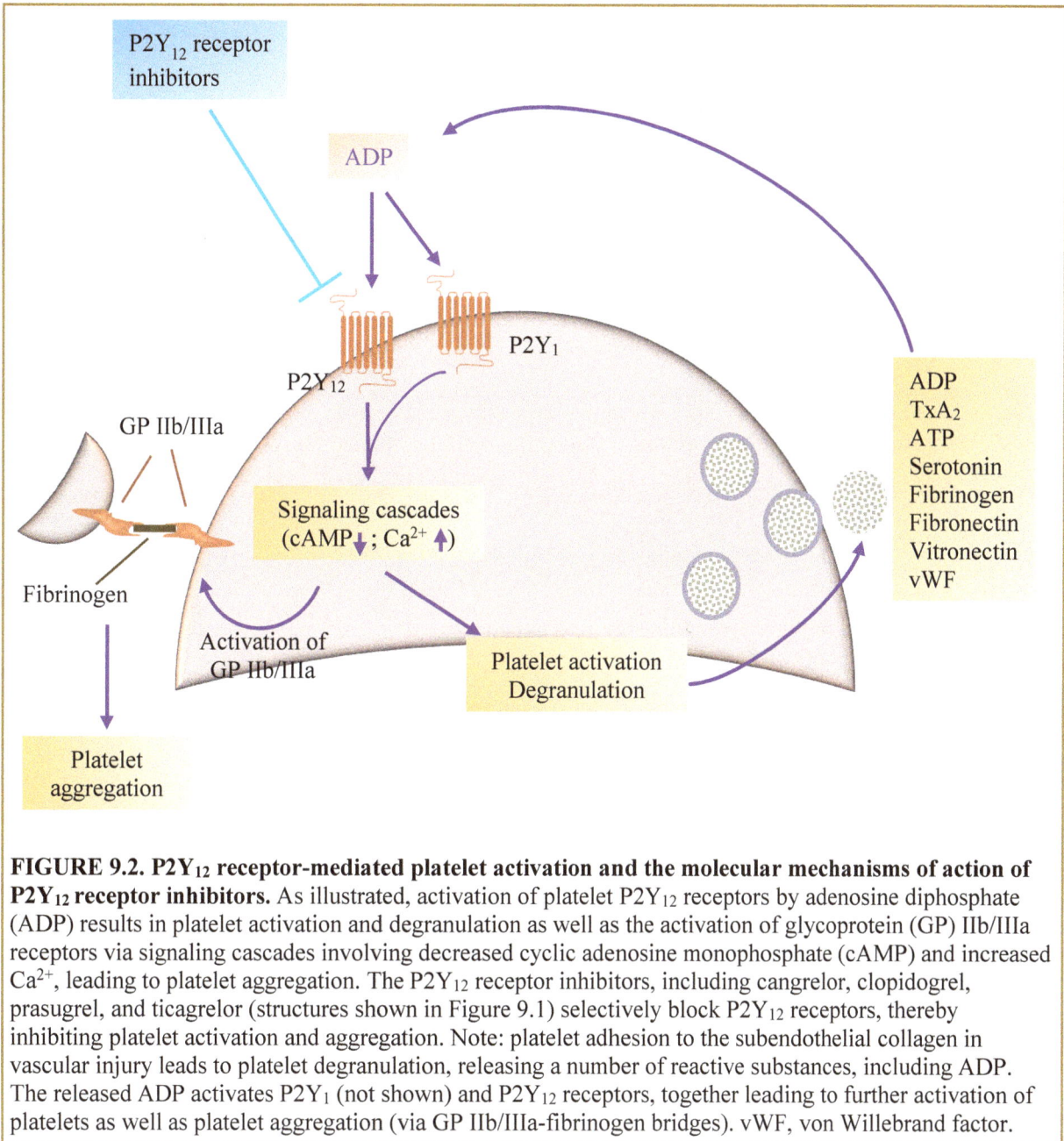

FIGURE 9.2. P2Y$_{12}$ receptor-mediated platelet activation and the molecular mechanisms of action of P2Y$_{12}$ receptor inhibitors. As illustrated, activation of platelet P2Y$_{12}$ receptors by adenosine diphosphate (ADP) results in platelet activation and degranulation as well as the activation of glycoprotein (GP) IIb/IIIa receptors via signaling cascades involving decreased cyclic adenosine monophosphate (cAMP) and increased Ca^{2+}, leading to platelet aggregation. The P2Y$_{12}$ receptor inhibitors, including cangrelor, clopidogrel, prasugrel, and ticagrelor (structures shown in Figure 9.1) selectively block P2Y$_{12}$ receptors, thereby inhibiting platelet activation and aggregation. Note: platelet adhesion to the subendothelial collagen in vascular injury leads to platelet degranulation, releasing a number of reactive substances, including ADP. The released ADP activates P2Y$_1$ (not shown) and P2Y$_{12}$ receptors, together leading to further activation of platelets as well as platelet aggregation (via GP IIb/IIIa-fibrinogen bridges). vWF, von Willebrand factor.

2.3. Molecular Mechanisms and Pharmacological Effects

As noted earlier, activation of platelet P2Y$_{12}$ receptors by ADP plays an important role in platelet activation and aggregation, leading to thrombogenesis. All the four drugs selectively inhibit ADP-mediated P2Y$_{12}$ receptor activation and the subsequent activation of the glycoprotein (GP) IIb/IIIa complex, thereby inhibiting platelet aggregation, a critical event in thrombogenesis (**Figure 9.2**). Both cangrelor and ticagrelor (and the active metabolite of ticagrelor) are reversible inhibitors of P2Y$_{12}$ receptors. Ticagrelor and its active metabolite are approximately equipotent. On the other hand, clopidogrel and prasugrel are prodrugs and the inhibition of platelet activation and aggregation occurs through the irreversible binding of their active metabolites to the $P2Y_{12}$ receptors.

Cangrelor is currently the only $P2Y_{12}$ inhibitor that is given intravenously (iv). The other three $P2Y_{12}$ inhibitors are given orally. Following iv infusion of cangrelor, platelet inhibition occurs within 2 min. After discontinuation of the infusion, the anti-platelet effect decreases rapidly, and platelet function returns to normal within 1 h. **Table 9.2** compares the major pharmacodynamic properties of the four $P2Y_{12}$ receptor inhibitors.

TABLE 9.2. Pharmacodynamic properties of cangrelor and the other $P2Y_{12}$ receptor inhibitors

Drug	Nature of receptor inhibition	Time course of platelet inhibition
Cangrelor	Reversible (mediated by parent drug)	Significant platelet inhibition occurs within 2 min after intravenous injection. Platelet function returns to normal within 1 h after drug discontinuation
Clopidogrel	Irreversible (mediated by active metabolite)	Significant platelet inhibition occurs 2 h after oral administration. Platelet function returns to normal in about 5 days after drug discontinuation
Prasugrel	Irreversible (mediated by active metabolite)	Significant platelet inhibition occurs 1 h after oral administration. Platelet function returns to normal in 5–9 days after drug discontinuation
Ticagrelor	Reversible (mediated by parent drug and active metabolite)	Significant platelet inhibition occurs 1 h after oral administration. Platelet function returns to normal in 5 days after drug discontinuation

2.4. Clinical Uses

Cangrelor and the other three $P2Y_{12}$ receptor inhibitors are approved for use in the management of ACS. Clopidogrel is also approved for use in patients with a history of recent MI, recent stroke, or established peripheral arterial disease (EPAD). The US FDA-approved indications of cangrelor as well as clopidogrel, prasugrel, and ticagrelor are summarized in **Table 9.3**.

2.5. Therapeutic Dosages

The dosage forms and strengths of cangrelor and the other three $P2Y_{12}$ receptor inhibitors are given below. The recommended dosage regimens are provided in **Table 9.4**.

- Cangrelor: iv, single-use 10 ml vial containing 50 mg cangrelor as a lyophilized powder for reconstitution
- Clopidogrel: oral, 75 mg tablets

- Prasugrel: oral, 5, 10 mg tablets
- Ticagrelor: oral, 90 mg tablets

TABLE 9.3. Clinical indications of cangrelor and the other P2Y$_{12}$ receptor inhibitors

Drug	Indication	Description and benefit
Cangrelor	ACS	Cangrelor is used as an adjunct to PCI to reduce the risk of periprocedural MI, repeat coronary revascularization, and stent thrombosis in patients who have not been treated with a P2Y$_{12}$ receptor inhibitor and are not being given a glycoprotein IIb/IIIa inhibitor
Clopidogrel	ACS (UA/NSTEMI, STEMI)	For patients with UA/NSTEMI or STEMI, clopidogrel reduces the rate of MI and stroke
	Recent MI, recent stroke, or EPAD	For patients with recent MI, stroke, or EPAD, clopidogrel reduces the rate of MI and stroke
Prasugrel	ACS (UA/NSTEMI, STEMI)	Prasugrel is used to reduce thrombotic cardiovascular events (including stent thrombosis) in patients with ACS who are to be managed with PCI as follows: (1) patients with UA or NSTEMI; or (2) patients with STEMI when managed with primary or delayed PCI
Ticagrelor	ACS (UA/NSTEMI, STEMI)	Ticagrelor is used to reduce the rate of cardiovascular death, MI, and stroke in patients with ACS or a history of MI. It also reduces the rate of stent thrombosis in patients who have been stented for the treatment of ACS

Note: ACS, acute coronary syndromes; EPAD, established peripheral arterial disease; MI, myocardial infarction; NSTEMI, non-ST elevation myocardial infarction; PCI, percutaneous coronary intervention; STEMI, ST elevation myocardial infarction; UA, unstable angina.

2.6. Adverse Effects and Drug Interactions

2.6.1. Adverse Effects

Bleeding, including life-threatening and fatal bleeding, is the most commonly reported adverse effect shared by cangrelor and the other P2Y$_{12}$ receptor inhibitors (clopidogrel, prasugrel, and ticagrelor). Cangrelor may also decrease renal function and cause dyspnea. Serious thrombotic thrombocytopenic purpura (TTP) may also occur with clopidogrel and prasugrel. Ticagrelor can also cause dyspnea and ventricular pauses (bradycardia).

2.6.2. Drug Interactions

2.6.2.1. CANGRELOR

Cangrelor strongly inhibits the binding of the active metabolites of clopidogrel and prasugrel to P2Y$_{12}$ receptors, resulting in a negative pharmacodynamic interaction. If clopidogrel or prasugrel is administered during cangrelor infusion, they will have no antiplatelet effect

TABLE 9.4. The recommended dosage regimens of cangrelor and the other P2Y$_{12}$ receptor inhibitors

Drug	Indication	Dosage regimen
Cangrelor	ACS	A 30 µg (mcg)/kg iv bolus followed immediately by a 4 µg (mcg)/kg/min iv infusion. Initiate the bolus infusion prior to PCI. The maintenance infusion should ordinarily be continued for at least 2 h or for the duration of PCI, whichever is longer. To maintain platelet inhibition after discontinuation of cangrelor infusion, an oral P2Y$_{12}$ inhibitor should be administered (180 mg ticagrelor at any time during cangrelor infusion or immediately after its discontinuation; or 60 mg prasugrel immediately after discontinuation of cangrelor; or 600 mg clopidogrel immediately after discontinuation of cangrelor; note: do not give prasugrel or clopidogrel prior to discontinuation of cangrelor)
Clopidogrel	UA/NSTEMI	A single 300 mg loading dose followed by 75 mg once daily, in combination with aspirin (75–325 mg once daily)
	STEMI	75 mg once daily, in combination with aspirin (75–325 mg once daily), with or without a loading dose
	Recent MI, recent stroke, or EPAD	75 mg once daily
Prasugrel	ACS	Initiate prasugrel treatment as a single 60 mg oral loading dose and then continue at 10 mg orally once daily. Patients taking prasugrel should also take aspirin (75–325 mg) daily
Ticagrelor	ACS	In the management of ACS, initiate ticagrelor treatment with a 180 mg loading dose. Administer 90 mg twice daily during the first year after an ACS event. After one year, administer 60 mg twice daily. Use ticagrelor with a daily maintenance dose of aspirin of 75–100 mg. Do not administer ticagrelor with another oral P2Y$_{12}$ inhibitor

Note: ACS, acute coronary syndromes; EPAD, established peripheral arterial disease; MI, myocardial infarction; NSTEMI, non-ST elevation myocardial infarction; PCI, percutaneous coronary intervention; STEMI, ST elevation myocardial infarction; UA, unstable angina.

until the next dose is administered. Clopidogrel and prasugrel, therefore, should not be administered until cangrelor infusion is discontinued. In contrast, ticagrelor given before or during infusion of cangrelor did not attenuate the pharmacodynamic effects of cangrelor. The pharmacodynamic effects of ticagrelor were preserved when ticagrelor was given during infusion of cangrelor. As such, this oral P2Y$_{12}$ receptor inhibitor may be administered before, during, or after treatment with cangrelor [6, 7] (also see **Table 9.4**). Because cangrelor does not affect liver enzymes, drug interaction is much less significant with cangrelor than with the other P2Y$_{12}$ receptor inhibitors.

2.6.2.2. CLOPIDOGREL

- Clopidogrel is metabolized to its active metabolite in part by CYP2C19. Concomitant use of drugs (e.g., the proton pump inhibitors omeprazole and esomeprazole) that inhibit the activity of this enzyme results in reduced plasma concentrations of the active metabolite of clopidogrel and a reduction in platelet inhibition. Likewise, individuals with inactive CYP2C19 gene (CYP2C19 poor metabolizers) show a reduced drug effect.

- Co-administration of clopidogrel with warfarin or nonsteroidal anti-inflammatory drugs (NSAIDs) as well as drugs that affect platelet activation (e.g., selective serotonin reuptake inhibitors and serotonin norepinephrine reuptake inhibitors) increases the risk of bleeding.
- The acyl-β-glucuronide metabolite of clopidogrel is a strong inhibitor of CYP2C8. Clopidogrel can increase the systemic exposure to drugs that are primarily cleared by CYP2C8 (e.g., the antidiabetic drug repaglinide).

2.6.2.3. PRASUGREL

- Co-administration of prasugrel with warfarin or NSAIDs increases the risk of bleeding.
- Although prasugrel is metabolized by CYP3A4, CYP2B6, CYP2C9, and CYP2C19, co-administration with inhibitors or inducers of these enzymes (e.g., ketoconazole, rifampin) does not significantly alter the pharmacodynamics of prasugrel. As such, prasugrel can be administered with drugs that are inducers or inhibitors of CYP enzymes.

2.6.2.4. TICAGRELOR

- Since ticagrelor is predominantly metabolized by CYP3A4 and to a lesser extent by CYP3A5, and is also a P-glycoprotein substrate, drug interactions may become clinically significant.
- Concomitant treatment with strong inhibitors of CYP3A (e.g., ketoconazole, itraconazole, voriconazole, clarithromycin, nefazodone, ritonavir, saquinavir, nelfinavir, indinavir, atazanavir, and telithromycin) or potent inducers of CYP3A (e.g., rifampin, dexamethasone, phenytoin, carbamazepine, and phenobarbital) should be avoided.
- Because simvastatin and lovastatin are metabolized also by CYP3A4, co-treatment with ticagrelor increases the plasma concentrations of these statins.
- Because of the inhibition of P-glycoprotein by ticagrelor, P-glycoprotein-mediated elimination of digoxin may be reduced. As such, digoxin levels should be monitored with initiation of or any change in ticagrelor therapy.
- Based on clinical studies, concomitant use of ticagrelor with maintenance doses of aspirin above 100 mg decreases the effectiveness of ticagrelor. As such, after the initial loading dose of aspirin, use ticagrelor with a maintenance dose of aspirin of 75–100 mg (also see **Table 9.4**)

2.6.3. Contraindications and FDA Pregnancy Category

The contraindications and FDA pregnancy category of cangrelor and the other three $P2Y_{12}$ receptor inhibitors are listed in **Table 9.5**.

TABLE 9.5. The contraindications and FDA pregnancy category of cangrelor and the other P2Y$_{12}$ receptor inhibitors

Drug	Contraindications	Pregnancy category
Cangrelor	(1) Significant active bleeding; (2) hypersensitivity to cangrelor or any component of the product	B
Clopidogrel	(1) Active bleeding (e.g., peptic ulcer, intracranial hemorrhage); (2) hypersensitivity to clopidegrel or any component of the product	B
Prasugrel	(1) Active bleeding (e.g., peptic ulcer, intracranial hemorrhage); (2) prior transient ischemic attack or stroke; (3) hypersensitivity to prasugrel or any component of the product	Unknown
Ticagrelor	(1) Active bleeding (e.g., peptic ulcer, intracranial hemorrhage); (2) history of intracranial hemorrhage; (3) hypersensitivity to ticagrelor or any component of the product	C

2.7. Comparison with Existing Members and New Development since the US FDA Approval

2.7.1. Cangrelor versus the Oral P2Y$_{12}$ Receptor Inhibitors

The oral P2Y$_{12}$ receptor inhibitors (clopidogrel, prasugrel, and ticagrelor) have several limitations such as delayed onset and offset of action, and only oral availability. As an intravenous, fast-onset, direct-acting P2Y$_{12}$ receptor inhibitor, cangrelor offers potent platelet inhibition that is rapidly reversible. It is most useful in ACS patients undergoing PCI, who require an immediate, profound, and predictable level of P2Y$_{12}$ receptor inhibition, which is then maintained by giving an oral P2Y$_{12}$ receptor inhibitor, typically for at least 12 months [8–10].

   In large randomized trials, cangrelor has shown substantial reduction in ischemic events with no increase in severe bleeding compared with clopidogrel among patients undergoing PCI, and thus may offer greater net clinical benefit than clopidogrel [5, 11]. More recently, based on a pooled analysis from the three phase 3 CHAMPION trials, cangrelor alone was found to be associated with similar ischemic risk and lower risk-adjusted bleeding risk compared with clopidogrel plus glycoprotein IIb/IIIa inhibitor (GPI) [12]. Furthermore, Cangrelor's efficacy in reducing ischemic complications in patients undergoing PCI was found to be maintained irrespective of GP IIb/IIIa inhibitor administration [13].

2.7.2. Comparison among the Oral P2Y$_{12}$ Receptor Inhibitors

Among the oral inhibitors, prasugrel and ticagrelor have relatively more prompt, potent, and predictable antiplatelet effects than clopidogrel, and compared with clopidogrel, prasugrel and ticagrelor result in further reduced ischemic outcomes in patients with ACS, albeit at the expense of an increased risk of bleeding [10, 14]. A more recent meta-analysis of nine randomized controlled trials involving 106,288 patients with ACS suggested that among the three oral inhibitors, ticagrelor has the best net efficacy and safety profile in reducing myocardial ischemic events, whereas prasugrel is the least safe, and clopidogrel is the least efficacious [15]. When added to low-dose aspirin, ticagrelor not only reduces the risk of adverse cardiovascular events, but also decreases the risk of stroke in patients with prior MI [16]. Notably, in patients with MI more than one year previously, long-term treatment (a median of 33 months) with ticagrelor on a background therapy of low-dose aspirin significantly reduces the risk of cardiovascular death, MI, or stroke though at the expense of an increased risk of major bleeding [17].

3. THE THROMBIN RECEPTOR ANTAGONIST: VORAPAXAR (ZONTIVITY)

3.1. Overview

Antiplatelet drugs commonly used in ACS target two important platelet activation pathways, i.e., (1) cyclooxygenase (COX)-1-mediated thromboxane A_2 (TxA_2) synthesis and the activation of platelets via TxA_2 receptors, and (2) ADP signaling via activating the $P2Y_{12}$ receptors. Despite the efficacy of low-dose aspirin (a COX-1 inhibitor) and of a growing family of $P2Y_{12}$ receptor antagonists, major cardiovascular events continue to occur in patients with ischemic heart disease, suggesting the involvement of other platelet activation pathway(s). In this context, thrombin, a serine protease, is considered one of the most potent platelet activators and plays a central role in blood coagulation.

Platelet responses to thrombin are mediated by surface G-protein-coupled receptors known as protease-activated receptors (PARs) or thrombin receptors. In humans, there are 4 known subtypes of PARs, which display wide tissue distribution. PAR-1, PAR-3, and PAR-4 are activated by thrombin, whereas PAR-2 is activated by trypsin and trypsin-like proteases and not by thrombin. Thrombin-mediated platelet activation in humans is shown to occur through PAR-1 and PAR-4, especially PAR-1. Indeed, PAR-1 acts as the principal thrombin receptor on human platelets and mediates platelet activation by subnanomolar thrombin concentrations, whereas PAR-4 requires higher concentration of thrombin for activation [18–20]. It should be noted that PAR-1 is also activated by other factors, such as metalloprotease-1 and -2, enzymes involved in thrombogenesis [21, 22].

Thrombin-mediated PAR-1 cleavage results in the activation of heterotrimeric G proteins of the $G\alpha12/13$, $G\alpha q$, and $G\alpha i/z$ families that interconnect several intracellular signaling pathways to the various phenotypic effects of thrombin on platelets. These include TxA_2 production, ADP release, serotonin and epinephrine release, activation/mobilization of P-selectin and CD40 ligand, integrin activation, and platelet aggregation. Notably, PAR-1 activation also stimulates platelet procoagulant activity, leading to enhanced thrombin formation, and the consequent generation of fibrin from fibrinogen [18–20] (**Figure 9.3**).

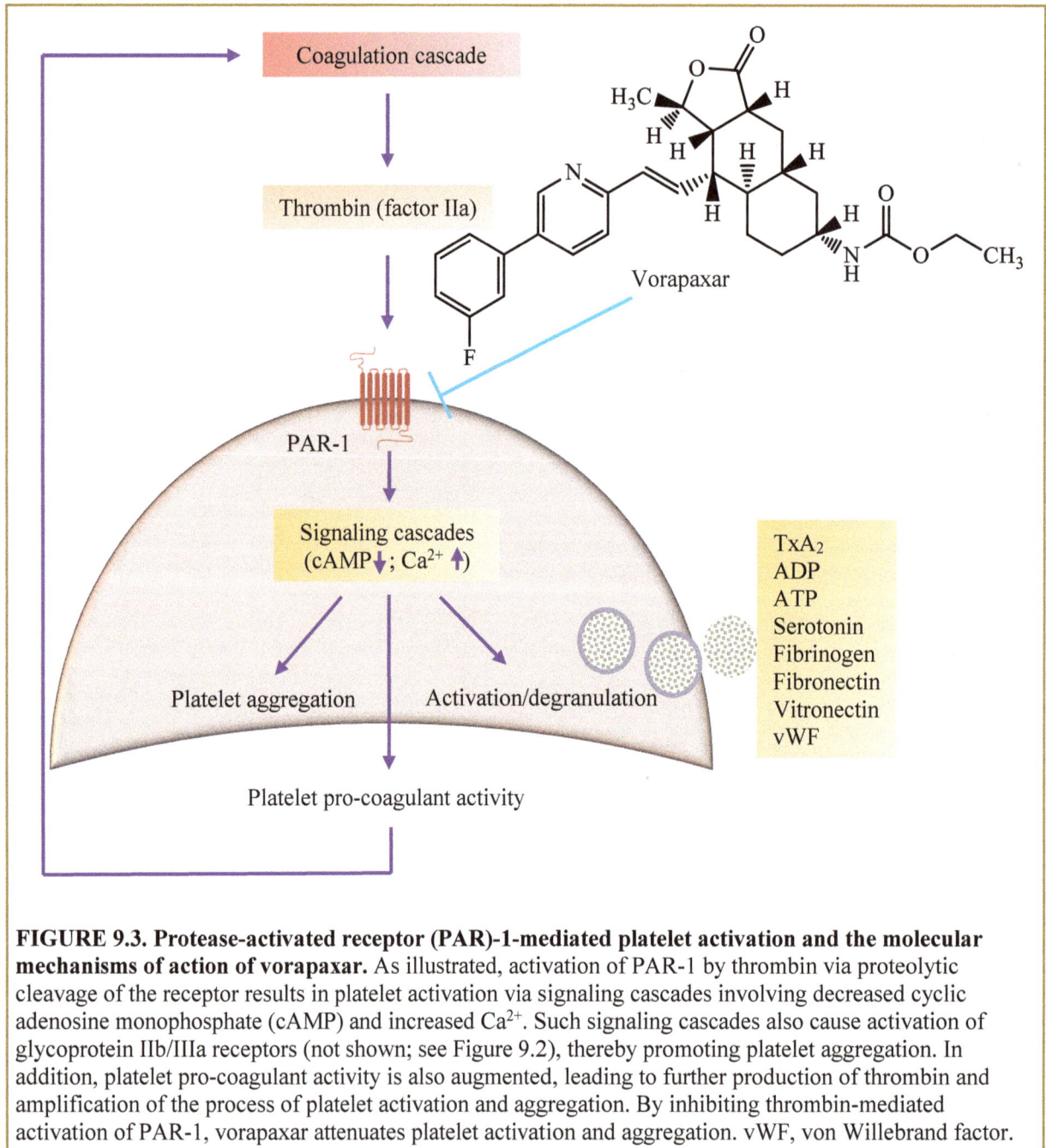

FIGURE 9.3. Protease-activated receptor (PAR)-1-mediated platelet activation and the molecular mechanisms of action of vorapaxar. As illustrated, activation of PAR-1 by thrombin via proteolytic cleavage of the receptor results in platelet activation via signaling cascades involving decreased cyclic adenosine monophosphate (cAMP) and increased Ca^{2+}. Such signaling cascades also cause activation of glycoprotein IIb/IIIa receptors (not shown; see Figure 9.2), thereby promoting platelet aggregation. In addition, platelet pro-coagulant activity is also augmented, leading to further production of thrombin and amplification of the process of platelet activation and aggregation. By inhibiting thrombin-mediated activation of PAR-1, vorapaxar attenuates platelet activation and aggregation. vWF, von Willebrand factor.

The understanding of the critical role of PAR-1 signaling in platelet activation and thrombogenesis has led to the development of a novel class of antiplatelet agents able to specifically block PAR-1. Two PAR-1 antagonists, vorapaxar and atopaxar, have recently undergone clinical investigations [23–26], and vorapaxar received approval on May 8, 2014 by the US FDA for clinical use. The US FDA approval of vorapaxar was based on a randomized controlled trial (TRA 2P-TIMI 50) involving 26,449 patients who had a history of MI, ischemic stroke, or peripheral arterial disease. The trial demonstrated that inhibition of PAR-1 with vorapaxar reduced the risk of cardio-vascular death or ischemic events in patients with stable atheroscle-rosis who were receiving standard therapy. However, it increased the risk of moderate or severe bleeding, including intracranial hemor-rhage [23, 24, 27].

3.2. Chemistry and Pharmacokinetics

Vorapaxar is a synthetic tricyclic himbacine-derivative (structure shown in **Figure 9.3**). The drug is readily absorbed following oral administration, with a bioavailability of nearly 100%. Vorapaxar is widely distributed and highly bound to plasma proteins with a vol-ume of distribution of ~424 L/70 kg body weight. It is metabolized by CYP3A4 and CYP2J2 (the monohydroxy metabolite also inhibits PAR-1), and eliminated mainly in the feces, and to a lesser extent in the urine. The terminal elimination half-life of vorapaxar is ~8 days.

3.3. Molecular Mechanisms and Pharmacological Effects

3.3.1. Molecular Mechanisms

Vorapaxar is a reversible antagonist of PAR-1 expressed on platelets, but its long half-life makes the inhibition effectively irreversible (**Figure 9.3**). Vorapaxar inhibits thrombin- and thrombin receptor ag-onist peptide (TRAP)-induced platelet aggregation. Vorapaxar does not inhibit platelet aggregation induced by ADP, collagen, or TxA_2. PAR-1 is also expressed in a wide variety of cell types, including endothelial cells, neurons, and smooth muscle cells, but the pharma-codynamic effects of vorapaxar in these cell types remain unknown.

3.3.2. Pharmacological Effects

At the recommended dose, vorapaxar causes $\geq 80\%$ inhibition of TRAP-induced platelet aggregation within one week of initiation of treatment. The duration of platelet inhibition is dose- and concentra-tion-dependent. Significant inhibition of TRAP-induced platelet ag-gregation remains 4 weeks after discontinuation of vorapaxar, consistent with the long terminal elimination half-life of the drug ($t_{1/2}$ = ~8 days).

3.4. Clinical Uses

Vorapaxar is indicated for the reduction of thrombotic cardiovascular events in patients with a history of MI or with peripheral arterial dis-ease (PAD). It has been shown to reduce the rate of a combined end-point of cardiovascular death, MI, stroke, and urgent coronary revascularization in this population [23, 24].

3.5. Therapeutic Dosages

Listed below are the dosage form and strength of vorapaxar.

- Vorapaxar: oral, 2.08 mg (2.5 mg vorapaxar sulfate) tablets

> **Thrombin receptor agonist peptide (TRAP)**
> Thrombin (also known as factor IIa) is a protease that cleaves the N-terminus of the PAR-1 receptor (a G protein-coupled receptor). This cleavage exposes a segment of the extracellular domain of the PAR-1 receptor, and this segment acts as a tethered ligand to interact with the extracellular portions of the transmembrane domains of the receptor, causing its activation (refer to Figure 9.3 for the different domains of the PAR-1 receptor). Synthetic peptides that mimic the amino acid sequence of the tethered ligand also cause activation of the PAR-1 receptor, and those peptides are known as thrombin receptor agonist peptides (TRAPs). TRAPs are frequently used as model activators of PAR-1 receptors to investigate the biological responses of the receptor activation.

The recommended dosage regimen of vorapaxar for the indication stated above (Section 3.4) is one tablet (2.08 mg) orally once daily, with or without food.

3.6. Adverse Effects and Drug Interactions

3.6.1. Adverse Effects

Bleeding, including life-threatening and fatal bleeding, is the most commonly reported adverse effect of vorapaxar therapy. Other rare adverse effects may include anemia, depression, rashes, eruptions, and exanthemas.

3.6.2. Drug Interactions

As noted earlier, vorapaxar is metabolized by CYP3A4 and CYP2J2. Drugs that are strong CYP3A4 inhibitors (e.g., ketoconazole, itraconazole, posaconazole, clarithromycin, nefazodone, ritonavir, saquinavir, nelfinavir, indinavir, boceprevir, telaprevir, telithromycin, conivaptan) or strong CYP3A4 inducers (e.g., rifampin, carbamazepine, phenytoin, and St. John's wort) can significant affect the drug disposition and its pharmacological and adverse effects. As such, concomitant use of vorapaxar with these CYP3A4-modulating drugs should be avoided.

3.6.3. Contraindications and FDA Pregnancy Category

- Vorapaxar is contraindicated in patients with a history of stroke, transient ischemic attack, or intracranial hemorrhage (ICH) due to an increased risk of ICH in this population.
- Vorapaxar is contraindicated in patients with active pathological bleeding such as ICH or peptic ulcer.
- FDA pregnancy category: B

3.7. Comparison with Existing Members and New Development since the US FDA Approval

Vorapaxar is the first-in-class and presently the only member of the thrombin receptor antagonist drug class, that has received the US FDA approval for the reduction of thrombotic cardiovascular events in patients with a history of MI or with PAD. Recently, the drug has also been studied in several other specific patient populations. For example, subgroup analysis from the TRACER trial [25] suggested that in UA/NSTEMI patients undergoing coronary artery bypass grafting (CABG), vorapaxar therapy was associated with a significant reduction in ischemic events and no significant increase in major CABG-related bleeding [28]. As noted above, because of an increased risk of intracranial hemorrhage, vorapaxar is contraindicated in patients with a history of stroke. Subsequent studies (TRA 2°P-TIMI 50) indicated that treatment with vorapaxar reduced ischemic stroke in patients with MI or PAD and no known cerebrovascular disease. Although primary hemorrhagic stroke was increased, vorapaxar reduced the total incidence of stroke [29].

In patients with previous MI and diabetes, the addition of vorapaxar to standard therapy significantly reduced the risk of major vascular events with greater potential for absolute benefit in this group at high risk of recurrent ischemic events [30]. Vorapaxar treatment reduced cardiovascular death, MI, or stroke in stable patients with a history of previous MI, whether treated concomitantly with a thienopyridine P2Y$_{12}$ receptor inhibitor (e.g., clopidogrel, prasugrel) or not. The relative risk of moderate or severe bleeding was similarly increased irrespective of thienopyridine use. These results suggested that the efficacy and safety of antiplatelet therapy with vorapaxar was not modified by concurrent thienopyridine P2Y$_{12}$ receptor-inhibiting therapy [27]. A more recent study reported that in stable patients with symptomatic atherosclerosis, more intensive antiplatelet therapy (vorapaxar plus ticagrelor) significantly reduced the risk of venous thromboembolism by 29% compared with background antiplatelet therapy [31]. Collectively, these new findings implicate that vorapaxar may become an important addition to the tools for effectively reducing cardiovascular events and mortality.

In addition to its benefits in ischemic heart disease, vorapaxar therapy also reduced acute limb ischemia in patients with symptomatic PAD with consistency across different types, including PAD resulting from surgical graft thrombosis and in situ thrombosis [32]. In patients with known PAD, vorapaxar treatment decreased the need for peripheral revascularization [33].

4. SELF-ASSESSMENT QUESTIONS

4.1. A 67-year-old woman with an acute myocardial infraction undergoes percutaneous coronary intervention. A decision is made to administer a newly approved antiplatelet drug intravenously to achieve a rapid inhibition of platelet function and suppress the ongoing thrombogenesis. Which of the following is most likely the drug administered?

A. Cangrelor
B. Clopidogrel
C. Prasugrel
D. Ticagrelor
E. Ticlopidine

4.2. Following the successful management of a non-ST elevation myocardial infarction, a 51-year-old man is put on a dual antiplatelet therapy (DAPT) to prevent recurrence of cardiovascular events. One of the DAPT drugs acts via irreversibly blocking platelet P2Y$_{12}$ receptor-mediated signaling. Which of the following is most likely the drug?

A. Aspirin
B. Cangrelor
C. Prasugrel
D. Ticagrelor
E. Vorapaxar

4.3. A 65-year-old woman with an acute coronary syndrome has been treated successfully with percutaneous coronary intervention with stent placement. She is also prescribed low-dose aspirin and ticagrelor to reduce stent thrombosis. Which of the following pairs are the most likely molecular targets of this dual antiplatelet therapy?

A. Cyclooxygenase-2/protease-activated receptor-1
B. Cyclooxygenase-1/cyclooxygenase-2
C. Cyclooxygenase-1/P2Y$_{12}$ receptor
D. Cyclooxygenase-1/protease-activated receptor-4
E. Cyclooxygenase-2/ P2Y$_{12}$ receptor

4.4. A 54-year-old woman is diagnosed with peripheral arterial disease. A decision is made to treat her with an oral drug targeting the protease-activated receptors on platelets to reduce the risk of thrombotic cardiovascular events. Which of the following conditions would prohibit the use of this oral drug in the patient?

A. A history of migraine headache
B. A history of myocardial infarction
C. A history of rheumatoid arthritis
D. A history of stable angina
E. A history of stroke

4.5. In a recently completed clinical trial, a newly approved drug inhibiting thrombin-induced platelet aggregation via G-protein-coupled receptor signaling was shown to reduce acute limb ischemia in patient with symptomatic peripheral arterial disease. Which of the following is most likely the molecular target of this new drug?

A. Cyclooxygenase-1
B. P2Y$_{12}$ receptor
C. Phosphodiesterase-3
D. Protease-activated receptor-1
E. Protease-activated receptor-2

ANSWERS AND EXPLANATIONS

4.1. The correct answer is A. Among the five P2Y$_{12}$ receptor inhibitors listed, only cangrelor is given intravenously as an adjunct to percutaneous coronary intervention (PCI) to reduce the risk of periprocedural myocardial infarction, repeat coronary revascularization, and stent thrombosis in patients who have not been treated with a P2Y$_{12}$ receptor inhibitor and are not being given a glycoprotein IIb/IIIa inhibitor. It should be noted that ticlopidine is rarely used due to serious adverse effects.

4.2. The correct answer is C. Among the drugs listed, only cangrelor, prasugrel, and ticagrelor are P2Y$_{12}$ receptor inhibitors. Among them, only prasugrel causes irreversible inhibition of the P2Y$_{12}$ receptors via its active metabolite. Cangrelor and ticagrelor are reversible inhibitors of P2Y$_{12}$ receptors.

4.3. The correct answer is C. The molecular target of low-dose aspirin is cyclooxygenase-1 in platelets, whereas the molecular target for ticagrelor is platelet $P2Y_{12}$ receptor.

4.4. The correct answer is E. Based on the molecular target, one can tell that the oral drug is vorapaxar. Vorapaxar is contraindicated in patients with a history of stroke, transient ischemic attack, or intracranial hemorrhage (ICH) due to an increased risk of ICH in this subpopulation of patients.

4.5. The correct answer is D. Based on the mechanism of action, one can tell that drug is mostly likely vorapaxar, which is a selective inhibitor of protease-activated receptor-1.

REFERENCES

1. Mega JL, Simon T. Pharmacology of antithrombotic drugs: an assessment of oral antiplatelet and anticoagulant treatments. *Lancet* 2015; 386(9990):281–91.
2. Wiviott SD, Steg PG. Clinical evidence for oral antiplatelet therapy in acute coronary syndromes. *Lancet* 2015; 386(9990):292–302.
3. Franchi F, Rollini F, Angiolillo DJ. Antithrombotic therapy for patients with STEMI undergoing primary PCI. *Nat Rev Cardiol* 2017; 14(6):361–79.
4. Patrono C, Morais J, Baigent C, Collet JP, Fitzgerald D, Halvorsen S, Rocca B, Siegbahn A, Storey RF, Vilahur G. Antiplatelet agents for the treatment and prevention of coronary atherothrombosis. *J Am Coll Cardiol* 2017; 70(14):1760–76.
5. Bhatt DL, Stone GW, Mahaffey KW, Gibson CM, Steg PG, Hamm CW, Price MJ, Leonardi S, Gallup D, Bramucci E, Radke PW, Widimsky P, et al. Effect of platelet inhibition with cangrelor during PCI on ischemic events. *N Engl J Med* 2013; 368(14):1303–13.
6. Schneider DJ, Agarwal Z, Seecheran N, Keating FK, Gogo P. Pharmacodynamic effects during the transition between cangrelor and ticagrelor. *JACC Cardiovasc Interv* 2014; 7(4):435–42.
7. Rollini F, Franchi F, Thano E, Faz G, Park Y, Kureti M, Cho JR, Been L, Bass TA, Angiolillo DJ. In vitro pharmacodynamic effects of cangrelor on platelet $P2Y_{12}$ receptor-mediated signaling in ticagrelor-treated patients. *JACC Cardiovasc Interv* 2017; 10(13):1374–5.
8. Leonardi S, Bhatt DL. Practical considerations for cangrelor use in patients with acute coronary syndromes. *Eur Heart J Acute Cardiovasc Care* 2017:2048872617707960.
9. Levine GN, Bates ER, Bittl JA, Brindis RG, Fihn SD, Fleisher LA, Granger CB, Lange RA, Mack MJ, Mauri L, Mehran R, Mukherjee D, et al. 2016 ACC/AHA guideline focused update on duration of dual antiplatelet therapy in patients with coronary artery disease: a report of the American College of Cardiology/American Heart Association Task Force on Clinical Practice Guidelines. *J Am Coll Cardiol* 2016; 68(10):1082–115.
10. Angiolillo DJ, Rollini F, Storey RF, Bhatt DL, James S, Schneider DJ, Sibbing D, So DYF, Trenk D, Alexopoulos D, Gurbel PA, Hochholzer W, et al. International expert consensus on switching platelet $P2Y_{12}$ receptor-inhibiting therapies. *Circulation* 2017; 136(20):1955–75.
11. O'Donoghue ML, Bhatt DL, Stone GW, Steg PG, Gibson CM, Hamm CW, Price MJ, Prats J, Liu T, Deliargyris EN, Mahaffey KW, White HD, et al. Efficacy and safety of cangrelor in women versus men during percutaneous coronary intervention: insights from the cangrelor versus standard therapy to achieve optimal management of platelet inhibition (CHAMPION PHOENIX) trial. *Circulation* 2016; 133(3):248–55.
12. Vaduganathan M, Harrington RA, Stone GW, Deliargyris EN, Steg PG, Gibson CM, Hamm CW, Price MJ, Menozzi A, Prats J, Elkin S, Mahaffey KW, et al. Evaluation of ischemic and bleeding risks associated with 2 parenteral antiplatelet strategies comparing cangrelor with glycoprotein IIb/IIIa inhibitors: an exploratory analysis from the CHAMPION trials. *JAMA Cardiol* 2017; 2(2):127–35.
13. Vaduganathan M, Harrington RA, Stone GW,

Deliargyris EN, Steg PG, Gibson CM, Hamm CW, Price MJ, Menozzi A, Prats J, Elkin S, Mahaffey KW, et al. Cangrelor with and without glycoprotein IIb/IIIa inhibitors in patients undergoing percutaneous coronary intervention. *J Am Coll Cardiol* 2017; 69(2):176–85.

14. Rollini F, Franchi F, Angiolillo DJ. Switching P2Y$_{12}$-receptor inhibitors in patients with coronary artery disease. *Nat Rev Cardiol* 2016; 13(1):11–27.

15. Shah R, Rashid A, Hwang I, Fan TM, Khouzam RN, Reed GL. Meta-analysis of the relative efficacy and safety of oral P2Y$_{12}$ inhibitors in patients with acute coronary syndrome. *Am J Cardiol* 2017; 119(11):1723–8.

16. Bonaca MP, Goto S, Bhatt DL, Steg PG, Storey RF, Cohen M, Goodrich E, Mauri L, Ophuis TO, Ruda M, Spinar J, Seung KB, et al. Prevention of stroke with ticagrelor in patients with prior myocardial infarction: insights from PEGASUS-TIMI 54 (Prevention of Cardiovascular Events in Patients With Prior Heart Attack Using Ticagrelor Compared to Placebo on a Background of Aspirin-Thrombolysis in Myocardial Infarction 54). *Circulation* 2016; 134(12):861–71.

17. Bonaca MP, Bhatt DL, Cohen M, Steg PG, Storey RF, Jensen EC, Magnani G, Bansilal S, Fish MP, Im K, Bengtsson O, Oude Ophuis T, et al. Long-term use of ticagrelor in patients with prior myocardial infarction. *N Engl J Med* 2015; 372(19):1791–800.

18. Angiolillo DJ, Capodanno D, Goto S. Platelet thrombin receptor antagonism and atherothrombosis. *Eur Heart J* 2010; 31(1):17–28.

19. O'Brien PJ, Molino M, Kahn M, Brass LF. Protease activated receptors: theme and variations. *Oncogene* 2001; 20(13):1570–81.

20. Nieman MT. Protease-activated receptors in hemostasis. *Blood* 2016; 128(2):169–77.

21. Trivedi V, Boire A, Tchernychev B, Kaneider NC, Leger AJ, O'Callaghan K, Covic L, Kuliopulos A. Platelet matrix metalloprotease-1 mediates thrombogenesis by activating PAR1 at a cryptic ligand site. *Cell* 2009; 137(2):332–43.

22. Sebastiano M, Momi S, Falcinelli E, Bury L, Hoylaerts MF, Gresele P. A novel mechanism regulating human platelet activation by MMP-2-mediated PAR1 biased signaling. *Blood* 2017; 129(7):883–95.

23. Morrow DA, Braunwald E, Bonaca MP, Ameriso SF, Dalby AJ, Fish MP, Fox KA, Lipka LJ, Liu X, Nicolau JC, Ophuis AJ, Paolasso E, et al. Vorapaxar in the secondary prevention of atherothrombotic events. *N Engl J Med* 2012; 366(15):1404–13.

24. Scirica BM, Bonaca MP, Braunwald E, De Ferrari GM, Isaza D, Lewis BS, Mehrhof F, Merlini PA, Murphy SA, Sabatine MS, Tendera M, Van de Werf F, et al. Vorapaxar for secondary prevention of thrombotic events for patients with previous myocardial infarction: a prespecified subgroup analysis of the TRA 2 degrees P-TIMI 50 trial. *Lancet* 2012; 380(9850):1317–24.

25. Tricoci P, Huang Z, Held C, Moliterno DJ, Armstrong PW, Van de Werf F, White HD, Aylward PE, Wallentin L, Chen E, Lokhnygina Y, Pei J, et al. Thrombin-receptor antagonist vorapaxar in acute coronary syndromes. *N Engl J Med* 2012; 366(1):20–33.

26. Wiviott SD, Flather MD, O'Donoghue ML, Goto S, Fitzgerald DJ, Cura F, Aylward P, Guetta V, Dudek D, Contant CF, Angiolillo DJ, Bhatt DL, et al. Randomized trial of atopaxar in the treatment of patients with coronary artery disease: the lessons from antagonizing the cellular effect of Thrombin-Coronary Artery Disease trial. *Circulation* 2011; 123(17):1854–63.

27. Bohula EA, Aylward PE, Bonaca MP, Corbalan RL, Kiss RG, Murphy SA, Scirica BM, White H, Braunwald E, Morrow DA. Efficacy and safety of vorapaxar with and without a thienopyridine for secondary prevention in patients with previous myocardial infarction and no history of stroke or transient ischemic attack: results from TRA 2 degrees P-TIMI 50. *Circulation* 2015; 132(20):1871–9.

28. Whellan DJ, Tricoci P, Chen E, Huang Z, Leibowitz D, Vranckx P, Marhefka GD, Held C, Nicolau JC, Storey RF, Ruzyllo W, Huber K, et al. Vorapaxar in acute coronary syndrome patients undergoing coronary artery bypass graft surgery: subgroup analysis from the TRACER trial (Thrombin Receptor Antagonist for Clinical Event Reduction in Acute Coronary Syndrome). *J Am Coll Cardiol* 2014; 63(11):1048–57.

29. Bonaca MP, Scirica BM, Braunwald E, Wiviott SD, Goto S, Nilsen DW, Bonarjee V, Murphy SA, Morrow DA. New ischemic stroke and outcomes with vorapaxar versus placebo: results from the TRA 2 degrees P-TIMI 50 trial. *J Am Coll Cardiol* 2014; 64(22):2318–26.

30. Cavender MA, Scirica BM, Bonaca MP,

Angiolillo DJ, Dalby AJ, Dellborg M, Morais J, Murphy SA, Ophuis TO, Tendera M, Braunwald E, Morrow DA. Vorapaxar in patients with diabetes mellitus and previous myocardial infarction: findings from the thrombin receptor antagonist in secondary prevention of atherothrombotic ischemic events-TIMI 50 trial. *Circulation* 2015; 131(12):1047–53.

31. Cavallari I, Morrow DA, Creager MA, Olin J, Bhatt DL, Steg PG, Storey RF, Cohen M, Scirica BS, Piazza G, Goodrich EL, Braunwald E, et al. Frequency, predictors and impact of combined antiplatelet therapy on venous thromboembolism in patients with symptomatic atherosclerosis. *Circulation* 2018; 137(7):684–92.

32. Bonaca MP, Gutierrez JA, Creager MA, Scirica BM, Olin J, Murphy SA, Braunwald E, Morrow DA. Acute limb ischemia and outcomes with vorapaxar in patients with peripheral artery disease: results from the Trial to Assess the Effects of Vorapaxar in Preventing Heart Attack and Stroke in Patients With Atherosclerosis-Thrombolysis in Myocardial Infarction 50 (TRA2 degrees P-TIMI 50). *Circulation* 2016; 133(10):997–1005.

33. Bonaca MP, Creager MA, Olin J, Scirica BM, Gilchrist IC, Jr., Murphy SA, Goodrich EL, Braunwald E, Morrow DA. Peripheral revascularization in patients with peripheral artery disease with vorapaxar: insights from the TRA 2 degrees P-TIMI 50 trial. *JACC Cardiovasc Interv* 2016; 9(20):2157–64.

CHAPTER 10

New Drugs for Other Thromboembolic Disorders

CHAPTER HIGHLIGHTS

- In addition to acute coronary syndromes, thromboembolic disorders, including deep vein thrombosis (DVT), pulmonary embolism (PE), and thromboembolic stroke also cause significant morbidity and mortality. As such, effective management of these disorders has great impact on human health.
- Drug therapy of thromboembolic disorders primarily involves the use of anticoagulants, which are classified into vitamin K antagonists, heparins, selective factor Xa (SFXa) inhibitors, and direct thrombin inhibitors.
- Over the past five years, the United States Food and Drug Administration (US FDA) has approved two new oral anticoagulants, namely, betrixaban and edoxaban, both belonging to the SFXa inhibitor drug class, which currently consists of five members.
- Betrixaban is indicated for the prophylaxis of venous thromboembolism in adult patients hospitalized for an acute medical illness who are at risk for thromboembolic complications.
- Edoxaban is approved for reducing the risk of stroke and systemic embolism in patients with nonvalvular atrial fibrillation and for treating DVT and PE following the initial therapy with a parenteral anticoagulant.

KEYWORDS | Apixaban; Betrixaban; Deep vein thrombosis; Edoxaban; Fondaparinux; Nonvalvular atrial fibrillation; Pulmonary embolism; Rivaroxaban; Selective factor Xa inhibitor; Stroke; Venous thromboembolism

CITATION | *Li YR. Cardiovascular Medicine: New Therapeutic Drugs Approved by the US FDA (2013–2017). Cell Med Press, Raleigh, NC, USA. 2018. http://dx.doi.org/10.20455/ndcvd.2018.10*

ABBREVIATIONS | CrCL, creatinine clearance; CYP, cytochrome P450; DVT, deep vein thrombosis; NVAF, nonvalvular atrial fibrillation; PE, pulmonary embolism; P-gp, P-glycoprotein; SFXa, selective factor Xa; US FDA, the United States Food and Drug Administration; VTE, venous thromboembolism

CHAPTER AT A GLANCE

1. INTRODUCTION

Thrombotic disorders result from thrombus formation in either the arterial or venous system, with the former including myocardial infarction and atherosclerotic stroke, and the latter including deep vein thrombosis (DVT). Thromboembolic disorders, on the other hand, result from the occlusion of a vessel by a detached thrombus that is initially formed elsewhere and carried by the blood stream to the inflicted vessel. Pulmonary thromboembolism (or simply called pulmonary embolism [PE]) in patients with DVT is an example of thromboembolic disorders. Another example is ischemic stroke caused by a blood clot initially formed in the atria of patients with atrial fibrillation. Although DVT is a thrombotic disorder, it is considered under thromboembolic conditions because it causes PE.

Management of thromboembolic disorders involves the use of various drugs, especially anticoagulants. Anticoagulants act on the different steps of the coagulation cascades (**Figure 10.1**). They inhibit either the action of coagulation factors or interfere with their biosynthesis. Currently, there are 15 anticoagulants approved by the United States Food and Drug Administration (US FDA) for clinical use, which are classified into four groups (also see Chapter 8), as outlined below:

(1) Vitamin K antagonists
(2) Heparins
(3) Selective factor Xa inhibitors
(4) Direct thrombin inhibitors

Over the past five years, the US FDA has approved two new anticoagulants, namely betrixaban (Bevyxxa) (approved on June 23, 2017) and edoxaban (Savaysa) (approved on January 8, 2015). Both belong to the selective factor Xa (SFXa)-inhibiting drug class, which currently consists of five members. This chapter focuses on these two new SFXa inhibitors, and comparisons with the other three old members (i.e., apixaban, fondaparinux, and rivaroxaban) are also made. **Table 10.1** lists the US FDA approval dates for the five SFXa inhibitors in reverse chronological order.

2. EDOXABAN AND BETRIXABAN

2.1. Overview

Because of its central role in coagulation, factor Xa is an attractive target for the design of new anticoagulants that selectively inhibit it. In this context, two types of SFXa inhibitors are available: direct and indirect SFXa inhibitors. The synthetic pentasaccharide fondaparinux, the first-in-class drug, is an indirect SFXa inhibitor that has been in clinical use for more than a decade. A limitation of its long-term use for thromboembolic prevention is the route of administration by subcutaneous injection. On the other hand, the recently approved ones (betrixaban, edoxaban, apixaban and rivaroxaban) are oral agents that directly inhibit factor Xa.

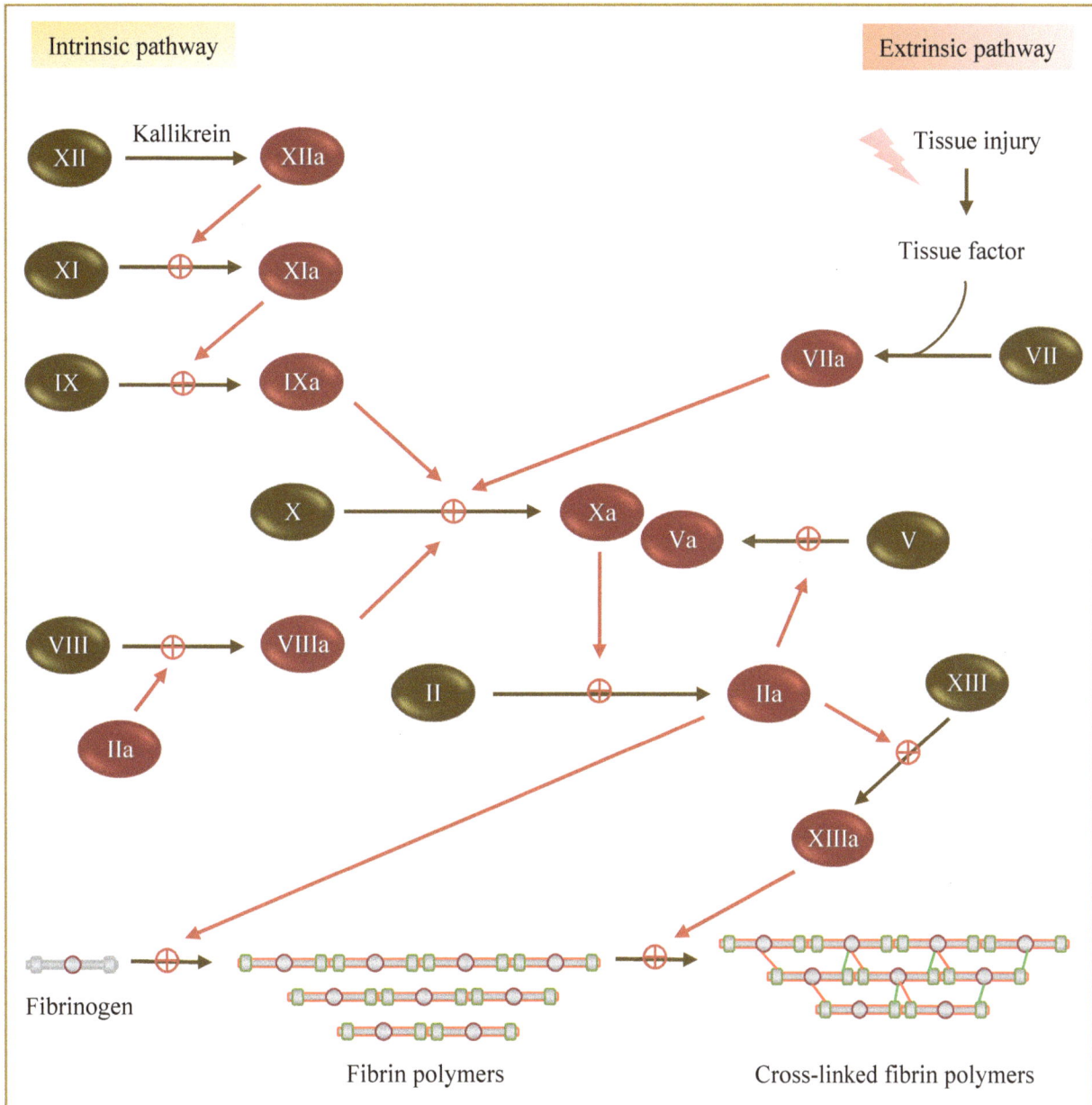

FIGURE 10.1. **Blood coagulation cascades and the targeting sites of anticoagulants.** As illustrated, the intrinsic and extrinsic pathways of coagulation converge with the activation of factor X and the subsequent formation of thrombin (also known as factor IIa), which in turn catalyzes the formation of fibrin, leading to the fibrin clot formation. Vitamin K antagonists (e.g., warfarin) inhibit the functional maturation of factors II, VII, IX, and X. On the other hand, heparins, selective factor Xa inhibitors (e.g., betrixaban, edoxaban), and direct thrombin inhibitors (e.g., dabigatran) either indirectly or directly inhibit factor Xa and/or factor IIa. The plus sign in a circle indicates stimulation of the conversion. The Roman numeral followed by an "a" denotes the activated form of the coagulation factor.

TABLE 10.1. SFXa inhibitors and their US FDA approval date

Drug	FDA approval date
Betrixaban (Bevyxxa)	June 23, 2017
Edoxaban (Savaysa)	January 8, 2015
Apixaban (Eliquis)	December 28, 2012
Rivaroxaban (Xarelto)	July 1, 2011
Fondaparinux (Arixtra)	December 7, 2001

Approval of betrixaban (Portola Pharmaceuticals, South San Francisco, CA, USA) by the US FDA was based on a randomized controlled trial (APEX), involving 7,513 patients who were hospitalized for acute medical illnesses and at high risk for venous thromboembolism (VTE). The study compared extended duration of betrixaban (35 to 42 days) to short duration of enoxaparin (6 to 14 days) in the prevention of venous thromboembolic events. Analysis of the trial data concluded that betrixaban caused increased improvement in symptomatic events including symptomatic DVT, non-fatal PE, or VTE-related death [1–3].

Approval of edoxaban (Daiichi Sankyo, Tokyo, Japan) by the US FDA was based on two randomized controlled trials, namely, ENGAGE AF-TIMI 48 and Hokusai VTE, which involved 21,105 patients with moderate-to-high-risk atrial fibrillation and 8,240 patients with acute VTE, respectively. The ENGAGE AF-TIMI 48 trial demonstrated that edoxaban was noninferior to warfarin with respect to the prevention of stroke or systemic embolism and was associated with significantly lower rates of bleeding and death from cardiovascular causes [4]. The Hokusai VTE trial revealed that edoxaban was noninferior to warfarin therapy and caused significantly less bleeding in a broad spectrum of patients with VTE, including those with severe PE [5].

2.2. Chemistry and Pharmacokinetics

SFXa inhibitors are chemically diverse (structures shown in **Figure 10.2**). Betrixaban is chemically described as N-(5-chloropyridin-2-yl)-2-[4-(N,N-dimethylcarbamimidoyl)-benzoylamino]-5-methoxybenzamide maleate, whereas edoxaban as N-(5-chloropyridin-2-yl)-N'-[(1S,2R,4S)-4-(N,N-dimethylcarbamoyl)-2-(5-methyl-4,5,6,7-tetrahydro[1,3]thiazolo[5,4-c]pyridine-2-carboxamido)cyclohexyl] oxamide mono (4-methylbenzenesulfonate) monohydrate. As noted earlier, fondaparinux is a synthetic pentasaccharide molecule that contains the sequence of five essential carbohydrates necessary for binding to antithrombin III and inducing the conformational change in antithrombin III required for conjugation to factor Xa. Apixaban and rivaroxaban are carboxamide derivatives. The major pharmacokinetic properties of betrixaban and edoxaban as well as the other three SFXa inhibitors are summarized in **Table 10.2.**

> **Antithrombin III**
> Antithrombin III, more formally called antithrombin, is a glycoprotein of 432 amino acids synthesized in the liver and secreted into the plasma. As the name indicates, antithrombin III binds to and inhibits thrombin (also known as factor IIa) as well as other coagulation factors such as factors Xa and IXa. Inhibition of the above coagulation factors by antithrombin III is greatly enhanced by heparins.

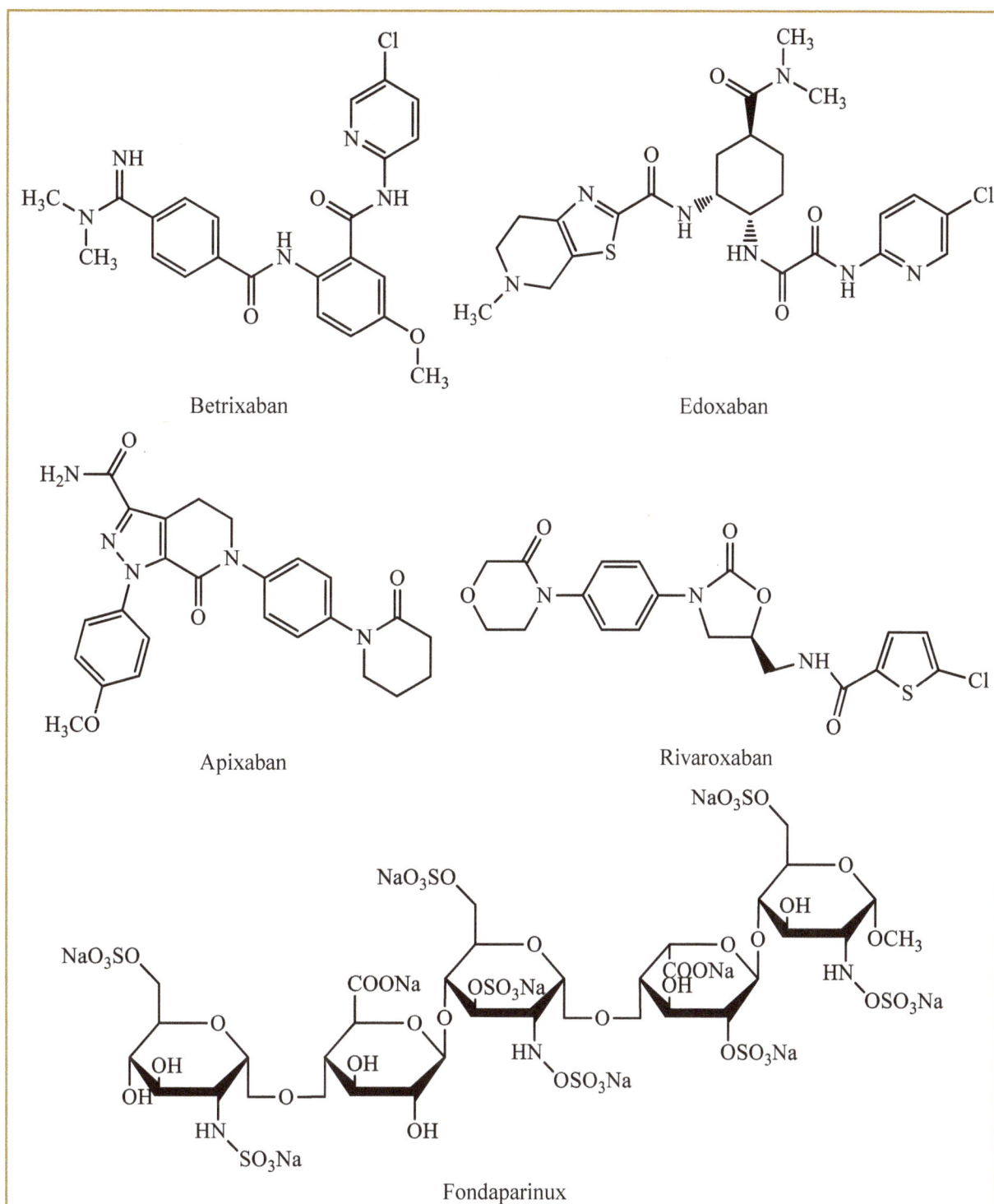

FIGURE 10.2. Structures of betrixaban and edoxaban as well as the other three SFXa inhibitors. As shown, although SFXa inhibitors are chemically diverse compounds, the newly approved betrixaban and edoxaban share some similar structural components (e.g., "5-chloropyridin-2-yl"). Both apixaban and rivaroxaban are considered as carboxamide derivatives. Different from the above oral SFXa inhibitors, fondaparinux is a sodium salt of a pentasaccharide molecule, which needs to be administered subcutaneously.

TABLE 10.2. Major pharmacokinetic properties of betrixaban, edoxaban, and other SFXa inhibitors

Drug	BA	t_{max}	Vd	Metabolism and excretion	$t_{1/2}$
Betrixaban	34%	3–4 h	2240 L	>80% unchanged; eliminated in feces (major) and urine (minor); a substrate of P-gp	19–27 h
Edoxaban	62%	1–2 h	107 L	>90% unchanged; eliminated as unchanged drug in urine; a substrate of P-gp	10–14 h
Apixaban	50%	3–4 h	21 L	Metabolized (~25%) by CYP3A4; eliminated in urine and feces; a substrate of P-gp	12 h
Rivaroxaban	66–100%	2–4 h	50 L	Metabolized (~51%) by CYP3A4/5 and CYP2J2; eliminated in urine and feces; a substrate of P-gp	5–9 h
Fondaparinux	100% (sc)	2 h	7–11 L	Excreted in the urine as unchanged form	17–21 h

Note: BA, bioavailability; CYP, cytochrome P450; sc, subcutaneous; P-gp, P-glycoprotein; $t_{1/2}$, elimination half-life; t_{max}, the time when the maximum plasma concentration is reached; Vd, volume of distribution per 70 kg body weight.

2.3. Molecular Mechanisms and Pharmacological Effects

Like apixaban and rivaroxaban, both betrixaban and edoxaban are oral SFXa inhibitors that directly block the active site of factor Xa and do not require a cofactor (such as antithrombin III) for activity. Betrixaban and edoxaban, as well as the other two oral SFXa inhibitors inhibit free factor Xa and prothrombinase activity. By inhibiting factor Xa, these drugs decrease thrombin generation. Although oral SFXa inhibitors have no direct effects on platelet aggregation, they indirectly inhibit platelet aggregation induced by thrombin, thereby leading to decreased thrombus formation (**Figure 10.3**).

In contrast, the antithrombotic activity of fondaparinux is the result of antithrombin III-mediated selective inhibition of factor Xa. By selectively binding to antithrombin III, fondaparinux potentiates (about 300 times) the innate neutralization of factor Xa by antithrombin III. Neutralization of factor Xa leads to decreased thrombin formation and consequently diminished thrombus development (**Figure 10.3**).

> **Prothrombinase**
> This term refers to a complex consisting of factor Xa, factor Va, phospholipids, and Ca^{2+} with factor Xa being the active center of the complex. As the name indicates, prothrombinase is responsible for converting factor II (also known as prothrombin) to factor IIa (thrombin).

2.4. Clinical Uses

All SFXa inhibitors are indicated in the management of DVT. Many are also used in patients with atrial fibrillation to reduce the risk of thromboembolic stroke. The US FDA-approved indications of betrixaban and edoxaban, as well as the other three SFXa inhibitors are summarized in **Table 10.3**.

2.5. Therapeutic Dosages

Listed below are the dosage forms and strengths of betrixaban and edoxaban, as well as the other three SFXa inhibitors.

- Betrixaban: oral, 40 mg and 80 mg capsules
- Edoxaban: oral, 15, 30, 60 mg tablets
- Apixaban: oral, 2.5, 5 mg tablets
- Rivaroxaban: oral, 10, 15, 20 mg tablets
- Fondaparinux: subcutaneous injection, single-dose, prefilled syringes containing 2.5, 5, 7.5, or 10 mg of fondaparinux

The recommended dosage regimens of betrixaban and edoxaban, as well as the other three SFXa inhibitors in the management of DVT and atrial fibrillation are given in **Table 10.4**.

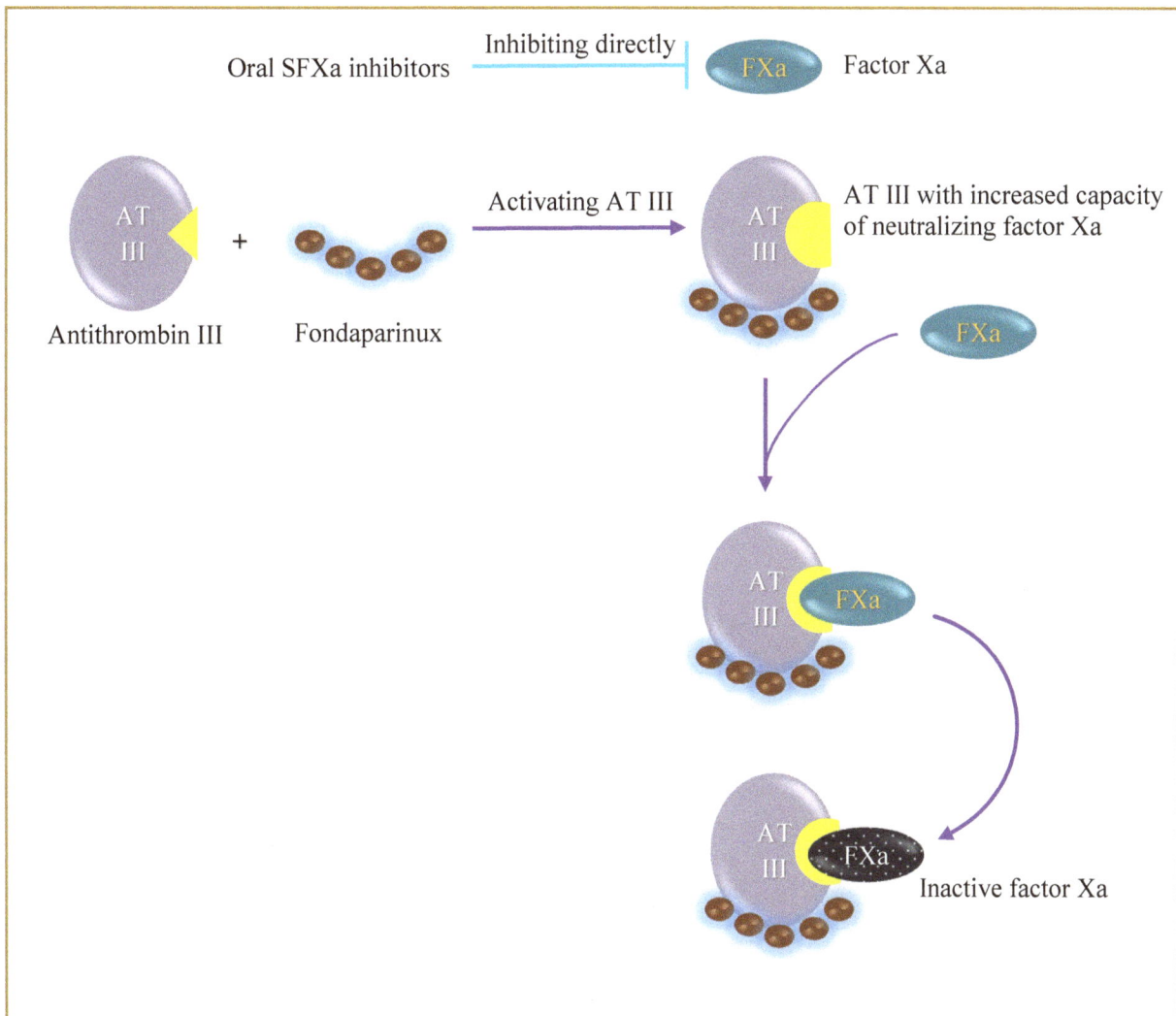

FIGURE 10.3. Molecular mechanisms of action of oral SFXa inhibitors and the indirect SFXa inhibitor fondaparinux. As illustrated, the oral SFXa inhibitors (betrixaban, edoxaban, apixaban, and rivaroxaban) directly inhibit factor Xa and block factor Xa-catalyzed coagulation cascade reaction (i.e., the conversion of factor II to factor IIa). In contrast, fondaparinux does not directly inhibit factor Xa. Instead, it binds to antithrombin III (AT III) and greatly enhances the activity of AT III to neutralize factor Xa. AT III is an endogenous protease that neutralizes factors Xa and IIa. Fondaparinux selectively enhances AT III-mediated inactivation of Xa, while heparins enhance AT III-mediated inactivation of both Xa and IIa.

TABLE 10.3. The US FDA-approved indications of betrixaban, edoxaban, and other SFXa inhibitors

Drug	Indication	Description and benefits
Betrixaban	VTE	Prophylaxis of VTE in adult patients hospitalized for an acute medical illness who are at risk for thromboembolic complications due to moderate or severe restricted mobility and other risk factors for VTE
Edoxaban	NVAF	Reduction in the risk of stroke and systemic embolism in patients with NVAF
	DVT, PE	Treatment of DVT and PE following 5 to 10 days of initial therapy with a parenteral anticoagulant
Apixaban	NVAF	Reduction in the risk of stroke and systemic embolism in patients with NVAF
	DVT, PE	(1) Prophylaxis of DVT, which may lead to PE, in patients who have undergone hip or knee replacement surgery; (2) treatment of DVT and PE; (3) reduction in the risk of recurrent DVT and PE following initial therapy
Rivaroxaban	NVAF	Reduction in the risk of stroke and systemic embolism in patients with NVAF
	DVT, PE	(1) Prophylaxis of DVT, which may lead to PE, in patients who have undergone hip or knee replacement surgery; (2) treatment of DVT and PE; (3) reduction in the risk of recurrent DVT and/or PE after completion of initial treatment lasting at least 6 months
Fondaparinux	DVT, PE	(1) Prophylaxis of DVT in patients undergoing hip fracture, hip replacement, knee replacement, or abdominal surgery who are at risk for thromboembolic complications; (2) treatment of acute DVT or acute PE when administered in conjunction with warfarin

Note: DVT, deep vein thrombosis; NVAF, nonvalvular atrial fibrillation; PE, pulmonary embolism; VTE, venous thromboembolism.

TABLE 10.4. The recommended dosage regimens of betrixaban, edoxaban, and other SFXa inhibitors

Drug	Indication	Dosage regimen
Betrixaban	VTE	For prophylaxis of VTE in adult patients hospitalized for an acute medical illness, (1) an initial single dose of 160 mg, followed by 80 mg once daily for 35–42 days; (2) an initial single dose of 80 mg, followed by 40 mg once daily for patients with severe renal impairment or patients on P-gp inhibitors
Edoxaban	NVAF	For reduction in the risk of stroke and systemic embolism in patients with NVAF, (1) 60 mg once daily in patients with CrCL >50 to ≤95 ml/min; (2) do not use it in patients with CrCL >95 ml/min due to potentially decreased efficacy and an increased risk of stroke compared with warfarin (in those patients another anticoagulant should be used); (3) reduce dose to 30 mg once daily in patients with CrCL of 15–50 ml/min
	DVT, PE	For treating DVT and PE, (1) 60 mg once daily following 5–10 days of initial therapy with a parenteral anticoagulant; (2) 30 mg once daily for patients with CrCL of 15–50 ml/min or body weight ≤60 kg or who use certain P-gp inhibitors

TABLE 10.4. (*continued*)

Drug	Indication	Dosage regimen
Apixaban	NVAF	For reduction in the risk of stroke and systemic embolism in patients with NVAF, (1) 5 mg twice daily; (2) 2.5 mg twice daily in patients with at least 2 of the following characteristics: age ≥80 years, body weight ≤60 kg, or serum creatinine ≥1.5 mg/dl
	DVT, PE	(1) For prophylaxis of DVT following hip or knee replacement surgery, 2.5 mg twice daily in patients following the replacement procedure; taken 12–24 h after surgery and for 35 days (hip surgery) or 12 days (knee replacement surgery); (2) for treating DVT/PE, 10 mg twice daily for the first 7 days of therapy. After 7 days, 5 mg twice daily; (3) for reduction in the risk of recurrence of DVT and PE, 2.5 mg twice daily after at least 6 months of treatment for DVT or PE
Rivaroxaban	NVAF	For reduction in the risk of stroke in NVAF, (1) 20 mg once daily with the evening meal (see Note below for the rationale) in patients with CrCL >50 ml/min; (2) 15 mg once daily with the evening meal in patients with CrCL of 15–50 ml/min
	DVT, PE	(1) For prophylaxis of DVT following hip or knee replacement surgery, 10 mg once daily for 35 days (hip replacement) or 12 days (knee replacement); (2) for treating DVT or PE, 15 mg twice daily with food for the first 21 days followed by 20 mg once daily with food for the remaining treatment; (3) for reduction in the risk of recurrence of DVT and/or PE in patients at continued risk for DVT and/or PE, 10 mg once daily, after at least 6 months of standard anticoagulant treatment
Fondaparinux	DVT, PE	(1) For DVT prophylaxis in patients undergoing hip fracture, hip replacement, knee replacement surgery, or abdominal surgery, 2.5 mg subcutaneously once daily after hemostasis has been established. The initial dose should be given no earlier than 6–8 h after surgery and continued for 5–9 days. For patients undergoing hip fracture surgery, extended prophylaxis up to 24 additional days is recommended; (2) for treating DVT and PE, 5 mg (body weight <50 kg), 7.5 mg (50–100 kg), or 10 mg (>100 kg) subcutaneously once daily in patients with acute symptomatic DVT and in patients with acute symptomatic PE. Treatment should continue for at least 5 days until an INR of 2–3 achieved with warfarin (concomitant treatment with warfarin should be initiated as soon as possible, usually within 72 h)

Note: CrCL, renal creatinine clearance; DVT, deep vein thrombosis; INR, international normalized ratio; NVAF, nonvalvular atrial fibrillation; PE, pulmonary embolism; P-gp, P-glycoprotein; VTE, venous thromboembolism. Taking rivaroxaban (15 and 20 mg dose) with food leads to increased bioavailability, and as such, the drug at the above doses should be taken with meal.

2.6. Adverse Effects and Drug Interactions

2.6.1. Adverse Effects

The most common adverse effects of betrixaban and edoxaban as well as the other three SFXa inhibitors are bleeding complications, including epidural or spinal hematomas in patients who are receiving neuraxial anesthesia or undergoing spinal puncture. Edoxaban treatment may also cause rash, increased serum levels of liver enzymes, and anemia. Premature discontinuation of edoxaban, apixaban, or rivaroxaban may increase the risk of thromboembolic stroke in patients with nonvalvular atrial fibrillation (NVAF). Mild local irritation (injection site bleeding, rash, and pruritus), anemia, and thrombocytopenia may occur following subcutaneous injection of fondaparinux.

2.6.2. Drug Interactions

The shared drug interaction for all five SFXa inhibitors is that their co-administration with anticoagulants, antiplatelet drugs, and thrombolytics may increase the risk of bleeding. In addition, as summarized below, various drug interactions may also occur with different SFXa inhibitors.

2.6.2.1. BETRIXABAN AND EDOXABAN

Betrixaban is a substrate of P-glycoprotein (P-gp) and concomitant use of P-gp inhibitors (e.g., amiodarone, azithromycin, verapamil, ketoconazole, clarithromycin) results in an increased exposure to betrixaban. As such, dose reduction of betrixaban is required for patients receiving or starting concomitant P-gp inhibitors.

Edoxaban is also a substrate of P-gp; however, no dose reduction of edoxaban is recommended for concomitant P-gp inhibitor use, due to the unlikely change of edoxaban exposure in patients with concomitant P-gp inhibitor therapy (based on clinical experience from the ENGAGE AF-TIMI 48 study). On the other hand, concomitant use of edoxaban with P-gp inducers (e.g., rifampin) should be avoided due to markedly decreased drug exposure and consequent diminished efficacy.

2.6.2.2. APIXABAN, RIVAROXABAN, AND FONDAPARINUX

Since apixaban and rivaroxaban are metabolized by cytochrome P450 (CYP) enzymes and substrates of P-gp, pharmacokinetic drug interactions can be significant. In this regard, strong dual inhibitors of CYP3A4 and P-gp (e.g., ketoconazole, ritonavir, clarithromycin, erythromycin, fluconazole) increase blood levels of apixaban and rivaroxaban. On the other hand, simultaneous use of strong dual inducers of CYP3A4 and P-gp (e.g., carbamazepine, phenytoin, rifampin, St. John's wort) reduces blood levels of apixaban and rivaroxaban. In contrast to apixaban and rivaroxaban, fondaparinux does not affect CYP enzymes, and as such, pharmacokinetic drug interactions with fondaparinux are typically insignificant.

2.6.3. Contraindications and FDA Pregnancy Category

The contraindications and FDA pregnancy category of betrixaban and edoxaban, as well as the other three SFXa inhibitors are summarized in **Table 10.5**.

> **Nonvalvular atrial fibrillation (NVAF)**
> Currently, there is no universal definition for NVAF. According to the 2014 ACCF/AHA/HRS guideline (*J Am Coll Cardiol* 2014; 64:e1–e76), NVAF refers to atrial fibrillation in the absence of rheumatic mitral stenosis, a mechanical or bioprosthetic heart valve, or mitral valve repair. Conversely, valvular atrial fibrillation may be defined as atrial fibrillation in the presence of rheumatic mitral stenosis, a mechanical or bioprosthetic heart valve, or mitral valve repair.

TABLE 10.5. Contraindications and FDA pregnancy category of betrixaban, edoxaban, and other SFXa inhibitors

Drug	Contraindication	Pregnancy category
Betrixaban	(1) Active pathological bleeding; (2) severe hypersensitivity reaction to betrixaban	Not known
Edoxaban	Active pathological bleeding	Not known
Apixaban	Active pathological bleeding	B
Rivaroxaban	(1) Active pathological bleeding; (2) severe hypersensitivity reaction to rivaroxaban (e.g., anaphylactic reactions)	Not known
Fondaparinux	(1) Severe renal impairment (due to decreased clearance); (2) active major bleeding; (3) bacterial endocarditis (due to lack of benefits, see Note); (4) thrombocytopenia associated with a positive in vitro test for anti-platelet antibody in the presence of fondaparinux; (5) body weight <50 kg (VTE prophylaxis only, due to increased risk of bleeding); (6) history of serious hypersensitivity reaction (e.g., angioedema, anaphylactoid/anaphylactic reactions) to fondaparinux	Not known

Note: The available limited data do not establish a benefit from fondaparinux in reducing the risk of embolism in patients with bacterial endocarditis, and as such, this drug is contraindicated in this clinical setting. VTE, venous thromboembolism.

2.7. Comparison with Existing Members and New Development since the US FDA Approval

2.7.1. Comparison with Existing Members

Betrixaban, edoxaban, apixaban, and rivaroxaban are the oral SFXa inhibitors approved by the US FDA over the past seven years, with betrixaban approved in 2017. While betrixaban therapy is more efficacious than enoxaparin [1, 2, 6, 7], and edoxaban, apixaban, and rivaroxaban generally show better or as least similar efficacy as compared with the classical vitamin K antagonist—warfarin [8–14], direct head-to-head comparative trials of the efficacy and safety among the oral SFXa inhibitors are currently lacking. Nevertheless, indirect comparisons based on data from separate clinical trials suggest that the oral SFXa inhibitors have an overall similar efficacy in reducing the risk of stroke in patients with NVAF and in the management of VTE. Indirect comparative analyses also suggest that the major adverse effect—bleeding varies among different oral SFXa inhibitors, with apixaban showing a better safety profile [10, 13, 15–19].

2.7.2. New Development

As noted earlier, the US FDA approval of betrixaban was based on the APEX trial demonstrating increased improvement in symptomatic events including symptomatic DVT, non-fatal PE, or VTE-related death in patients who were hospitalized for acute medical ill-nesses and at high risk for VTE, as compared with standard-dose enoxaparin therapy [1]. Recently, an APEX trial substudy demon-strated that among hospitalized medically ill patients, extended-dura-tion betrixaban therapy significantly reduced all-cause stroke and ischemic stroke through 77 days of follow-up with an over 50% greater reduction than enoxaparin [2]. Even in high-risk patients with congestive heart failure or ischemic stroke, betrixaban therapy caused an approximately 25% greater reduction in all-cause stroke and is-chemic stroke than enoxaparin therapy [2]. Another APEX substudy reported that among hospitalized medically ill patients, extended-du-ration betrixaban treatment demonstrated an ~30% greater reduction in fatal or irreversible ischemic or bleeding events compared with standard enoxaparin therapy, suggesting a much better efficacy and safety profile for betrixaban [6]. More recently, a post-hoc analysis of the APEX trial also revealed that extended-duration betrixaban, compared with enoxaparin therapy, was associated with a much lower risk of VTE-related rehospitalization among acutely ill hospi-talized medical patients [7]. This finding may have important quality of life and health economic implications.

The past two years have also witnessed new developments regard-ing clinical use of edoxaban, another relatively new oral SFXa inhib-itor. One notable development is the similar efficacy and safety of edoxaban therapy and possibly other SFXa inhibitors in reducing the risk of stroke and systemic embolism in AF patients with and without valvular heart disease [20–24]. In addition, edoxaban may be as ef-fective as warfarin or dalteparin for the treatment of cancer-associ-ated VTE [25, 26]. As mentioned earlier (**Table 10.4**), according to the US FDA-approved drug labeling, edoxaban is not indicated in patients with renal creatinine clearance (CrCL) >95 ml/min due to potentially decreased efficacy and an increased risk of stroke as com-pared with warfarin. However, a post-hoc analysis of the ENGAGE AF-TIMI 48 trial suggested that although there was an apparent de-crease in relative efficacy to prevent arterial thromboembolism in the upper range of CrCL, the safety and net clinical benefit of edoxaban compared with warfarin were consistent across the range of re-nal function [27]. A post-hoc analysis of the ENSURE-AF study (edoxaban versus warfarin in subjects undergoing cardioversion of atrial fibrillation) also reported no effects of renal function on the ef-ficacy and safety of edoxaban therapy [28, 29].

As oral SFXa inhibitors may cause serious bleeding, reversal of the drug action with specific antidotes is critically important. While the US FDA has approved a monoclonal antibody fragment drug—ida-rucizumab as a specific reversal agent for dabigatran (a direct throm-bin inhibitor) [30], currently, there is no specific antidote for any of the five SFXa inhibitors [31, 32]. Several drugs are currently under development for specific reversal of SFXa inhibitor therapy, among which andexanet alfa has received much attention. Andexanet alfa is a modified recombinant factor Xa molecule (catalytically inactive) that competitively binds SFXa inhibitors, including betrixaban, edox-aban, apixaban, and rivaroxaban, and reverses the SFXa inhibitor-mediated inhibition of the native factor Xa and decreases the conse-quent major bleeding [33, 34]. Before the specific antidotes become

clinically available, prothrombin complex concentrates will continue to be the mainstay of therapy for treating patients with life-threatening bleeding due to the use of SFXa inhibitors [32].

3. SELF-ASSESSMENT QUESTIONS

3.1. A 65-year-old woman is diagnosed with deep vein thrombosis (DVT). History reveals that she has stable ischemic heart disease of 7 years of duration and diabetes of 12 years of duration, and is on a number of medications. In designing a treatment regimen for her DVT, an oral drug with less extensive drug interactions is considered as a first-line therapy. Which of the following drugs will be most likely given?

A. Apixaban
B. Betrixaban
C. Fondaparinux
D. Heparin
E. Warfarin

3.2. A 49-year-old woman with hyperlipidemia undergoes a knee replacement surgery. Following the procedure, an oral anticoagulant is given to prevent deep vein thrombosis and pulmonary embolism. Which of the following molecules is most likely the molecular target of the drug?

A. Antithrombin III
B. Factor Xa
C. HMG-CoA reductase
D. $P2Y_{12}$ receptor
E. P-Glycoprotein

3.3. In designing a treatment regimen for a 59-year-old man with nonvalvular atrial fibrillation to reduce the risk of ischemic stroke, a selective factor Xa (SFXa) inhibitor is considered as a possible candidate. If the patient's renal creatinine clearance is 100 ml/min, which of the following oral SFXa inhibitors is most unlikely prescribed in line with the US FDA-approved product labelling?

A. Apixaban
B. Dabigatran
C. Edoxaban
D. Fondaparinux
E. Rivaroxaban

3.4. A serious bleeding occurs in a 62-year-old man with deep vein thrombosis following treatment with an oral selective factor Xa inhibitor. Which of the following agents should be given to reverse the drug's action?

A. Andexanet alfa
B. Fondaparinux

C. Idarucizumab
D. Prothrombin complex concentrate
E. Warfarin

3.5. A 67-year-old woman with osteoporosis receives a pentasaccharide anticoagulant subcutaneously following a hip replacement surgery for prophylaxis of venous thromboembolism. This drug acts most likely via directly affecting the activity of which of the following molecules?

A. Antithrombin III
B. Factor IIa
C. Factor Xa
D. Protease-activated receptor-1
E. Vitamin K 2,3-epoxide reductase

ANSWERS AND EXPLANATIONS

3.1. The correct answer is A. Among the drugs listed, only apixaban, betrixaban, and warfarin are given orally. Warfarin suffers from extensive drug interactions, whereas drug interactions for apixaban and betrixaban are less extensive. Currently, betrixaban is not indicated for treating DVT.

3.2. The correct answer is B. Among the molecular targets listed, only antithrombin III and factor Xa serve as targets for anticoagulants. Antithrombin III is the molecular target for parenteral anticoagulants, such as heparins and fondaparinux. Thus, the oral drug is most likely an oral selective factor Xa inhibitor (e.g., apixaban, edoxaban, or rivaroxaban).

3.3. The correct answer is C. Among the drugs listed, only apixaban, edoxaban, and rivaroxaban are oral SFXa inhibitors. Among these three oral SFXa inhibitors, edoxaban is not indicated in patients with renal creatinine clearance >95 ml/min due to potentially decreased efficacy and an increased risk of stroke compared with warfarin. Thus, if an oral SFXa needs to be used, choose apixaban or rivaroxaban.

3.4. The correct answer is D. Currently, there is no specific antidote approved by the US FDA for reversing selective factor Xa inhibitor-associated severe bleeding. Prothrombin complex concentrate (PCC) is typically used as a reversal agent. Idarucizumab is a US FDA-approved reversal agent for dabigatran (a direct thrombin inhibitor). Andexanet alfa is currently an investigational drug with promising results from clinical trials. Fondaparinux and warfarin are themselves anticoagulants that cause bleeding.

3.5. The correct answer is A. Based on the pentasaccharide nature and the route of administration, the drug is fondaparinux. It directly stimulates the activity of antithrombin III (an inhibitor of factor Xa), and thereby indirectly causes inhibition of factor Xa. Factor IIa is the direct molecular target for direct thrombin inhibitors (e.g., dabigatran). Factor Xa is the direct molecular target for oral selective Xa inhibitors (e.g., apixaban).

REFERENCES

1. Cohen AT, Harrington RA, Goldhaber SZ, Hull RD, Wiens BL, Gold A, Hernandez AF, Gibson CM, APEX Investigators. Extended thromboprophylaxis with betrixaban in acutely ill medical patients. *N Engl J Med* 2016; 375(6):534–44.

2. Gibson CM, Chi G, Halaby R, Korjian S, Daaboul Y, Jain P, Arbetter D, Goldhaber SZ, Hull R, Hernandez AF, Gold A, Bandman O, et al. Extended-duration betrixaban reduces the risk of stroke versus standard-dose enoxaparin among hospitalized medically ill patients: an APEX trial substudy (Acute Medically Ill Venous Thromboembolism Prevention With Extended Duration Betrixaban). *Circulation* 2017; 135(7):648–55.

3. Gibson CM, Halaby R, Korjian S, Daaboul Y, Arbetter DF, Yee MK, Goldhaber SZ, Hull R, Hernandez AF, Lu SP, Bandman O, Leeds JM, et al. The safety and efficacy of full- versus reduced-dose betrixaban in the Acute Medically Ill VTE (Venous Thromboembolism) Prevention With Extended-Duration Betrixaban (APEX) trial. *Am Heart J* 2017; 185:93–100.

4. Giugliano RP, Ruff CT, Braunwald E, Murphy SA, Wiviott SD, Halperin JL, Waldo AL, Ezekowitz MD, Weitz JI, Spinar J, Ruzyllo W, Ruda M, et al. Edoxaban versus warfarin in patients with atrial fibrillation. *N Engl J Med* 2013; 369(22):2093–104.

5. Hokusai VTEI, Buller HR, Decousus H, Grosso MA, Mercuri M, Middeldorp S, Prins MH, Raskob GE, Schellong SM, Schwocho L, Segers A, Shi M, et al. Edoxaban versus warfarin for the treatment of symptomatic venous thromboembolism. *N Engl J Med* 2013; 369(15):1406–15.

6. Gibson CM, Korjian S, Chi G, Daaboul Y, Jain P, Arbetter D, Goldhaber SZ, Hull R, Hernandez AF, Lopes RD, Gold A, Cohen AT, et al. Comparison of fatal or irreversible events with extended-duration betrixaban versus standard dose enoxaparin in acutely ill medical patients: an APEX trial substudy. *J Am Heart Assoc* 2017; 6(7):e006015.

7. Chi G, Yee MK, Amin AN, Goldhaber SZ, Hernandez AF, Hull RD, Cohen AT, Harrington RA, Gibson CM. Extended-duration betrixaban reduces the risk of rehospitalization associated with venous thromboembolism among acutely ill hospitalized medical patients: findings from the APEX trial (Acute Medically Ill Venous Thromboembolism Prevention With Extended Duration Betrixaban Trial). *Circulation* 2018; 137(1):91–4.

8. Ruff CT, Giugliano RP, Braunwald E, Hoffman EB, Deenadayalu N, Ezekowitz MD, Camm AJ, Weitz JI, Lewis BS, Parkhomenko A, Yamashita T, Antman EM. Comparison of the efficacy and safety of new oral anticoagulants with warfarin in patients with atrial fibrillation: a meta-analysis of randomised trials. *Lancet* 2014; 383(9921):955–62.

9. Larsen TB, Skjoth F, Nielsen PB, Kjaeldgaard JN, Lip GY. Comparative effectiveness and safety of non-vitamin K antagonist oral anticoagulants and warfarin in patients with atrial fibrillation: propensity weighted nationwide cohort study. *BMJ* 2016; 353:i3189.

10. Hernandez I, Zhang Y, Saba S. Comparison of the effectiveness and safety of apixaban, dabigatran, rivaroxaban, and warfarin in newly diagnosed atrial fibrillation. *Am J Cardiol* 2017; 120(10):1813–9.

11. Coleman CI, Peacock WF, Bunz TJ, Alberts MJ. Effectiveness and safety of apixaban, dabigatran, and rivaroxaban versus warfarin in patients with nonvalvular atrial fibrillation and previous stroke or transient ischemic attack. *Stroke* 2017; 48(8):2142–9.

12. Jun M, Lix LM, Durand M, Dahl M, Paterson JM, Dormuth CR, Ernst P, Yao S, Renoux C, Tamim H, Wu C, Mahmud SM, et al. Comparative safety of direct oral anticoagulants and warfarin in venous thromboembolism: multicentre, population based, observational study. *BMJ* 2017; 359:j4323.

13. Lopez-Lopez JA, Sterne JAC, Thom HHZ, Higgins JPT, Hingorani AD, Okoli GN, Davies PA, Bodalia PN, Bryden PA, Welton NJ, Hollingworth W, Caldwell DM, et al. Oral anticoagulants for prevention of stroke in atrial fibrillation: systematic review, network meta-analysis, and cost effectiveness analysis. *BMJ* 2017; 359:j5058.

14. Almutairi AR, Zhou L, Gellad WF, Lee JK,

Slack MK, Martin JR, Lo-Ciganic WH. Effectiveness and safety of non-vitamin k antagonist oral anticoagulants for atrial fibrillation and venous thromboembolism: a systematic review and meta-analyses. *Clin Ther* 2017; 39(7):1456–78 e36.

15. Schneeweiss S, Gagne JJ, Patrick AR, Choudhry NK, Avorn J. Comparative efficacy and safety of new oral anticoagulants in patients with atrial fibrillation. *Circ Cardiovasc Qual Outcomes* 2012; 5(4):480–6.

16. Cohen AT, Hamilton M, Mitchell SA, Phatak H, Liu X, Bird A, Tushabe D, Batson S. Comparison of the novel oral anticoagulants apixaban, dabigatran, edoxaban, and rivaroxaban in the initial and long-term treatment and prevention of venous thromboembolism: systematic review and network meta-analysis. *PLoS One* 2015; 10(12):e0144856.

17. Cohen AT, Hamilton M, Bird A, Mitchell SA, Li S, Horblyuk R, Batson S. Comparison of the non-VKA oral anticoagulants apixaban, dabigatran, and rivaroxaban in the extended treatment and prevention of venous thromboembolism: systematic review and network meta-analysis. *PLoS One* 2016; 11(8):e0160064.

18. Noseworthy PA, Yao X, Abraham NS, Sangaralingham LR, McBane RD, Shah ND. Direct comparison of dabigatran, rivaroxaban, and apixaban for effectiveness and safety in nonvalvular atrial fibrillation. *Chest* 2016; 150(6):1302–12.

19. Ntaios G, Papavasileiou V, Makaritsis K, Vemmos K, Michel P, Lip GYH. Real-world setting comparison of nonvitamin-K antagonist oral anticoagulants versus vitamin-K Antagonists for stroke prevention in atrial fibrillation: a systematic review and meta-analysis. *Stroke* 2017; 48(9):2494–503.

20. De Caterina R, Renda G, Carnicelli AP, Nordio F, Trevisan M, Mercuri MF, Ruff CT, Antman EM, Braunwald E, Giugliano RP. Valvular heart disease patients on edoxaban or warfarin in the ENGAGE AF-TIMI 48 trial. *J Am Coll Cardiol* 2017; 69(11):1372–82.

21. Breithardt G. NOACs for stroke prevention in atrial fibrillation with valve disease: filling the gaps. *J Am Coll Cardiol* 2017; 69(11):1383–5.

22. Renda G, Ricci F, Giugliano RP, De Caterina R. Non-vitamin K antagonist oral anticoagulants in patients with atrial fibrillation and valvular heart disease. *J Am Coll Cardiol* 2017; 69(11):1363–71.

23. Pan KL, Singer DE, Ovbiagele B, Wu YL, Ahmed MA, Lee M. Effects of non-vitamin K antagonist oral anticoagulants versus warfarin in patients with atrial fibrillation and valvular heart disease: a systematic review and meta-analysis. *J Am Heart Assoc* 2017; 6(7):e005835.

24. Caldeira D, David C, Costa J, Ferreira JJ, Pinto FJ. Non-vitamin K antagonist oral anticoagulants in patients with atrial fibrillation and valvular heart disease: systematic review and meta-analysis. *Eur Heart J Cardiovasc Pharmacother* 2018 (in press).

25. Raskob GE, van Es N, Segers A, Angchaisuksiri P, Oh D, Boda Z, Lyons RM, Meijer K, Gudz I, Weitz JI, Zhang G, Lanz H, et al. Edoxaban for venous thromboembolism in patients with cancer: results from a non-inferiority subgroup analysis of the Hokusai-VTE randomised, double-blind, double-dummy trial. *Lancet Haematol* 2016; 3(8):e379–87.

26. Raskob GE, van Es N, Verhamme P, Carrier M, Di Nisio M, Garcia D, Grosso MA, Kakkar AK, Kovacs MJ, Mercuri MF, Meyer G, Segers A, et al. Edoxaban for the treatment of cancer-associated venous thromboembolism. *N Engl J Med* 2018 (in press).

27. Bohula EA, Giugliano RP, Ruff CT, Kuder JF, Murphy SA, Antman EM, Braunwald E. Impact of renal function on outcomes with edoxaban in the ENGAGE AF-TIMI 48 trial. *Circulation* 2016; 134(1):24–36.

28. Goette A, Merino JL, Ezekowitz MD, Zamoryakhin D, Melino M, Jin J, Mercuri MF, Grosso MA, Fernandez V, Al-Saady N, Pelekh N, Merkely B, et al. Edoxaban versus enoxaparin-warfarin in patients undergoing cardioversion of atrial fibrillation (ENSURE-AF): a randomised, open-label, phase 3b trial. *Lancet* 2016; 388(10055):1995–2003.

29. Lip GYH, Al-Saady N, Ezekowitz MD, Banach M, Goette A. The relationship of renal function to outcome: a post hoc analysis from the EdoxabaN versus warfarin in subjectS UndeRgoing cardiovErsion of Atrial Fibrillation (ENSURE-AF) study. *Am Heart J* 2017; 193:16–22.

30. Pollack CV, Jr., Reilly PA, van Ryn J, Eikelboom JW, Glund S, Bernstein RA, Dubiel R, Huisman MV, Hylek EM, Kam CW, Kamphuisen PW, Kreuzer J, et al. Idarucizumab for dabigatran reversal: full cohort analysis. *N Engl J Med* 2017; 377(5):431–41.

31. Ruff CT, Giugliano RP, Antman EM.

Management of bleeding with non-vitamin K antagonist oral anticoagulants in the era of specific reversal agents. *Circulation* 2016; 134(3):248–61.

32. Levy JH, Douketis J, Weitz JI. Reversal agents for non-vitamin K antagonist oral anticoagulants. *Nat Rev Cardiol* 2018 (in press).

33. Connolly SJ, Milling TJ, Jr., Eikelboom JW, Gibson CM, Curnutte JT, Gold A, Bronson MD, Lu G, Conley PB, Verhamme P, Schmidt J, Middeldorp S, et al. Andexanet alfa for acute major bleeding associated with factor Xa inhibitors. *N Engl J Med* 2016; 375(12):1131–41.

34. Siegal DM, Curnutte JT, Connolly SJ, Lu G, Conley PB, Wiens BL, Mathur VS, Castillo J, Bronson MD, Leeds JM, Mar FA, Gold A, et al. Andexanet alfa for the reversal of factor Xa inhibitor activity. *N Engl J Med* 2015; 373(25):2413–24.

UNIT V

HEART FAILURE

CHAPTER 11

Overview of Heart Failure and Drug Therapy

CHAPTER HIGHLIGHTS

- Heart failure (HF) is a complex clinical syndrome that can result from any structural or functional impairment of ventricular filling or ejection of blood. Based on the changes in left ventricular ejection fraction, HF is classified into HF with reduced ejection fraction (HFrEF), HF with preserved ejection fraction (HFpEF), and HF with mid-range ejection fraction (HFmrEF).
- While the etiology and pathophysiology of HF are complex, dysregulated activity of the sympathetic nervous system (SNS) and the renin-angiotensin-aldosterone system (RAAS) plays a critical role in the development and progression of HFrEF. In contrast, the pathophysiology of HFpEF and HFmrEF remains poorly defined.
- Effective drugs for treating HFrEF have been developed over the past decades to primarily target the SNS and RAAS, which include β-blockers, angiotensin-converting enzyme (ACE) inhibitors, angiotensin receptor blockers (ARBs), and aldosterone receptor antagonists (ARAs), as well as the newly approved angiotensin receptor-neprilysin inhibitor (ARNI) sacubitril/valsartan and the I_f channel inhibitor ivabradine.
- The drugs effective for HFrEF are largely ineffective for treating HFpEF and HFmrEF, whose management is primarily based on the treatment of symptoms and comorbidities. The high prevalence and mortality rate of HF in both developed and developing nations necessitate further investigations to develop more effective medical therapeutics including gene and stem cell therapies for this complex clinical syndrome.

KEYWORDS | Aldosterone receptor antagonist; Angiotensin receptor blocker; Angiotensin receptor-neprilysin inhibitor; Angiotensin-converting enzyme inhibitor; β-Blocker; Gene therapy; Heart failure disease-modifying drug; Heart failure symptom-relieving drug; Heart failure with mid-range ejection fraction; Heart failure with preserved ejection fraction; Heart failure with reduced ejection fraction; Heart failure; I_f channel inhibitor; Stem cell therapy

CITATION | *Li YR. Cardiovascular Medicine: New Therapeutic Drugs Approved by the US FDA (2013–2017). Cell Med Press, Raleigh, NC, USA. 2018. http://dx.doi.org/10.20455/ndcvd.2018.11*

ABBREVIATIONS | ACC, the American College of Cardiology; ACE, angiotensin-converting enzyme; AHA, the American Heart Association; AHFS, acute heart failure syndromes; ARA, aldosterone receptor antagonist; ARB, angiotensin receptor blocker; ARNI, angiotensin receptor-neprilysin inhibitor; CAD, coronary artery disease; CRT, cardiac-resynchronization therapy; ESC, the European Society of Cardiology; HF, heart failure; HFbEF, heart failure with borderline ejection fraction; HFmrEF, heart failure with mid-range ejection fraction; HFpEF, heart failure with preserved ejection fraction; HFrEF, heart failure with reduced ejection fraction; HFSA, the Heart Failure Society of America; LVEF, left ventricular ejection fraction; NYHA, the New York Heart Association; PDE5, phosphodiesterase type 5; RAAS, renin-angiotensin-aldosterone system; SGLT2, sodium-glucose cotransporter 2; SNS, sympathetic nervous system; US FDA, the United States Food and Drug Administration

CHAPTER AT A GLANCE

1. INTRODUCTION

Heart failure (HF) is a common clinical syndrome representing the end-stage of a number of different cardiac diseases. It can result from any structural or functional cardiac disorder that impairs the ability of the ventricle to fill with or eject blood. HF is a serious condition, and currently, there is no cure for it. Many people with HF may live a reasonably good quality of life when the condition is appropriately managed with evidence-based medications along with healthy lifestyle changes. This chapter provides an overview of HF, including its definitions, classifications, and epidemiology. The chapter also examines the molecular pathophysiology of HF, which serves as a basis for drug targeting and pharmacotherapy. Finally, the chapter outlines the commonly used drugs for treating HF to set a stage for the subsequent discussion of the newly approved drugs for HF in Chapter 12.

2. MOLECULAR MEDICINE OF HF

2.1. Definitions

There is no universal definition for HF. The American College of Cardiology Foundation/American Heart Association (ACCF/AHA) simply defines HF as a complex clinical syndrome that can result from any structural or functional impairment of ventricular filling or ejection of blood [1]. On the other hand, the European Society of Cardiology (ESC) defines HF comprehensively as a clinical syndrome characterized by typical symptoms (e.g., breathlessness, ankle swelling, and fatigue) that may be accompanied by signs (e.g., elevated jugular venous pressure, pulmonary crackles, and peripheral edema) caused by a structural and/or functional cardiac abnormality, resulting in a reduced cardiac output and/or elevated intracardiac pressures at rest or during stress [2]. Regardless of the comprehensiveness, both definitions confine themselves to stages at which clinical symptoms are apparent. Before clinical symptoms become apparent, patients can present with asymptomatic structural or functional cardiac abnormalities, which are considered as precursors of

HF. Recognition of these precursors is important because they are related to poor outcomes, and starting treatment at the precursor stage may more effectively reduce mortality and prolong survival [2].

As noted above, the cardinal manifestations of HF are dyspnea and fatigue (which may limit exercise tolerance) and fluid retention (which may lead to pulmonary congestion and peripheral edema). Both abnormalities can impair the functional capacity and quality of life of the affected individuals, but they do not necessarily dominate the clinical picture at the same time. It is important to note that HF is not equivalent to cardiomyopathy or to left ventricular dysfunction; these latter terms describe possible structural or functional reasons for the development of HF [1]. Instead, as aforementioned, HF is defined as a clinical syndrome characterized by specific symptoms (dyspnea and fatigue) in the medical history and signs (edema, rales) on the physical examination. There is no single diagnostic test for HF because it is largely a clinical diagnosis that is based on a careful history and physical examination along with cardiac imaging and other diagnostic tests [1, 2].

2.2. Classifications

HF can be classified in various ways [3, 4]. The classification schemes may be based on the time-course of the syndrome, the systolic or diastolic function, the side of the heart involved, the left ventricular ejection fraction, and the severity of the symptoms and others.

2.2.1. Classification Based on the Time Course

Based on the time course of the disease process, HF is classified into acute and chronic HF. Patients who have had HF for some time are often said to have chronic HF. A treated patient with symptoms and signs, which have remained generally unchanged for at least a month, is said to be stable. If chronic stable HF deteriorates, the patient may be described as decompensated and this may happen suddenly, i.e., acutely, usually leading to hospital admission, an event of considerable prognostic importance.

New (de novo) HF may present acutely, for example, as a consequence of acute myocardial infarction or in a subacute (gradual) fashion, such as in a patient who has had asymptomatic cardiac dysfunction, often for an indeterminate period, and may persist or resolve (patients may become compensated). Acute HF is not a single disease, but rather a family of related disorders. Hence, the term "acute HF syndromes" (AHFS) is commonly used in the literature and clinical practice to describe these acute conditions. AHFS is defined as the new onset or recurrence of gradually or rapidly developing syndromes and signs of HF requiring urgent or emergent therapy and resulting in hospitalization [1].

2.2.2. Classification Based on the Side of the Heart

Based on the side of the heart affected, HF is classified into left-sided and right-sided HF. In left-sided or left ventricular HF, the ability of the left ventricle to fill with or eject blood is impaired. There are two

Cardiomyopathy

Cardiomyopathies are a heterogeneous group of diseases of the myocardium associated with mechanical and/or electrical dysfunction that usually (but not invariably) exhibit inappropriate ventricular hypertrophy or dilatation and are due to a variety of causes that frequently are genetic. Cardiomyopathies either are confined to the heart or are part of generalized systemic disorders, often leading to cardiovascular death or progressive heart failure-related disability. Cardiomyopathies are divided into two major groups based on predominant organ involvement: (1) primary cardiomyopathies (genetic, nongenetic, acquired) are those solely or predominantly confined to heart muscle and are relatively few in number; and (2) secondary cardiomyopathies show pathological myocardial involvement as part of a large number and variety of generalized systemic (multiorgan) disorders (AHA scientific statement: contemporary definitions and classification of the cardiomyopathies. *Circulation* 2006; 113:1807-1816).

types of left-sided HF: systolic and diastolic HF (see Section 2.2.3 below). Right-sided or right ventricular HF usually occurs as a result of left-sided HF. When the left ventricle fails, increased fluid pressure is, in effect, transferred back through the lungs, ultimately damaging the heart's right side. When the right side loses pumping power, blood backs up in the body's veins. This usually causes swelling in the legs and ankles.

2.2.3. Classification Based on the Systolic or Diastolic Function

Based on the impairment of systolic or diastolic function, HF is classified into systolic and diastolic HF. In systolic HF, the left ventricle loses its ability to contract normally. The heart cannot pump with sufficient force to push enough blood into circulation, and hence, the left ventricular ejection fraction (LVEF) is reduced. On the other hand, in diastolic HF, the left ventricle loses its ability to relax normally because the muscle has become stiff. As such, the heart cannot properly fill with blood during the resting period between each beat, and the LVEF is preserved or normal.

2.2.4. Classification Based on the Left Ventricular Ejection Fraction

Based on the LVEF, HF is classified into three types: (1) HF with reduced ejection fraction (HFrEF); (2) HF with preserved ejection fraction (HFpEF); and (3) HF with mid-range ejection fraction (HFmrEF) (**Table 11.1**). HFrEF is typically defined as the clinical diagnosis of HF and LVEF <40% (or <0.4). HFrEF is seen in systolic HF, and thus, it is also loosely referred to as systolic HF in the literature and medical practice. HFpEF is typically defined as clinical diagnosis of HF and LVEF ≥50% (or ≥0.5). HFpEF is seen in diastolic HF, and as such, it is also loosely referred to as diastolic HF. HFmrEF is also known as HF with borderline ejection fraction (HFbEF) and defined as clinical diagnosis of HF with LVEF ranging from 40% to 49% (or 0.4 to 0.49) [1, 2]. The exact proportion of the above three types of HF remains to be defined. It is estimated that HFrEF and HFpEF each accounts for ~46% and HFmrEF for the remaining ~8% of all HF cases, and that all the three types of HF have a similarly poor 5-year survival with a median survival of 2.1 years [5]. Although there are effective disease-modifying drugs (i.e., drugs that retard disease progression and reduce mortality) for patients with HFrEF (see below), no drugs thus far show measurable survival benefits in patients with HFpEF [5, 6]. Likewise, effective drug therapies for HFmrEF remain to be established [5, 7, 8].

2.2.5. Classification Based on the Severity of the Symptoms

HF is frequently classified based on the severity of the patients' symptoms and functional limitations. **Table 11.2** below outlines the most commonly used classification system—the New York Heart Association (NYHA) functional classification. It places patients in one of four categories (classes I–IV) based on how much they are limited during physical activity.

TABLE 11.1. Definition and characteristics of HFrEF, HFpEF, and HFmrEF

HF	LVEF	Proportion	Also (loosely) known as
HFrEF	<40%	~46%	Systolic HF
HFpEF	≥50%	~46%	Diastolic HF
HFmrEF	40–49%	~8%	HF with borderline ejection fraction (HFbEF)

TABLE 11.2. The NYHA functional classification of HF

NYHA class	Description
Class I (mild)	No limitation of physical activity; ordinary physical activity does not cause undue fatigue, palpitation, or dyspnea
Class II (mild)	Slight limitation of physical activity; comfortable at rest, but ordinary physical activity results in fatigue, palpitation, or dyspnea
Class III (moderate)	Marked limitation of physical activity; comfortable at rest, but less than ordinary activity results in fatigue, palpitation, or dyspnea
Class IV (severe)	Unable to carry on any physical activity without discomfort; symptoms present at rest, and if any physical activity is undertaken, discomfort is increased

TABLE 11.3. The ACC/AHA stage classification of HF and its relationship to the NYHA functional classification

ACC/AHA stage	Description	Equivalent to NYHA class
Stage A	At high risk for HF; no identified structural or functional abnormality; no signs or symptoms	None
Stage B	Structural heart disease but without signs or symptoms of HF	Class I
Stage C	Structural heart disease with prior or current signs or symptoms of HF	Classes II–IV
Stage D	Advanced structural heart disease and marked symptoms of HF at rest despite maximal medical therapy; refractory HF requiring specialized interventions	Class IV

2.2.6. The ACC/AHA Stage Classification

The American College of Cardiology (ACC) and AHA jointly released a guideline for the evaluation and management of chronic HF in 2001, in which a new classification system was first described, which is now commonly known as the ACC/AHA stage classification. As outlined in **Table 11.3**, HF is classified into four stages (A–D);

however, only stages C and D qualify for the traditional clinical diagnosis of HF. The ACC/AHA stage classification system was developed to emphasize both the evolution and the progression of chronic HF and to implement early preventive and therapeutic interventions to ultimately reduce HF morbidity and mortality [9]. The AHA/ACC stage classification system is intended to complement rather than replace the NYHA functional classification.

2.2.7. Congestive HF

In addition to the above terminologies on HF, another term that is sometimes still used, particularly in the United States, is congestive HF. This term may describe acute or chronic HF with evidence of congestion (i.e., sodium and water retention). Because of HF, blood flowing out of the heart slows down and blood returning to the heart through the veins backs up, causing congestion in the body's tissues, which is manifested as peripheral edema (e.g., edema in the legs and ankles). Sometimes fluid collects in the lungs and interferes with breathing, causing shortness of breath, especially when a person is lying down. This is known as pulmonary edema, and if left untreated, can cause respiratory distress. HF also affects the kidneys' ability to dispose of sodium and water. This retained water further aggravates edema in the body's tissues. Because some patients present without signs or symptoms of volume overload, the term "heart failure" is preferred over "congestive HF" [1]. Indeed, regardless of the presence or absence of congestion, HF patients should receive evidence-based therapies to retard the underlying disease progression and thereby prolong survival.

2.3. Epidemiology

HF is a major global public health issue [10–14] and it was estimated to affect ~38 million people worldwide [15, 16]. Approximately 1–2% of the population in developed countries has HF with the prevalence rising to 10% or more among persons 70 years of age and older [3]. There are many causes of HF, and these vary in different parts of the world. The most common cause of HF is ischemic heart disease (myocardial infarction). Other causes include dilated cardiomyopathies, familial cardiomyopathies, diabetic cardiomyopathy, and toxic cardiomyopathy. The major risk factors for HF include hypertension, diabetes, metabolic syndrome, and atherosclerotic cardiovascular diseases [1, 11, 17–19].

As noted earlier, about one half of the patients with HF have a low LVEF (i.e., HFrEF). HFrEF is the best understood type of HF in terms of pathophysiology and treatment, and is also the focus of the current guidelines on HF management. Coronary artery disease (CAD) is the cause of approximately two-thirds of all cases of HFrEF, although hypertension and diabetes are probable contributing factors in many cases. On the other hand, HFpEF seems to have a different epidemiological and etiological profile from HFrEF. Patients with HFpEF are older and more often female and obese than those with HFrEF. They are less likely to have CAD and more likely to have hypertension and atrial fibrillation. Indeed, hypertension remains the most important cause of HFpEF, with a prevalence of 60% to 89% from large controlled clinical trials, epidemiological studies, and HF registries [1].

In the United States, it is estimated that ~6.5 million Americans ≥20 years of age have HF. Projections show that the prevalence of HF will increase 46% from 2012 to 2030, resulting in >8 million people ≥18 years of age with HF [19]. Currently, there are 960,000 new HF cases annually in the United States, and the incidence approaches 2.1% of the population after 65 years of age. Overall, at age 45 years through age 95 years, the lifetime risks of developing HF range from 20% to 45%. Survival after HF diagnosis has improved over time along with declining risk of sudden death [20]. However, the death rate remains high: ~50% of people diagnosed with HF will die within 5 years. The number of any mention deaths attributable to HF was estimated to be 309,000 in 2014. HF is not only highly prevalent, but also highly costly. The total costs for HF were estimated to be $30.7 billion in 2012. Projections show that by 2030, the total costs of HF will increase almost 127% to ~$70 billion from 2012 [19]. Hence, HF is also a major issue of public health in the United States.

2.4. Pathophysiology

2.4.1. Pathophysiology of HFrEF

The mechanisms of HF, especially HFrEF have been investigated from a variety of perspectives during the past several decades [12, 21]. The pathophysiological process of HFrEF is typically initiated by a primary myocardial injury, most commonly myocardial infarction. This injury results in left ventricular systolic dysfunction. In patients with left ventricular systolic dysfunction, the maladaptive changes occurring in surviving myocytes and extracellular matrix after myocardial injury lead to pathological remodeling of the ventricle with dilatation and impaired contractility, one measure of which is a reduced LVEF [3, 22]. What characterizes untreated systolic dysfunction is progressive worsening of these changes over time, with increasing enlargement of the left ventricle and decline in LVEF, even though the patient may be symptomless initially. Two mechanisms are thought to account for this progression. The first is occurrence of further events leading to additional cardiomyocyte death (e.g., recurrent myocardial infarction). The other is the systemic responses induced by the decline in systolic function (i.e., a decreased cardiac output), especially the activation of the sympathetic nervous system (SNS) and the renin-angiotensin-aldosterone system (RAAS) (**Figure 11.1**).

The above neurohumoral adaptations, in the form of activation of the RAAS and SNS due to decreased cardiac output, can temporarily contribute to maintenance of perfusion of vital organs in two ways: (1) maintenance of systemic pressure by vasoconstriction, resulting in redistribution of blood flow to vital organs; and (2) restoration of cardiac output by increasing myocardial contractility and heart rate and by expansion of the extracellular fluid volume. Although some of the responses are initially compensatory, they eventually contribute to the further worsening of heart function and disease progression,

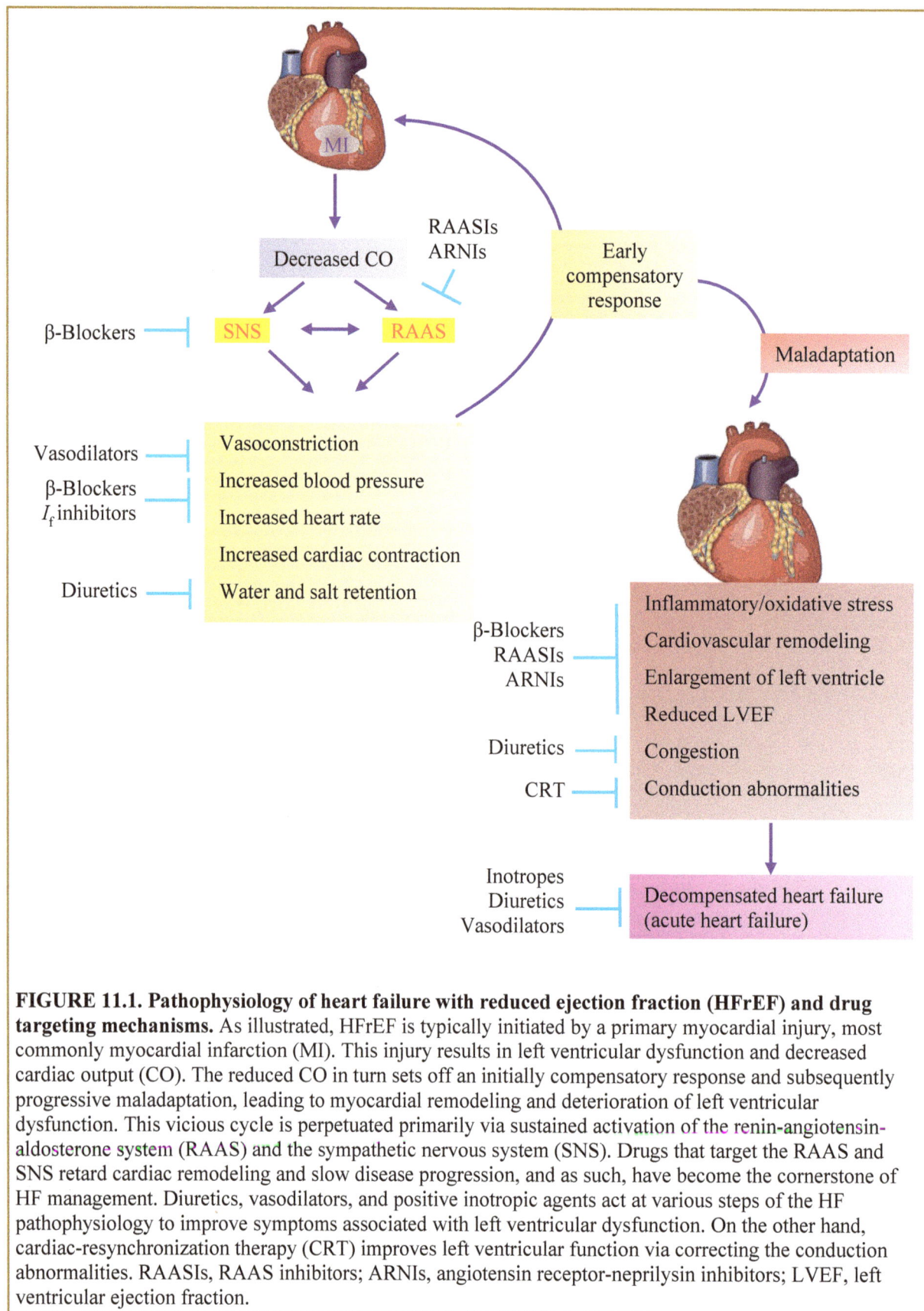

FIGURE 11.1. Pathophysiology of heart failure with reduced ejection fraction (HFrEF) and drug targeting mechanisms. As illustrated, HFrEF is typically initiated by a primary myocardial injury, most commonly myocardial infarction (MI). This injury results in left ventricular dysfunction and decreased cardiac output (CO). The reduced CO in turn sets off an initially compensatory response and subsequently progressive maladaptation, leading to myocardial remodeling and deterioration of left ventricular dysfunction. This vicious cycle is perpetuated primarily via sustained activation of the renin-angiotensin-aldosterone system (RAAS) and the sympathetic nervous system (SNS). Drugs that target the RAAS and SNS retard cardiac remodeling and slow disease progression, and as such, have become the cornerstone of HF management. Diuretics, vasodilators, and positive inotropic agents act at various steps of the HF pathophysiology to improve symptoms associated with left ventricular dysfunction. On the other hand, cardiac-resynchronization therapy (CRT) improves left ventricular function via correcting the conduction abnormalities. RAASIs, RAAS inhibitors; ARNIs, angiotensin receptor-neprilysin inhibitors; LVEF, left ventricular ejection fraction.

creating a pathophysiologically vicious cycle, accounting for many of the clinical features of the HF syndrome [3]. Interruption of the above processes, especially the SNS and the RAAS, is thus the basis of much of the effective treatment of systolic HF [21, 23]. In this context, as discussed next, the mainstay of therapy of HFrEF includes the use of β-blockers and the RAAS inhibitors (**Figure 11.1**).

Clinically, the aforementioned changes are associated with the development of symptoms and worsening of the symptoms over time. In this regard, the elevation in diastolic pressures of the failing heart is transmitted to the atria and to the pulmonary and systemic venous circulations, and the ensuing elevation in capillary pressures promotes the development of pulmonary congestion and peripheral edema. On the other hand, the increase in left ventricular afterload induced by the rise in peripheral resistance can both directly depress cardiac function and enhance the rate of deterioration of myocardial function via pathological remodeling. Moreover, activation of the RAAS and the SNS results in inflammatory and oxidative stress, contributing to pathological cardiac remodeling. Collectively, these deleterious effects due to maladaptation cause diminished quality of life, declining functional capacity, episodes of frank decompensation leading to hospital admission (which is often recurrent and costly to health services), and premature death, usually due to pump failure or a ventricular arrhythmia. The acute decompensated HF necessitates the use of (1) positive inotropic agents to augment myocardial contractility and hence improve cardiac output and the perfusion of vital organs, and (2) diuretics to alleviate edema, especially pulmonary edema, thereby reducing pulmonary congestion and alleviating dyspnea (**Figure 11.1**).

The limited cardiac reserve of such patients is also dependent on atrial contraction, synchronized contraction of the left ventricle, and a normal interaction between the right and left ventricles. Intercurrent events affecting any of these including the development of atrial fibrillation or conduction abnormalities (such as left bundle branch block) or imposing an additional hemodynamic load on the failing heart (e.g., anemia) can lead to acute decompensation. Indeed, HF patients frequently have conduction abnormalities which further aggravate left vetricular dysfunction. The established efficacy of cardiac-resynchronization therapy (CRT) in HF is consistent with the above electro-pathophysiological concept [24–27] (**Figure 11.1**).

2.4.2. Pathophysiology of HFpEF

HFpEF is estimated to account for about 50% of all HF cases (**Table 11.1**), and the prevalence and hospitalization related to HFpEF are rising. Indeed, HFpEF is increasing out of proportion to HFrEF, and its prognosis is worsening while that of HFrEF is improving. The health and economic impact of HFpEF is at least as great as that of HFrEF, with similar severity of chronic exercise intolerance, acute hospitalization rates, and substantial mortality [6, 28, 29].

In contrast to HFrEF, to date, there are no approved therapies to reduce hospitalization or mortality for HFpEF, largely due to the pathophysiological heterogeneity that exists within the broad spectrum of HFpEF. This syndrome was historically considered to be caused exclusively by left ventricular diastolic dysfunction due to hypertrophy and other remodeling processes that result in left ventricular stiffness. However, recent research has identified multiple other contributory factors, including: (1) decreased left ventricular systolic reserve; (2) systemic and pulmonary vascular dysfunction; (3) endothelial dysfunction, decreased nitric oxide bioavailability, and increased arterial stiffness; and (4) decreased right heart function and left atrial function [30, 31].

Multiple individual mechanisms frequently coexist within the same patient to cause symptomatic HF, but between patients with HFpEF, the extent to which each component is operative can differ widely, further confounding treatment approaches. In line with this notion, clinical trials on HFpEF therapies have been largely unsuccessful. These include the trials on RAAS inhibitors, digoxin, β-blockers, and phosphodiesterase type 5 (PDE5) inhibitors (e.g., sildenafil) [29]. Because of the lack of specific treatment, the management of HFpEF is currently limited to diuretics and treatment of comorbidities [29, 32].

2.4.3. Pathophysiology of HFmrEF

HFmrEF and HFbEF may be used interchangeably to refer to a subset of HF patients who belong to neither HFrEF nor HFpEF. HFbEF was first defined in 2013 in the ACC/AHA guideline as the presence of the typical symptoms of HF and a LVEF of 41–49% [1]. In 2016, the ESC proposed the term HFmrEF and defined it as LVEF of 40–49% [2]. HFmrEF is less well studied compared with HFrEF and HFpEF. Identifying HFmrEF as a separate group will stimulate research into the underlying molecular pathophysiology and treatment of this group of HF patients. Patients with HFmrEF most probably have primarily mild systolic dysfunction, but with features of diastolic dysfunction as well [1, 2].

3. OVERVIEW OF MECHANISTICALLY BASED DRUG THERAPY

Drugs for treating HF may be broadly classified into two categories (**Figure 11.2**): (1) symptom-relieving drugs and (2) disease-modifying drugs. Symptom-relieving drugs refer to those that are typically used on a short-term basis for simply alleviating the patient's symptoms (e.g., apnea caused by pulmonary congestion) and other phenotypes (e.g., peripheral edema, hypotension). These drugs primarily include diuretics and positive inotropic agents. Symptom-relieving drugs may reduce hospital admission and improve the quality of life of the HF patients, but they are generally considered to be incapable of reducing the mortality or prolonging survival, likely due to the inability of these drugs to retard the underlying disease progression. On the other hand, the disease-modifying drugs for HF target the fundamental pathophysiological processes of the disease, especially the heightened activities of the SNS and RAAS, and as such, are able to retard the disease progression and prolong patient's survival. Currently, the disease-modifying drugs for HF include β-blockers, angiotensin-converting enzyme (ACE) inhibitors, angiotensin receptor blockers (ARBs), and aldosterone receptor antagonists (ARAs), as well as the most recently developed angiotensin receptor-neprilysin inhibitors (ARNIs) [33]. The combination of isosorbide dinitrate and hydralazine (Bidil) is also effective in reducing the mortality in HF patients of African heritage [34, 35].

As discussed earlier, the efficacy of the HF disease-modifying drugs has been established only for HFrEF. Hence, this section primarily focuses on describing the mechanistically based drug therapy for HFrEF. Some recent promising findings on drug therapy of HFpEF are also introduced. It is worth mentioning that although many of the disease-modifying drugs lack the immediate action of alleviating the symptoms and congestion in HF patients, by retarding the disease process these drugs in the long run certainly contribute to the improvement of the symptoms and overall quality of life in addition to the prolongation of survival in patients with HFrEF.

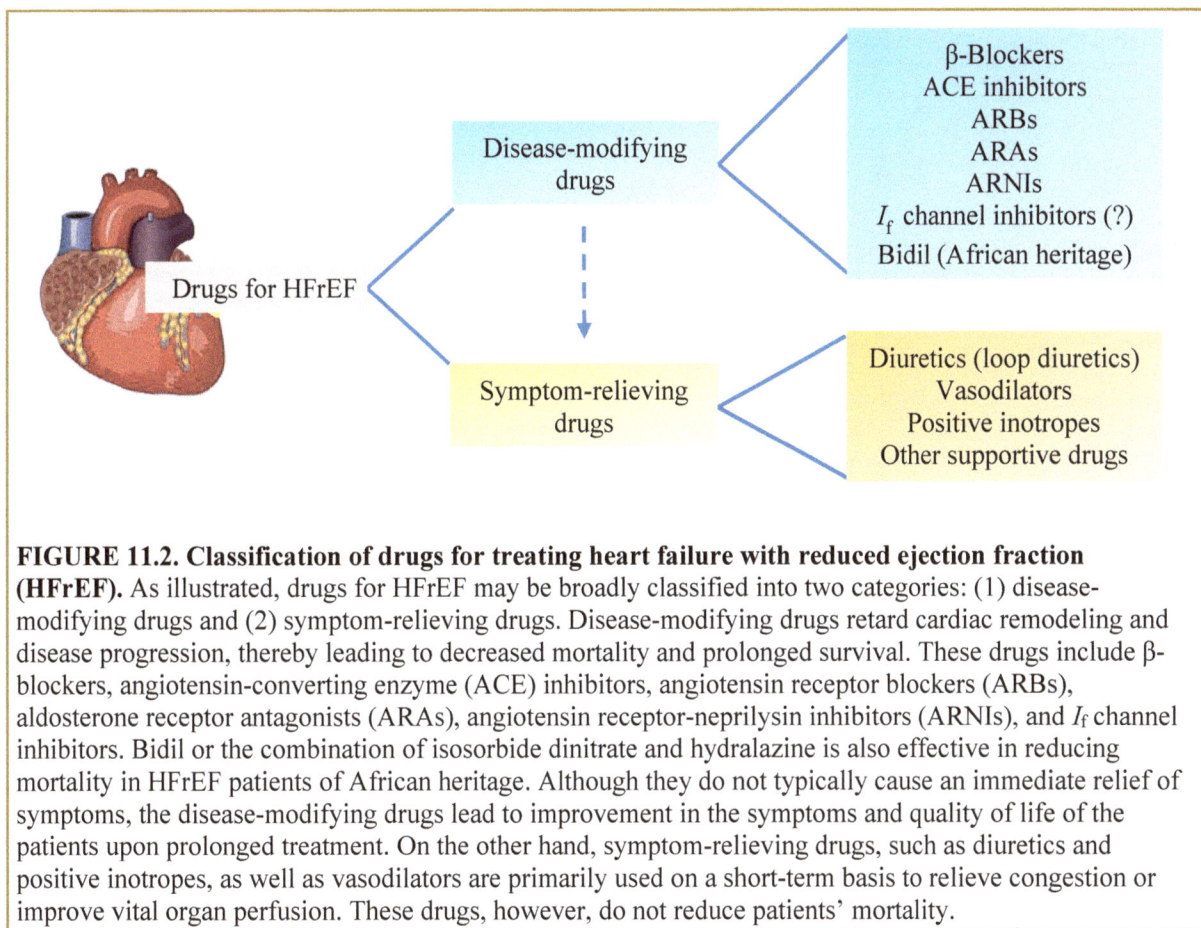

FIGURE 11.2. Classification of drugs for treating heart failure with reduced ejection fraction (HFrEF). As illustrated, drugs for HFrEF may be broadly classified into two categories: (1) disease-modifying drugs and (2) symptom-relieving drugs. Disease-modifying drugs retard cardiac remodeling and disease progression, thereby leading to decreased mortality and prolonged survival. These drugs include β-blockers, angiotensin-converting enzyme (ACE) inhibitors, angiotensin receptor blockers (ARBs), aldosterone receptor antagonists (ARAs), angiotensin receptor-neprilysin inhibitors (ARNIs), and I_f channel inhibitors. Bidil or the combination of isosorbide dinitrate and hydralazine is also effective in reducing mortality in HFrEF patients of African heritage. Although they do not typically cause an immediate relief of symptoms, the disease-modifying drugs lead to improvement in the symptoms and quality of life of the patients upon prolonged treatment. On the other hand, symptom-relieving drugs, such as diuretics and positive inotropes, as well as vasodilators are primarily used on a short-term basis to relieve congestion or improve vital organ perfusion. These drugs, however, do not reduce patients' mortality.

3.1. Overview of Disease-Modifying Drugs for HFrEF

Table 11.4 summarizes the currently available disease-modifying drugs for HFrEF and their US FDA approval date and major pharmacological/clinical effects in the management of HFrEF.

TABLE 11.4. Disease-modifying drugs for treating HFrEF

Drug	FDA approval date	Pharmacological/clinical effects and others
β-Blockers		
Bisoprolol (Zebeta)	July 1992	(1) By suppressing the heightened SNS activity and cardiac remodeling, β-blockers lessen symptoms, improve quality of life, and reduce mortality in patients with HFrEF; (2) bisoprolol, carvedilol, and sustained-release metoprolol succinate are the only β-blockers approved by the US FDA for treating HFrEF and recommended by the ACC/AHA and the ESC guidelines [1, 2]
Carvedilol (Coreg)	September 1995	
Metoprolol succinate-ER (Toprol XL)	January 1992	
Angiotensin-converting enzyme (ACE) inhibitors		
Captopril (Capoten)	Prior to January 1, 1982	(1) ACE inhibitors decrease ACE-catalyzed conversion of angiotensin I to angiotensin II and suppress cardiac remodeling. These drugs can reduce the risk of death and decrease hospitalization in patients with HFrEF; (2) the benefits of ACE inhibitor therapy are seen in patients with mild, moderate, or severe symptoms of HFrEF and in patients with or without coronary artery disease; (3) the listed eight members are the only ACE inhibitors approved by the US FDA for treating HFrEF and recommended by the ACC/AHA and the ESC guidelines [1, 2]
Enalapril (Vasotec)	February 1988	
Fosinopril (Monopril)	May 1991	
Lisinopril (Prinivil, Zestril)	December 1987	
Perindopril (Aceon)	December 1993	
Quinapril (Accupril)	November 1991	
Ramipril (Altace)	January 1991	
Trandolapril (Mavik)	April 1996	
Angiotensin receptor blockers (ARBs)		
Candesartan (Atacand)	June 1998	(1) ARBs block angiotensin II type 1 (AT-1) receptor-mediated cardiovascular adverse effects including cardiac remodeling, and these drugs reduce hospitalization and mortality in patients with HFrEF; (2) candesartan and valsartan are the only ARBs approved by the US FDA for treating HFrEF; (3) although not approved by the US FDA for HFrEF, losartan is also widely used for treating HFrEF and recommended by the ACC/AHA and the ESC guidelines [1, 2]
Losartan (Cozaar)	April 1995	
Valsartan (Diovan)	December 1996	
Aldosterone receptor antagonists (ARAs)		
Eplerenone (Inspra)	September 2002	(1) By blocking aldosterone receptors (also known as mineralocorticoid receptors), ARAs suppress aldosterone-mediated cardiovascular adverse effects, including cardiac remodeling, and these drugs reduce hospitalization and mortality in patients with HFrEF; (2) ARAs may cause hyperkalemia, and as such, caution should be exercised when these drugs are used in patients with impaired renal function and in those with serum potassium levels >5.0 mM [1, 2]
Spironolactone (Aldactone)	Prior to January 1, 1982	

TABLE 11.4. (*continued*)

Drug	FDA approval date	Pharmacological/clinical effects and others
Angiotensin receptor-neprilysin inhibitors (ARNIs)		
Sacubitril/valsartan (Entresto)	July 2015	(1) ARNIs represent a newly developed drug class for treating HFrEF, and Entresto is the first-in-class member and a fixed-dose combination of equal molar sacubitril and valsartan (also see Chapter 12); (2) sacubitril inhibits neprilysin, an enzyme responsible for degrading vasoprotective peptides, such as the natriuretic peptide system, whereas valsartan is an ARB blocking angiotensin II type 1 receptors; (3) Entresto therapy is more effective than ACE inhibitor therapy in reducing hospitalization and mortality in patients with HFrEF [2]
I_f channel inhibitors		
Ivabradine (Corlanor)	April 2015	(1) I_f channel inhibitors represent a newly developed drug class for HFrEF, and ivabradine is the first-in-class member (also see Chapter 12); (2) ivabradine slows the heart rate via inhibiting the I_f channels in the pacemaker cells of the sinus node (also known as the sinoatrial node), and the drug can reduce hospitalization and possibly improve survival in patients with HFrEF and with a resting heart rate ≥70 beats per minute
Isosorbide dinitrate and hydralazine		
Fixed-dose combination (Bidil)	June 2005	(1) Isosorbide dinitrate is a venodilator whereas hydralazine primarily causes arterial vasodilation; (2) addition of isosorbide dinitrate/hydralazine to standard therapy (β-blocker, ACE inhibitor, and ARA) further reduces hospitalization and mortality in black patients with HFrEF; (3) the efficacy of isosorbide dinitrate/hydralazine in treating HFrEF in patients among other ethical groups remains to be established; (4) Bidil is more convenient for administration as two drugs are combined in one pill
Isosorbide dinitrate (Isordil) and hydralazine (Apresoline)	September 1986 (isosorbide dinitrate); prior to January 1, 1982 (hydralazine)	

3.2. Overview of Symptom-Relieving Drugs for HFrEF

The major symptom-improving drugs for HFrEF and their US FDA approval date and major pharmacological/clinical effects are summarized in **Table 11.5**.

3.3. Overview of Drugs for HFpEF and HFmrEF

In contrast to HFrEF, there are currently no specific therapies for HFpEF. Randomized controlled trials using comparable and efficacious agents for HFrEF have generally been disappointing when used in patients with HFpEF [6, 29, 30, 32, 36–39]. Current treatment of HFpEF remains largely empirical and focuses on the management of

TABLE 11.5. Major symptom-relieving drugs for HFrEF

Drug	FDA approval date	Pharmacological/clinical effects
Diuretics (loop diuretics)		
Bumetanide (Bumex)	February 1983	(1) Loop diuretics are potent diuretic drugs used to reduce the signs and symptoms of congestion (e.g., pulmonary edema and peripheral edema) in patients with HFrEF, but their effects on morbidity and mortality have not been established; (2) besides loop diuretics, the less potent thiazide diuretics (e.g., hydrochlorothiazide, metolazone, and indapamide) may also be used in patients with mild congestion
Furosemide (Lasix)	Prior to January 1, 1982	
Torsemide (Demadex)	August 1993	
Positive inotropic agents		
Digoxin (Lanoxin)	Prior to January 1, 1982	(1) Digoxin inhibits Na^+/K^+-ATPase, causing increased cytosolic Ca^{2+} in cardiomyocytes and consequently augmented contractility; (2) digoxin can alleviate the symptoms, increase exercise tolerance, and decrease the rate of hospitalization, but it does not prolong survival in patients with HFrEF; (2) besides digoxin, there are several other positive inotropic agents (e.g., dobutamine, dopamine, norepinephrine, milrinone), and these drugs are used only for short-term support of circulation in hypotensive patients with HFrEF to improve vital organ perfusion
Vasodilators		
Nitroglycerin (Nitrostat)	Prior to January 1, 1982	(1) Nitroglycerine, isosorbide dinitrate, and nitroprusside all give rise to nitric oxide, a cardiovascular protective molecule; (2) nesiritide is a recombinant human B-type natriuretic peptide; (3) vasodilators reduce cardiac preload and/or afterload, improving the symptoms of patients with acute heart failure, and they are used on a short-term basis
Isosorbide dinitrate (Isordil)	September 1986	
Nitroprusside (Nitropress)	Prior to January 1, 1982	
Nesiritide (Natrecor)	August 2001	

symptoms and comorbidities as well as risk factor modifications. These include : (1) control of systolic and diastolic hypertension; (2) control of ventricular rate in patients with atrial fibrillation; (3) control of pulmonary congestion and peripheral edema with diuretics and nitrates; and (4) treatment of myocardial ischemia (including coronary revascularization) and control of diabetes to prevent left ventricular remodeling that predisposes to diastolic dysfunction and increased ventricular stiffness [1, 2].

As HFpEF and HFmrEF together account for over 50% of all HF cases (**Table 11.1**), increasing attention has recently been drawn on developing specific drug therapies for them. In this context, the post-hoc analyses of the multinational TOPCAT (Treatment of Preserved Cardiac Function Heart Failure With an Aldosterone Antagonist) trial suggested an efficacy (a 17% reduction of a combined endpoint of death, aborted cardiac death, and HF hospitalization) for spironolactone in patients with HFpEF in the Americas, but not in the Russia/Georgia [40]. A recent small trial showed that spironolactone also improved exercise tolerance in patients with HFpEF [41]. More recently, a large-scale trial, known as Spironolactone Initiation Registry Randomized Interventional Trial in Heart Failure with Preserved Ejection Fraction (SPIRRIT) has been initiated involving ~3,500 patients with HFpEF to further determine the efficacy for aldosterone antagonism in treating HFpEF (https://clinicaltrials.gov/ct2/show/NCT02901184). In view of the existing data suggesting a potential efficacy, the 2017 ACC/AHA/HFSA updated guideline recommends that in appropriately selected patients with HFpEF (with LVEF ≥45%, elevated B-type natriuretic peptide levels or HF admission within one year, estimated glomerular filtration rate >30 ml/min, creatinine <2.5 mg/dl, potassium <5.0 mM), ARAs might be considered to decrease hospitalizations [42].

Currently, there is no evidence supporting an efficacy for β-blocker therapy (i.e., bisoprolol, carvedilol, metoprolol succinate) in treating HFpEF. Several clinical trials with nebivolol, a unique β-blocker that also increases nitric oxide production in cardiovascular system, demonstrated that in older patients with HFrEF, HFpEF, or HFmrEF, nebivolol treatment reduced the combined endpoint of death and cardiovascular hospitalization, and such an efficacy was independent of LVEF [43–46].

3.4. Overview of Emerging Medical Therapies for HF

As discussed above, the management of HF, especially HFrEF, has been advanced substantially over the past two decades due to a better understanding of the underlying pathophysiology and the development of mechanistically based therapies with β-blockers, RAAS inhibitors, and ARNIs, among others. However, the 5-year-mortality rate of HF patients remains unacceptably high, and furthermore, specific medical therapies for HFpEF or HFmrEF are currently lacking. This has necessitated the continued searching for more effective therapeutic modalities for HF patients. In this context, as described below, a number of novel pharmacological agents for HF have emerged and undergone randomized controlled clinical trials, yielding promising results.

3.4.1. Sildenafil

Sildenafil is a PDE5 inhibitor that is effective for treating erectile dysfunction and pulmonary arterial hypertension (also see Chapter 6). This PDE5 inhibitor was found to also improve functional capacity and clinical status in patients with HFrEF [47, 48], but not in patients with HFpEF [38, 49, 50].

3.4.2. Serelaxin

Serelaxin is a recombinant form of human relaxin-2, a vasoactive peptide hormone with many biological and hemodynamic effects, including vasodilation and stimulation of myocardial contraction [51].

The RELAX-AHF trial demonstrated that serelaxin treatment of patients with acute HF (with either preserved or reduced ejection fraction) was well-tolerated and associated with dyspnea relief and improvement in other clinical outcomes, including reduced mortality irrespective of ejection fraction [52–54]. RELAX-AHF-2 trial has been recently initiated to confirm the aforementioned serelaxin's efficacy in acute HF. RELAX-AHF-2 is a multicenter, randomized, double-blind, placebo-controlled, event-driven, phase 3 trial enrolling ~6,800 patients hospitalized for acute HF, and the results of the trial will provide data on the potential beneficial effect of serelaxin on cardiovascular mortality and worsening HF in selected patients with acute HF [55].

3.4.3. Interleukin-1 Inhibitors

Inflammatory stress plays a central role in cardiovascular diseases including acute coronary syndromes (ACS) (see Chapter 8) and HF [56–59]. Pilot clinical trials suggested an efficacy for interleukin-1 blockade by anakinra in improving the clinical outcomes in patients with recently decompensated systolic HF [60] as well as in reducing systemic inflammation and improving exercise capacity in patients with HFpEF [61].

3.4.4. Nitric Oxide-Based Therapies

Nitric oxide signaling has pleiotropic roles in biology and a crucial function in cardiovascular homeostasis, and enhancing nitric oxide signaling serves as an important therapeutic strategy for diverse cardiovascular disorders [62, 63]. Results from multiple small-scale clinical trials showed that acute sodium nitrite infusion or inhaled sodium nitrite favorably attenuated hemodynamic derangements of cardiac failure that developed at rest and/or during exercise in patients with HFpEF [64, 65]. It is noteworthy that nitrite can be converted into nitric oxide. In addition to nitrite, pilot clinical trials demonstrated that inorganic nitrate (which can be converted into nitrite by bacteria in the gastrointestinal system) also improved the exercise capacity and quality of life in patients with HFpEF [66, 67].

3.4.5. Sodium-Glucose Cotransporter 2 (SGLT2) Inhibitors

SGLT2 inhibitors are glucose-lowering drugs that have been shown to be associated with reduced HF hospitalization and mortality in patients with diabetes as compared with other classes of glucose-lowering drugs [68, 69]. SGLT2 inhibition promotes natriuresis and osmotic diuresis, leading to plasma volume contraction and reduced preload, and decreases in blood pressure, arterial stiffness, and afterload as well, thereby improving subendocardial blood flow in patients with HF. SGLT2 inhibition is also associated with preservation of renal function [70]. SGLT2 inhibitors may also inhibit sodium-hydrogen exchangers in the heart, vasculature, and kidneys, leading to a reduction in cardiac remodeling and systemic dysfunction [71, 72]. These favorable effects may collectively contribute to the efficacy of SGLT2 inhibitors (e.g., empagliflozin) in reducing the risk of

HF progression and mortality in patients with diabetes. Based on data from mechanistic studies and clinical trials, large clinical trials with SGLT2 inhibitors are now investigating the potential benefit of SGLT2 inhibition in patients who have HF (including HFpEF) with and without diabetes [70] (also see https://clinicaltrials.gov/ct2/show/NCT03057951).

3.4.6. Gene Therapy

The promise of cardiac gene therapy was exemplified with the notable success of a phase 2 first-in-human clinical gene therapy trial (CUPID) using an adeno-associated virus serotype 1 (AAV1) vector carrying the sarcoplasmic reticulum calcium ATPase gene (AAV1/SERCA2a) in patients with advanced HFrEF [73, 74]. Deficiency/dysfunction of SERCA2a, a protein involved in reloading sarcoplasmic reticulum with Ca^{2+} during systole is an important mechanism of systolic HF [75]. The CUPID trial involving 39 patients with advanced HF reported that the risk of prespecified recurrent cardiovascular events was reduced by 82% in the high-dose AAV1/SERCA2a group versus placebo group, and no safety concerns were noted during a 3-year follow-up [74]. The success of the CUPID study had prompted a phase 2b trial to further investigate the clinical efficacy and safety of intracoronary administration of AAV1/SERCA2a in patients with advanced HF, and this trial, known as CUPID 2, involving 250 patients with HFrEF, reported that AAV1/SERCA2a at the dose tested did not improve the clinical course of patients with HFrEF [76]. The failure of CUPID 2 is disappointing, but does not disapprove the conceptual validity of gene therapy in HF. Instead it points to the needs to re-evaluate current vectors, delivery systems, targets, endpoints, and patients' subpopulations, as well as search for new gene candidates, especially those involved in cardiac repair [77–80].

3.4.7. Stem Cell Therapy

Stem cell therapy is a promising treatment strategy for patients with HF though extensive further research is still needed before it can become routinely implemented in clinical practice [10, 81, 82]. The past few years have witnessed the rapid advancement in stem cell biology and clinical trials on the safety and efficacy, in treating HF, of various types of stem cells, including cardiopoietic cell produced through cardiogenic conditioning of patients' mesenchymal stem cells [83], embryonic stem cell-derived cardiovascular progenitors [84], and allogeneic mesenchymal stem cells [85], among others [86, 87]. Overall, the various stem cell-based therapies showed a good safety profile, and some provided benefits in improving cardiac function and/or reducing hospitalization in HF patients. For instance, in patients with stable HFrEF under optimal medical therapy, intravenous infusion of umbilical cord-derived mesenchymal stem cells was shown to be safe and lead to improvements in left ventricular function, functional status, and quality of life [88]. In the Congestive Heart Failure Cardiopoietic Regenerative Therapy (CHART-1) study involving 315 patients with advanced HFrEF, intramyocardial administration of

Gene therapy
Gene therapy is an experimental technique that uses genes to treat or prevent disease. Gene therapy may allow doctors to treat a disorder by inserting a gene into a patient's cells instead of using conventional drugs or surgery. Scientists are testing several approaches to gene therapy, including: (1) replacing a mutated gene that causes disease with a healthy copy of the gene; (2) inactivating, or "knocking out," a mutated gene that is functioning improperly; and (3) introducing a new gene into the body to help fight a disease. Currently, gene therapy is largely investigational and being tested only for disorders with no other cures (www.ghr.nlm.nih.gov).

Stem cell therapy
Stem cell therapy is a type of cell therapy in which the cells used are either "natural" stem cells (as in the case of bone marrow transplantation) or induced pluripotent stem cells (iPSCs) generated directly from adult cells. The term cell therapy refers to the administration of living whole cells to patients for treating and/or preventing diseases. The cells used in cell therapy can be either from the same individual (i.e., autologous cells) or from a different individual (allogeneic cells).

cardiopoietic stem cells led to reverse remodeling as evidenced by significant progressive decreases in both left ventricular end-diastolic volume (LVEDV) and end-systolic volume (LVESV) through the 52 weeks of follow-up [89].

Ixmyelocel-T is an expanded, multicellular therapy produced from a patient's own bone marrow by selectively expanding two key types of bone marrow mononuclear cells: CD90$^+$ mesenchymal stem cells and CD45$^+$/CD14$^+$ auto-fluorescent$^+$ activated macrophages. Early pilot trials suggested that intramyocardial delivery of ixmyelocel-T might improve clinical, functional, symptomatic, and quality-of-life outcomes in patients with HF due to ischemic dilated cardiomyopathy [90]. More recently, a phase 2b trial, involving 126 patients with NYHA class III and IV symptomatic HFrEF due to ischemic dilated cardiomyopathy, demonstrated that the transendocardial delivery of ixmyelocel-T resulted in a significant 37% reduction in adjudicated clinical cardiac events compared with placebo, leading to improved patient outcomes. The primary endpoint of clinical cardiac events was a composite of all-cause death, cardiovascular admission to hospital, and unplanned clinic visits to treat acute decompensated HF [86].

4. SELF-ASSESSMENT QUESTIONS

4.1. According to the 2013 ACCF/AHA guideline for the management of heart failure, heart failure with reduced ejection fraction (HFrEF) is defined as the clinical diagnosis of heart failure and reduced left ventricular ejection fraction (LVEF) of which of the following values?

A. ≤25%
B. ≤30%
C. ≤35%
D. ≤40%
E. ≤45%

4.2. A 65-year-old man is diagnosed with stable heart failure with reduced ejection fraction (HFrEF). A decision is made to put him on a combinational medical therapy including a β-blocker, an angiotensin-converting enzyme inhibitor, and an aldosterone receptor antagonist. Which of the following β-blockers is most likely the one in the combination regimen?

A. Atenolol
B. Carvedilol
C. Esmolol
D. Nebivolol
E. Propranolol

4.3. A 64-year-old Caucasian man living in the United States is diagnosed with heart failure with preserved ejection fraction (HFpEF). Blood tests of renal function and electrolytes are within the normal ranges while serum level of B-type natriuretic peptide is elevated.

Treatment with which of the following drugs will most likely improve the clinical outcomes of the patient?

A. Atenolol
B. Furosemide
C. Isosorbide dinitrate
D. Sildenafil
E. Spironolactone

4.4. Significant symptoms persist in a 61-year-old African American man with heart failure with reduced ejection fraction (HFrEF) following standard therapy with metoprolol succinate, lisinopril, spironolactone, and a diuretic. Which of the following drugs may be added to further reduce the morbidity and mortality in this patient?

A. Atenolol
B. Bidil
C. Captopril
D. Losartan
E. Sildenafil

4.5. Which of the following agents is not considered a disease-modifying drug for treating heart failure with reduced ejection fraction (HFrEF)?

A. Bisoprolol
B. Digoxin
C. Eplerenone
D. Fosinopril
E. Valsartan

ANSWERS AND EXPLANATIONS

4.1. The correct answer is D. HFrEF is defined, in the 2013 ACCF/AHA guideline, as the clinical diagnosis of HF and LVEF ≤40%. On the other hand, in the 2016 ESC guideline, HFrEF is defined as the clinical diagnosis of HF and LVEF <40%.

4.2. The correct answer is B. Currently, only three β-blockers are approved by the US FDA for treating HFrEF, and they are bisoprolol, carvedilol, and metoprolol succinate. Although nebivolol shows promising results in clinical trials, it is not approved by the US FDA for treating HF.

4.3. The correct answer is E. Although generally speaking, there is currently no effective medical therapy for HFpEF, the post-hoc analyses of the multinational TOPCAT (Treatment of Preserved Cardiac Function Heart Failure with an Aldosterone Antagonist) trial suggested an efficacy (a 17% reduction of a combined endpoint of death, aborted cardiac death, and HF hospitalization) for spironolactone in patients with HFpEF in the Americas. The 2017 ACC/AHA/HFSA updated guideline states that in appropriately selected patients with

HFpEF (with LVEF ≥45%, elevated B-type natriuretic peptide levels or HF admission within one year, estimated glomerular filtration rate >30 ml/min, creatinine <2.5 mg/dl, potassium <5.0 mM), aldosterone receptor antagonists might be considered to decrease hospitalizations. Currently, there is no evidence showing an efficacy in treating HFpEF for all the other drugs listed.

4.4. The correct answer is B. Adding Bidil (a fixed-dose combination of isosorbide dinitrite and hydralazine) to standard therapy can further reduce morbidity and mortality in HFrEF patients of African heritage. All the other drugs listed are not recommended due to lack of efficacy and/or increased adverse effects.

4.5. The correct answer is B. Among the drugs listed, digoxin therapy is not associated with prolongation of survival in patients with HFrEF though it reduces the rate of hospitalization. The other drugs listed have been shown to reduce mortality and prolong survival in patient with HFrEF due to their ability to suppress cardiac remodeling and disease progression.

REFERENCES

1. Yancy CW, Jessup M, Bozkurt B, Butler J, Casey DE, Jr., Drazner MH, Fonarow GC, Geraci SA, Horwich T, Januzzi JL, Johnson MR, Kasper EK, et al. 2013 ACCF/AHA guideline for the management of heart failure: a report of the American College of Cardiology Foundation/American Heart Association Task Force on Practice Guidelines. *J Am Coll Cardiol* 2013; 62(16):e147–239.

2. Ponikowski P, Voors AA, Anker SD, Bueno H, Cleland JG, Coats AJ, Falk V, Gonzalez-Juanatey JR, Harjola VP, Jankowska EA, Jessup M, Linde C, et al. 2016 ESC Guidelines for the diagnosis and treatment of acute and chronic heart failure: the Task Force for the diagnosis and treatment of acute and chronic heart failure of the European Society of Cardiology (ESC). Developed with the special contribution of the Heart Failure Association (HFA) of the ESC. *Eur J Heart Fail* 2016; 18(8):891–975.

3. McMurray JJ, Adamopoulos S, Anker SD, Auricchio A, Bohm M, Dickstein K, Falk V, Filippatos G, Fonseca C, Gomez-Sanchez MA, Jaarsma T, Kober L, et al. ESC Guidelines for the diagnosis and treatment of acute and chronic heart failure 2012: the Task Force for the Diagnosis and Treatment of Acute and Chronic Heart Failure 2012 of the European Society of Cardiology. Developed in collaboration with the Heart Failure Association (HFA) of the ESC. *Eur Heart J* 2012; 33(14):1787–847.

4. Hunt SA. ACC/AHA 2005 guideline update for the diagnosis and management of chronic heart failure in the adult: a report of the American College of Cardiology/American Heart Association Task Force on Practice Guidelines (Writing Committee to Update the 2001 Guidelines for the Evaluation and Management of Heart Failure). *J Am Coll Cardiol* 2005; 46(6):e1–82.

5. Shah KS, Xu H, Matsouaka RA, Bhatt DL, Heidenreich PA, Hernandez AF, Devore AD, Yancy CW, Fonarow GC. Heart failure with preserved, borderline, and reduced ejection fraction: 5-Year Outcomes. *J Am Coll Cardiol* 2017; 70(20):2476–86.

6. Redfield MM. Heart failure with preserved ejection fraction. *N Engl J Med* 2016; 375(19):1868–77.

7. Nauta JF, Hummel YM, van Melle JP, van der Meer P, Lam CSP, Ponikowski P, Voors AA. What have we learned about heart failure with mid-range ejection fraction one year after its introduction? *Eur J Heart Fail* 2017; 19(12):1569–73.

8. Hsu JJ, Ziaeian B, Fonarow GC. Heart failure with mid-range (borderline) ejection fraction: clinical implications and future directions. *JACC Heart Fail* 2017; 5(11):763–71.

9. Hunt SA, Baker DW, Chin MH, Cinquegrani MP, Feldman AM, Francis GS, Ganiats TG, Goldstein S, Gregoratos G, Jessup ML, Noble

RJ, Packer M, et al. ACC/AHA guidelines for the evaluation and management of chronic heart failure in the adult: executive summary. A report of the American College of Cardiology/American Heart Association Task Force on Practice Guidelines (Committee to revise the 1995 Guidelines for the Evaluation and Management of Heart Failure). *J Am Coll Cardiol* 2001; 38(7):2101–13.

10. Braunwald E. The war against heart failure: the Lancet lecture. *Lancet* 2015; 385(9970):812–24.

11. Ziaeian B, Fonarow GC. Epidemiology and aetiology of heart failure. *Nat Rev Cardiol* 2016; 13(6):368–78.

12. Metra M, Teerlink JR. Heart failure. *Lancet* 2017; 390(10106):1981–95.

13. Kievit RF, Gohar A, Hoes AW, Bots ML, van Riet EE, van Mourik Y, Bertens LC, Boonman-de Winter LJ, den Ruijter HM, Rutten FH, Queen of Hearts & RECONNECT consortium. Efficient selective screening for heart failure in elderly men and women from the community: a diagnostic individual participant data meta-analysis. *Eur J Prev Cardiol* 2018:2047487317749897.

14. Conrad N, Judge A, Tran J, Mohseni H, Hedgecott D, Crespillo AP, Allison M, Hemingway H, Cleland JG, McMurray JJV, Rahimi K. Temporal trends and patterns in heart failure incidence: a population-based study of 4 million individuals. *Lancet* 2018 (in press).

15. Bui AL, Horwich TB, Fonarow GC. Epidemiology and risk profile of heart failure. *Nat Rev Cardiol* 2011; 8(1):30–41.

16. Vos T, Flaxman AD, Naghavi M, Lozano R, Michaud C, Ezzati M, Shibuya K, Salomon JA, Abdalla S, Aboyans V, Abraham J, Ackerman I, et al. Years lived with disability (YLDs) for 1160 sequelae of 289 diseases and injuries 1990–2010: a systematic analysis for the Global Burden of Disease Study 2010. *Lancet* 2012; 380(9859):2163–96.

17. Mudd JO, Kass DA. Tackling heart failure in the twenty-first century. *Nature* 2008; 451(7181):919–28.

18. Jessup M, Brozena S. Heart failure. *N Engl J Med* 2003; 348(20):2007–18.

19. Benjamin EJ, Blaha MJ, Chiuve SE, Cushman M, Das SR, Deo R, de Ferranti SD, Floyd J, Fornage M, Gillespie C, Isasi CR, Jimenez MC, et al. Heart disease and stroke statistics–2017 update: a report from the American Heart Association. *Circulation* 2017; 135(10):e146–e603.

20. Shen L, Jhund PS, Petrie MC, Claggett BL, Barlera S, Cleland JGF, Dargie HJ, Granger CB, Kjekshus J, Kober L, Latini R, Maggioni AP, et al. Declining risk of sudden death in heart failure. *N Engl J Med* 2017; 377(1):41–51.

21. Braunwald E. Heart failure. *JACC Heart Fail* 2013; 1(1):1–20.

22. Heusch G, Libby P, Gersh B, Yellon D, Bohm M, Lopaschuk G, Opie L. Cardiovascular remodelling in coronary artery disease and heart failure. *Lancet* 2014; 383(9932):1933–43.

23. Lymperopoulos A, Rengo G, Koch WJ. Adrenergic nervous system in heart failure: pathophysiology and therapy. *Circ Res* 2013; 113(6):739–53.

24. Goldenberg I, Kutyifa V, Klein HU, Cannom DS, Brown MW, Dan A, Daubert JP, Estes NA, 3rd, Foster E, Greenberg H, Kautzner J, Klempfner R, et al. Survival with cardiac-resynchronization therapy in mild heart failure. *N Engl J Med* 2014; 370(18):1694–701.

25. Tang AS, Wells GA, Talajic M, Arnold MO, Sheldon R, Connolly S, Hohnloser SH, Nichol G, Birnie DH, Sapp JL, Yee R, Healey JS, et al. Cardiac-resynchronization therapy for mild-to-moderate heart failure. *N Engl J Med* 2010; 363(25):2385–95.

26. Holzmeister J, Leclercq C. Implantable cardioverter defibrillators and cardiac resynchronisation therapy. *Lancet* 2011; 378(9792):722–30.

27. Rogers JG, Pagani FD, Tatooles AJ, Bhat G, Slaughter MS, Birks EJ, Boyce SW, Najjar SS, Jeevanandam V, Anderson AS, Gregoric ID, Mallidi H, et al. Intrapericardial left ventricular assist device for advanced heart failure. *N Engl J Med* 2017; 376(5):451–60.

28. Kitzman DW, Upadhya B. Heart failure with preserved ejection fraction: a heterogenous disorder with multifactorial pathophysiology. *J Am Coll Cardiol* 2014; 63(5):457–9.

29. Butler J, Fonarow GC, Zile MR, Lam CS, Roessig L, Schelbert EB, Shah SJ, Ahmed A, Bonow RO, Cleland JG, Cody RJ, Chioncel O, et al. Developing therapies for heart failure with preserved ejection fraction: current state and future directions. *JACC Heart Fail* 2014; 2(2):97–112.

30. Sharma K, Kass DA. Heart failure with preserved ejection fraction: mechanisms, clinical features, and therapies. *Circ Res* 2014; 115(1):79–96.

31. Borlaug BA. The pathophysiology of heart failure with preserved ejection fraction. *Nat Rev Cardiol* 2014; 11(9):507–15.

32. Shah SJ, Kitzman DW, Borlaug BA, van Heerebeek L, Zile MR, Kass DA, Paulus WJ. Phenotype-specific treatment of heart failure with preserved ejection fraction: a multiorgan roadmap. *Circulation* 2016; 134(1):73–90.

33. Burnett H, Earley A, Voors AA, Senni M, McMurray JJ, Deschaseaux C, Cope S. Thirty years of evidence on the efficacy of drug treatments for chronic heart failure with reduced ejection fraction: a network meta-analysis. *Circ Heart Fail* 2017; 10: e003529.

34. Taylor AL, Ziesche S, Yancy C, Carson P, D'Agostino R, Jr., Ferdinand K, Taylor M, Adams K, Sabolinski M, Worcel M, Cohn JN, African-American Heart Failure Trial I. Combination of isosorbide dinitrate and hydralazine in blacks with heart failure. *N Engl J Med* 2004; 351(20):2049–57.

35. Ziaeian B, Fonarow GC, Heidenreich PA. Clinical effectiveness of hydralazine-isosorbide dinitrate in African-American patients with heart failure. *JACC Heart Fail* 2017; 5(9):632–9.

36. Edelmann F, Wachter R, Schmidt AG, Kraigher-Krainer E, Colantonio C, Kamke W, Duvinage A, Stahrenberg R, Durstewitz K, Loffler M, Dungen HD, Tschope C, et al. Effect of spironolactone on diastolic function and exercise capacity in patients with heart failure with preserved ejection fraction: the Aldo-DHF randomized controlled trial. *JAMA* 2013; 309(8):781–91.

37. Shah AM, Shah SJ, Anand IS, Sweitzer NK, O'Meara E, Heitner JF, Sopko G, Li G, Assmann SF, McKinlay SM, Pitt B, Pfeffer MA, et al. Cardiac structure and function in heart failure with preserved ejection fraction: baseline findings from the echocardiographic study of the Treatment of Preserved Cardiac Function Heart Failure with an Aldosterone Antagonist trial. *Circ Heart Fail* 2014; 7(1):104–15.

38. Redfield MM, Chen HH, Borlaug BA, Semigran MJ, Lee KL, Lewis G, LeWinter MM, Rouleau JL, Bull DA, Mann DL, Deswal A, Stevenson LW, et al. Effect of phosphodiesterase-5 inhibition on exercise capacity and clinical status in heart failure with preserved ejection fraction: a randomized clinical trial. *JAMA* 2013; 309(12):1268–77.

39. Pitt B, Pfeffer MA, Assmann SF, Boineau R, Anand IS, Claggett B, Clausell N, Desai AS, Diaz R, Fleg JL, Gordeev I, Harty B, et al. Spironolactone for heart failure with preserved ejection fraction. *N Engl J Med* 2014; 370(15):1383–92.

40. Pfeffer MA, Claggett B, Assmann SF, Boineau R, Anand IS, Clausell N, Desai AS, Diaz R, Fleg JL, Gordeev I, Heitner JF, Lewis EF, et al. Regional variation in patients and outcomes in the Treatment of Preserved Cardiac Function Heart Failure With an Aldosterone Antagonist (TOPCAT) trial. *Circulation* 2015; 131(1):34–42.

41. Kosmala W, Rojek A, Przewlocka-Kosmala M, Wright L, Mysiak A, Marwick TH. Effect of aldosterone antagonism on exercise tolerance in heart failure with preserved ejection fraction. *J Am Coll Cardiol* 2016; 68(17):1823–34.

42. Yancy CW, Jessup M, Bozkurt B, Butler J, Casey DE, Jr., Colvin MM, Drazner MH, Filippatos GS, Fonarow GC, Givertz MM, Hollenberg SM, Lindenfeld J, et al. 2017 ACC/AHA/HFSA focused update of the 2013 ACCF/AHA guideline for the management of heart failure: a report of the American College of Cardiology/American Heart Association Task Force on Clinical Practice Guidelines and the Heart Failure Society of America. *J Am Coll Cardiol* 2017; 70(6):776–803.

43. Flather MD, Shibata MC, Coats AJ, Van Veldhuisen DJ, Parkhomenko A, Borbola J, Cohen-Solal A, Dumitrascu D, Ferrari R, Lechat P, Soler-Soler J, Tavazzi L, et al. Randomized trial to determine the effect of nebivolol on mortality and cardiovascular hospital admission in elderly patients with heart failure (SENIORS). *Eur Heart J* 2005; 26(3):215–25.

44. Mulder BA, van Veldhuisen DJ, Crijns HJ, Bohm M, Cohen-Solal A, Babalis D, Roughton M, Flather MD, Coats AJ, Van Gelder IC. Effect of nebivolol on outcome in elderly patients with heart failure and atrial fibrillation: insights from SENIORS. *Eur J Heart Fail* 2012; 14(10):1171–8.

45. van Veldhuisen DJ, Cohen-Solal A, Bohm M, Anker SD, Babalis D, Roughton M, Coats AJ, Poole-Wilson PA, Flather MD, SENIOR Investigators. Beta-blockade with nebivolol in elderly heart failure patients with impaired and preserved left ventricular ejection fraction: data from SENIORS (Study of Effects of Nebivolol Intervention on Outcomes and Rehospitalization in Seniors With Heart Failure). *J Am Coll Cardiol* 2009; 53(23):2150–8.

46. Montero-Perez-Barquero M, Flather M, Roughton M, Coats A, Bohm M, Van Veldhuisen DJ, Babalis D, Solal AC, Manzano L. Influence of systolic blood pressure on clinical outcomes in elderly heart failure patients treated with nebivolol: data from the SENIORS trial. *Eur J Heart Fail* 2014; 16(9):1009–15.

47. Lewis GD, Shah R, Shahzad K, Camuso JM, Pappagianopoulos PP, Hung J, Tawakol A, Gerszten RE, Systrom DM, Bloch KD, Semigran MJ. Sildenafil improves exercise capacity and quality of life in patients with systolic heart failure and secondary pulmonary hypertension. *Circulation* 2007; 116(14):1555–62.

48. Guazzi M, Vicenzi M, Arena R, Guazzi MD. PDE5 inhibition with sildenafil improves left ventricular diastolic function, cardiac geometry, and clinical status in patients with stable systolic heart failure: results of a 1-year, prospective, randomized, placebo-controlled study. *Circ Heart Fail* 2011; 4(1):8–17.

49. Hussain I, Mohammed SF, Forfia PR, Lewis GD, Borlaug BA, Gallup DS, Redfield MM. Impaired right ventricular-pulmonary arterial coupling and effect of sildenafil in heart failure with preserved ejection fraction: an ancillary analysis from the Phosphodiesterase-5 Inhibition to Improve Clinical Status and Exercise Capacity in Diastolic Heart Failure (RELAX) trial. *Circ Heart Fail* 2016; 9(4):e002729.

50. Wang H, Anstrom K, Ilkayeva O, Muehlbauer MJ, Bain JR, McNulty S, Newgard CB, Kraus WE, Hernandez A, Felker GM, Redfield M, Shah SH. Sildenafil treatment in heart failure with preserved ejection fraction: targeted metabolomic profiling in the RELAX trial. *JAMA Cardiol* 2017; 2(8):896–901.

51. Bathgate RA, Halls ML, van der Westhuizen ET, Callander GE, Kocan M, Summers RJ. Relaxin family peptides and their receptors. *Physiol Rev* 2013; 93(1):405–80.

52. Teerlink JR, Cotter G, Davison BA, Felker GM, Filippatos G, Greenberg BH, Ponikowski P, Unemori E, Voors AA, Adams KF, Jr., Dorobantu MI, Grinfeld LR, et al. Serelaxin, recombinant human relaxin-2, for treatment of acute heart failure (RELAX-AHF): a randomised, placebo-controlled trial. *Lancet* 2013; 381(9860):29–39.

53. Metra M, Cotter G, Davison BA, Felker GM, Filippatos G, Greenberg BH, Ponikowski P, Unemori E, Voors AA, Adams KF, Jr., Dorobantu MI, Grinfeld L, et al. Effect of serelaxin on cardiac, renal, and hepatic biomarkers in the Relaxin in Acute Heart Failure (RELAX-AHF) development program: correlation with outcomes. *J Am Coll Cardiol* 2013; 61(2):196–206.

54. Filippatos G, Teerlink JR, Farmakis D, Cotter G, Davison BA, Felker GM, Greenberg BH, Hua T, Ponikowski P, Severin T, Unemori E, Voors AA, et al. Serelaxin in acute heart failure patients with preserved left ventricular ejection fraction: results from the RELAX-AHF trial. *Eur Heart J* 2014; 35(16):1041–50.

55. Teerlink JR, Voors AA, Ponikowski P, Pang PS, Greenberg BH, Filippatos G, Felker GM, Davison BA, Cotter G, Gimpelewicz C, Boer-Martins L, Wernsing M, et al. Serelaxin in addition to standard therapy in acute heart failure: rationale and design of the RELAX-AHF-2 study. *Eur J Heart Fail* 2017; 19(6):800–9.

56. Dick SA, Epelman S. Chronic heart failure and inflammation: what do we really know? *Circ Res* 2016; 119(1):159–76.

57. Zhang Y, Bauersachs J, Langer HF. Immune mechanisms in heart failure. *Eur J Heart Fail* 2017; 19(11):1379–89.

58. Hage C, Michaelsson E, Linde C, Donal E, Daubert JC, Gan LM, Lund LH. Inflammatory biomarkers predict heart failure severity and prognosis in patients with heart failure with preserved ejection fraction: a holistic proteomic approach. *Circ Cardiovasc Genet* 2017; 10: e001633.

59. Blyszczuk P, Kania G, Dieterle T, Marty RR, Valaperti A, Berthonneche C, Pedrazzini T, Berger CT, Dirnhofer S, Matter CM, Penninger JM, Luscher TF, et al. Myeloid differentiation factor-88/interleukin-1 signaling controls cardiac fibrosis and heart failure progression in inflammatory dilated cardiomyopathy. *Circ Res* 2009; 105(9):912–20.

60. Van Tassell BW, Canada J, Carbone S, Trankle C, Buckley L, Oddi Erdle C, Abouzaki NA, Dixon D, Kadariya D, Christopher S, Schatz A, Regan J, et al. Interleukin-1 blockade in recently decompensated systolic heart failure: results from REDHART (Recently Decompensated Heart Failure Anakinra Response Trial). *Circ Heart Fail* 2017; 10: e004373.

61. Van Tassell BW, Arena R, Biondi-Zoccai G, Canada JM, Oddi C, Abouzaki NA, Jahangiri A, Falcao RA, Kontos MC, Shah KB, Voelkel NF, Dinarello CA, et al. Effects of interleukin-1

blockade with anakinra on aerobic exercise capacity in patients with heart failure and preserved ejection fraction (from the D-HART pilot study). *Am J Cardiol* 2014; 113(2):321–7.

62. Lundberg JO, Gladwin MT, Weitzberg E. Strategies to increase nitric oxide signalling in cardiovascular disease. *Nat Rev Drug Discov* 2015; 14(9):623–41.

63. Farah C, Michel LYM, Balligand JL. Nitric oxide signalling in cardiovascular health and disease. *Nat Rev Cardiol* 2018 (in press).

64. Borlaug BA, Koepp KE, Melenovsky V. Sodium nitrite improves exercise hemodynamics and ventricular performance in heart failure with preserved ejection fraction. *J Am Coll Cardiol* 2015; 66(15):1672–82.

65. Borlaug BA, Melenovsky V, Koepp KE. Inhaled sodium nitrite improves rest and exercise hemodynamics in heart failure with preserved ejection fraction. *Circ Res* 2016; 119(7):880–6.

66. Zamani P, Rawat D, Shiva-Kumar P, Geraci S, Bhuva R, Konda P, Doulias PT, Ischiropoulos H, Townsend RR, Margulies KB, Cappola TP, Poole DC, et al. Effect of inorganic nitrate on exercise capacity in heart failure with preserved ejection fraction. *Circulation* 2015; 131(4):371–80.

67. Zamani P, Tan V, Soto-Calderon H, Beraun M, Brandimarto JA, Trieu L, Varakantam S, Doulias PT, Townsend RR, Chittams J, Margulies KB, Cappola TP, et al. Pharmacokinetics and pharmacodynamics of inorganic nitrate in heart failure with preserved ejection fraction. *Circ Res* 2017; 120(7):1151–61.

68. Zinman B, Wanner C, Lachin JM, Fitchett D, Bluhmki E, Hantel S, Mattheus M, Devins T, Johansen OE, Woerle HJ, Broedl UC, Inzucchi SE, et al. Empagliflozin, cardiovascular outcomes, and mortality in type 2 diabetes. *N Engl J Med* 2015; 373(22):2117–28.

69. Kosiborod M, Cavender MA, Fu AZ, Wilding JP, Khunti K, Holl RW, Norhammar A, Birkeland KI, Jorgensen ME, Thuresson M, Arya N, Bodegard J, et al. Lower risk of heart failure and death in patients initiated on sodium-glucose cotransporter-2 inhibitors versus other glucose-lowering drugs: the CVD-REAL study (Comparative Effectiveness of Cardiovascular Outcomes in New Users of Sodium-Glucose Cotransporter-2 Inhibitors). *Circulation* 2017; 136(3):249–59.

70. Lytvyn Y, Bjornstad P, Udell JA, Lovshin JA, Cherney DZI. sodium glucose cotransporter-2 inhibition in heart failure: potential mechanisms, clinical applications, and summary of clinical trials. *Circulation* 2017; 136(17):1643–58.

71. Packer M. Activation and inhibition of sodium-hydrogen exchanger is a mechanism that links the pathophysiology and treatment of diabetes mellitus with that of heart failure. *Circulation* 2017; 136(16):1548–59.

72. Packer M, Anker SD, Butler J, Filippatos G, Zannad F. Effects of sodium-glucose cotransporter 2 inhibitors for the treatment of patients with heart failure: proposal of a novel mechanism of action. *JAMA Cardiol* 2017; 2(9):1025–9.

73. Jessup M, Greenberg B, Mancini D, Cappola T, Pauly DF, Jaski B, Yaroshinsky A, Zsebo KM, Dittrich H, Hajjar RJ, Calcium upregulation by percutaneous administration of gene therapy in cardiac disease I. calcium upregulation by percutaneous administration of gene therapy in cardiac disease (CUPID): a phase 2 trial of intracoronary gene therapy of sarcoplasmic reticulum Ca^{2+}-ATPase in patients with advanced heart failure. *Circulation* 2011; 124(3):304–13.

74. Zsebo K, Yaroshinsky A, Rudy JJ, Wagner K, Greenberg B, Jessup M, Hajjar RJ. Long-term effects of AAV1/SERCA2a gene transfer in patients with severe heart failure: analysis of recurrent cardiovascular events and mortality. *Circ Res* 2014; 114(1):101–8.

75. Kho C, Lee A, Hajjar RJ. Altered sarcoplasmic reticulum calcium cycling: targets for heart failure therapy. *Nat Rev Cardiol* 2012; 9(12):717–33.

76. Greenberg B, Butler J, Felker GM, Ponikowski P, Voors AA, Desai AS, Barnard D, Bouchard A, Jaski B, Lyon AR, Pogoda JM, Rudy JJ, et al. Calcium upregulation by percutaneous administration of gene therapy in patients with cardiac disease (CUPID 2): a randomised, multinational, double-blind, placebo-controlled, phase 2b trial. *Lancet* 2016; 387(10024):1178–86.

77. Leach JP, Heallen T, Zhang M, Rahmani M, Morikawa Y, Hill MC, Segura A, Willerson JT, Martin JF. Hippo pathway deficiency reverses systolic heart failure after infarction. *Nature* 2017; 550(7675):260–4.

78. Chamuleau SAJ, van der Naald M, Climent AM, Kraaijeveld AO, Wever KE, Duncker DJ, Fernandez-Aviles F, Bolli R, Transnational

Alliance for Regenerative Therapies in Cardiovascular Syndromes (TACTICS) Group. Translational research in cardiovascular repair: a call for a paradigm shift. *Circ Res* 2018; 122(2):310–8.

79. Donahue JK. Cardiac gene therapy: a call for basic methods development. *Lancet* 2016; 387(10024):1137–9.

80. Madonna R, Van Laake LW, Davidson SM, Engel FB, Hausenloy DJ, Lecour S, Leor J, Perrino C, Schulz R, Ytrehus K, Landmesser U, Mummery CL, et al. Position paper of the European Society of Cardiology Working Group Cellular Biology of the Heart: cell-based therapies for myocardial repair and regeneration in ischemic heart disease and heart failure. *Eur Heart J* 2016; 37(23):1789–98.

81. Nguyen PK, Rhee JW, Wu JC. Adult stem cell therapy and heart failure, 2000 to 2016: a systematic review. *JAMA Cardiol* 2016; 1(7):831–41.

82. Yoshida Y, Yamanaka S. Induced pluripotent stem cells 10 years later: for cardiac applications. *Circ Res* 2017; 120(12):1958–68.

83. Bartunek J, Terzic A, Davison BA, Filippatos GS, Radovanovic S, Beleslin B, Merkely B, Musialek P, Wojakowski W, Andreka P, Horvath IG, Katz A, et al. Cardiopoietic cell therapy for advanced ischaemic heart failure: results at 39 weeks of the prospective, randomized, double blind, sham-controlled CHART-1 clinical trial. *Eur Heart J* 2017; 38(9):648–60.

84. Menasche P, Vanneaux V, Hagege A, Bel A, Cholley B, Parouchev A, Cacciapuoti I, Al-Daccak R, Benhamouda N, Blons H, Agbulut O, Tosca L, et al. Transplantation of human embryonic stem cell-derived cardiovascular progenitors for severe ischemic left ventricular dysfunction. *J Am Coll Cardiol* 2018; 71(4):429–38.

85. Florea V, Rieger AC, DiFede DL, El-Khorazaty J, Natsumeda M, Banerjee MN, Tompkins BA, Khan A, Schulman IH, Landin AM, Mushtaq M, Golpanian S, et al. Dose comparison study of allogeneic mesenchymal stem cells in patients with ischemic cardiomyopathy (The TRIDENT study). *Circ Res* 2017; 121(11):1279–90.

86. Patel AN, Henry TD, Quyyumi AA, Schaer GL, Anderson RD, Toma C, East C, Remmers AE, Goodrich J, Desai AS, Recker D, DeMaria A, et al. Ixmyelocel-T for patients with ischaemic heart failure: a prospective randomised double-blind trial. *Lancet* 2016; 387(10036):2412–21.

87. Gwizdala A, Rozwadowska N, Kolanowski TJ, Malcher A, Cieplucha A, Perek B, Seniuk W, Straburzynska-Migaj E, Oko-Sarnowska Z, Cholewinski W, Michalak M, Grajek S, et al. Safety, feasibility and effectiveness of first in-human administration of muscle-derived stem/progenitor cells modified with connexin-43 gene for treatment of advanced chronic heart failure. *Eur J Heart Fail* 2017; 19(1):148–57.

88. Bartolucci J, Verdugo FJ, Gonzalez PL, Larrea RE, Abarzua E, Goset C, Rojo P, Palma I, Lamich R, Pedreros PA, Valdivia G, Lopez VM, et al. Safety and efficacy of the intravenous infusion of umbilical cord mesenchymal stem cells in patients with heart failure: a phase 1/2 randomized controlled trial (RIMECARD trial [Randomized Clinical Trial of Intravenous Infusion Umbilical Cord Mesenchymal Stem Cells on Cardiopathy]). *Circ Res* 2017; 121(10):1192–204.

89. Teerlink JR, Metra M, Filippatos GS, Davison BA, Bartunek J, Terzic A, Gersh BJ, Povsic TJ, Henry TD, Alexandre B, Homsy C, Edwards C, et al. Benefit of cardiopoietic mesenchymal stem cell therapy on left ventricular remodelling: results from the Congestive Heart Failure Cardiopoietic Regenerative Therapy (CHART-1) study. *Eur J Heart Fail* 2017; 19(11):1520–9.

90. Henry TD, Traverse JH, Hammon BL, East CA, Bruckner B, Remmers AE, Recker D, Bull DA, Patel AN. Safety and efficacy of ixmyelocel-T: an expanded, autologous multi-cellular therapy, in dilated cardiomyopathy. *Circ Res* 2014; 115(8):730-7.

CHAPTER 12

New Drugs for Heart Failure

CHAPTER HIGHLIGHTS

- The high morbidity and mortality of heart failure (HF) demand continued search for more effective medical therapies to relieve symptoms, reduce hospitalization, improve quality of life, and prolong survival of the HF patients.
- Over the past five years, the United Stated Food and Drug Administration (US FDA) has approved two new drugs for HF: ivabradine and a fixed-dose combination of sacubitril and valsartan known as Entresto.
- Ivabradine is the first-in-class member of the I_f channel inhibitor drug class that reduces the sinus rate, whereas Entresto is the first-in-class member of the angiotensin receptor-neprilysin inhibitor (ARNI) drug class that causes simultaneous neprilysin inhibition and angiotensin II type 1 (AT1) receptor blockage.
- Ivabradine is indicated to reduce the risk of hospitalization for worsening HF in patients with stable, symptomatic chronic HF with left ventricular ejection fraction ≤35%, who are in sinus rhythm with resting heart rate ≥70 beats per minute and either are on maximally tolerated doses of β-blockers or have a contraindication to β-blocker use.
- Entresto is indicated to reduce the risk of cardiovascular death and hospitalization for HF in patients with chronic HF with reduced ejection fraction. It is typically given in conjunction with other HF therapies, as a replacement for an angiotensin-converting enzyme inhibitor or other AT1 receptor blocker.

KEYWORDS | Angiotensin receptor-neprilysin inhibitor; Entresto; Heart failure with preserved ejection fraction; Heart failure with reduced ejection fraction; Heart failure; I_f channel inhibitor; Ivabradine

CITATION | *Li YR. Cardiovascular Medicine: New Therapeutic Drugs Approved by the US FDA (2013–2017). Cell Med Press, Raleigh, NC, USA. 2018. http://dx.doi.org/10.20455/ndcvd.2018.12*

ABBREVIATIONS | Aβ, amyloid-β; ACE, angiotensin-converting enzyme; ANP, atrial natriuretic peptide; ARA, aldosterone receptor antagonist; ARB, angiotensin receptor blocker; ARNI, angiotensin receptor-neprilysin inhibitor; AT1, angiotensin II type 1 receptor; AV, atrioventricular; BNP, B-type natriuretic peptide; bpm, beats per minute; cGMP, cyclic guanosine monophosphate; CNP, C-type natriuretic peptide; CSF, cerebrospinal fluid; CYP, cytochrome P450; HCN, hyperpolarization-activated cyclic nucleotide-gated; HF, heart failure; HFpEF, heart failure with preserved ejection fraction; HFrEF, heart failure with reduced ejection fraction; I_f, "funny" pacemaker current; LVEF, left ventricular ejection fraction; NP, natriuretic peptide; NSAID, nonsteroidal anti-inflammatory drug; NYHA, the New York Heart Association; RAAS, renin-angiotensin-aldosterone system; US FDA, the United States Food and Drug Administration

CHAPTER AT A GLANCE

1. INTRODUCTION

The management of heart failure (HF), primarily HF with reduced ejection fraction (HFrEF), has been advanced substantially over the past two decades due to a better understanding of the underlying pathophysiology and the development of mechanistically based therapies with β-blockers and inhibitors of the renin-angiotensin-aldosterone system (RAAS). However, the 5-year mortality rate of HF remains unacceptably high. This has necessitated the continued searching for more effective therapeutic modalities. In this context, a number of novel pharmacological agents for HF have emerged and undergone randomized controlled trials with promising results. Indeed, the past two to three years have witnessed the approval of two new drugs by the United States Food and Drugs Administration (US FDA) for treating HFrEF. They are ivabradine (an I_f channel inhibitor) and a fixed-dose combination of sacubitril and valsartan (an angiotensin receptor-neprilysin inhibitor), approved on April 15, 2015 and July 7, 2015, respectively. Despite over 100 clinical trials on HF drugs, ivabradine and sacubitril/valsartan are the only two new drugs that have been approved by the US FDA for the treatment of chronic HF in more than a decade [1].

2. I_f CHANNEL INHIBITOR: IVABRADINE (CORLANOR)

2.1. Overview

Elevated heart rate is identified as a prognostic risk factor for increased morbidity and mortality in patients with HF [2, 3]. In HF patients, resting heart rate of ≥70 beats per minute (bpm) in sinus rhythm on hospital admission was associated with increased in-hospital mortality, and the resting heart rate on discharge predicted one-year rehospitalization and mortality [2–4]. These findings led to the development and approval of ivabradine for treating HFrEF. The US FDA approval of ivabradine (Amgen Inc., Thousand Oaks, CA,

USA) was based on a randomized controlled trial, namely, SHIFT. The SHIFT trial involved 6,558 adult patients with stable NYHA class II–IV HF (see Chapter 11 for HF classification), left ventricular ejection fraction (LVEF) ≤35%, and resting heart rate ≥70 bpm. Patients had to have been clinically stable for at least four weeks on an optimized and stable clinical regimen, which included maximally tolerated doses of β-blockers and, in most cases, angiotensin-converting enzyme (ACE) inhibitors or angiotensin receptor blockers (ARBs), spironolactone, and diuretics, with fluid retention and symptoms of congestion minimized. Patients had to have been hospitalized for HF within 12 months prior to study entry. The trial demonstrated that ivabradine treatment reduced the risk of the combined endpoint of hospitalization for worsening HF or cardiovascular death based on a time-to-event analysis. The treatment effect reflected only a reduction in the risk of hospitalization for worsening HF; there was no favorable effect on the mortality component of the primary endpoint. In the overall treatment population, ivabradine had no statistically significant benefit on cardiovascular death [5].

2.2. Chemistry and Pharmacokinetics

Ivabradine is a benzazepine derivative (structure shown in **Figure 12.1**). The major pharmacokinetic properties of ivabradine are summarized in **Table 12.1**.

2.3. Molecular Mechanisms and Pharmacological Effects

2.3.1. Molecular Mechanisms

Ivabradine is a specific inhibitor of hyperpolarization-activated cyclic nucleotide-gated (HCN) channels. HCN channels create the diastolic depolarization or "funny" pacemaker current (I_f) of the sinoatrial node, so termed because it is uniquely activated by the membrane hyperpolarization that follows systolic depolarization [6]. I_f was first discovered in animal studies in the 1970s, found to be primarily mediated in humans by abundant sinoatrial HCN4, and determined to be clinically relevant in part by genetic studies linking HCN4 mutations and asymptomatic bradycardia [7]. Ivabradine directly blocks HCN channels (also known as I_f channels) in a use-dependent manner, which decreases I_f and reduces the sinus rate in both healthy and diseased hearts at rest and with exertion [8] (**Figure 12.1**).

2.3.2. Pharmacological Effects

Ivabradine blocks cardiac pacemaker I_f current, which regulates heart rate. In clinical electrophysiology studies, the cardiac effects are most pronounced in the sinoatrial (SA) node, but prolongation of the atrioventricular (AV) node conduction interval may also occur. Ivabradine increases the uncorrected QT interval with heart rate slowing, but does not cause rate-corrected QT prolongation. It exerts no effects on ventricular repolarization and myocardial contractility.

Ivabradine causes a dose-dependent reduction in heart rate. The size of the effect is dependent on the baseline heart rate (i.e., greater

Use-dependent blockage
This refers to a phenomenon related to the blockage of ion channels (e.g., sodium channels) by drugs, in which the extent of inhibition of the ion channels by the drugs is proportional to the extent of the ion channel activities, i.e., more inhibition on more actively used channels.

TABLE 12.1. Major pharmacokinetic properties of ivabradine

Property	Description
Oral bioavailability	40%
t_{max}	1 h
Effect of food	Food delays absorption by ~1 h and increases plasma exposure by 20–40%; the drug should be taken with meals to increase its effectiveness
Plasma protein binding	70%
Vd	100 L
Metabolism	Extensively metabolized in the liver and intestines by CYP3A4-mediated oxidation
Elimination	Excreted via feces and urine to a similar extent
Clearance	24 L/h
$t_{1/2}$	6 h

Note: CYP, cytochrome P450; $t_{1/2}$, elimination half-life; t_{max}, the time when the maximum plasma concentration is reached; Vd, volume of distribution per 70 kg body weight.

heart rate reduction occurs in subjects with higher baseline heart rate). At recommended doses, heart rate reduction is approximately 10 bpm at rest and during exercise.

Ivabradine can also inhibit the retinal current I_h. I_h is involved in curtailing retinal responses to bright light stimuli. Under triggering circumstances (e.g., rapid changes in luminosity), partial inhibition of I_h by ivabradine may underlie the luminous phenomena experienced by patients. Luminous phenomena (phosphenes) are described as a transient enhanced brightness in a limited area of the visual field.

2.4. Clinical Uses

Ivabradine is indicated to reduce the risk of hospitalization for worsening HF in patients with stable, symptomatic chronic HF with LVEF ≤35%, who are in sinus rhythm with resting heart rate ≥70 bpm and either are on maximally tolerated doses of β-blockers or have a contraindication to β-blocker use.

2.5. Therapeutic Dosages

The dosage forms and strengths of ivabradine are listed below.

- Oral: 5, 7.5 mg tablets. The 5 mg tablet is scored and can be divided into equal halves to provide a 2.5 mg dose.

The recommended starting dose of ivabradine is 5 mg twice daily with meals (note: food delays absorption by about 1 h and increases plasma exposure by 20–40%, and as such, ivabradine should be taken

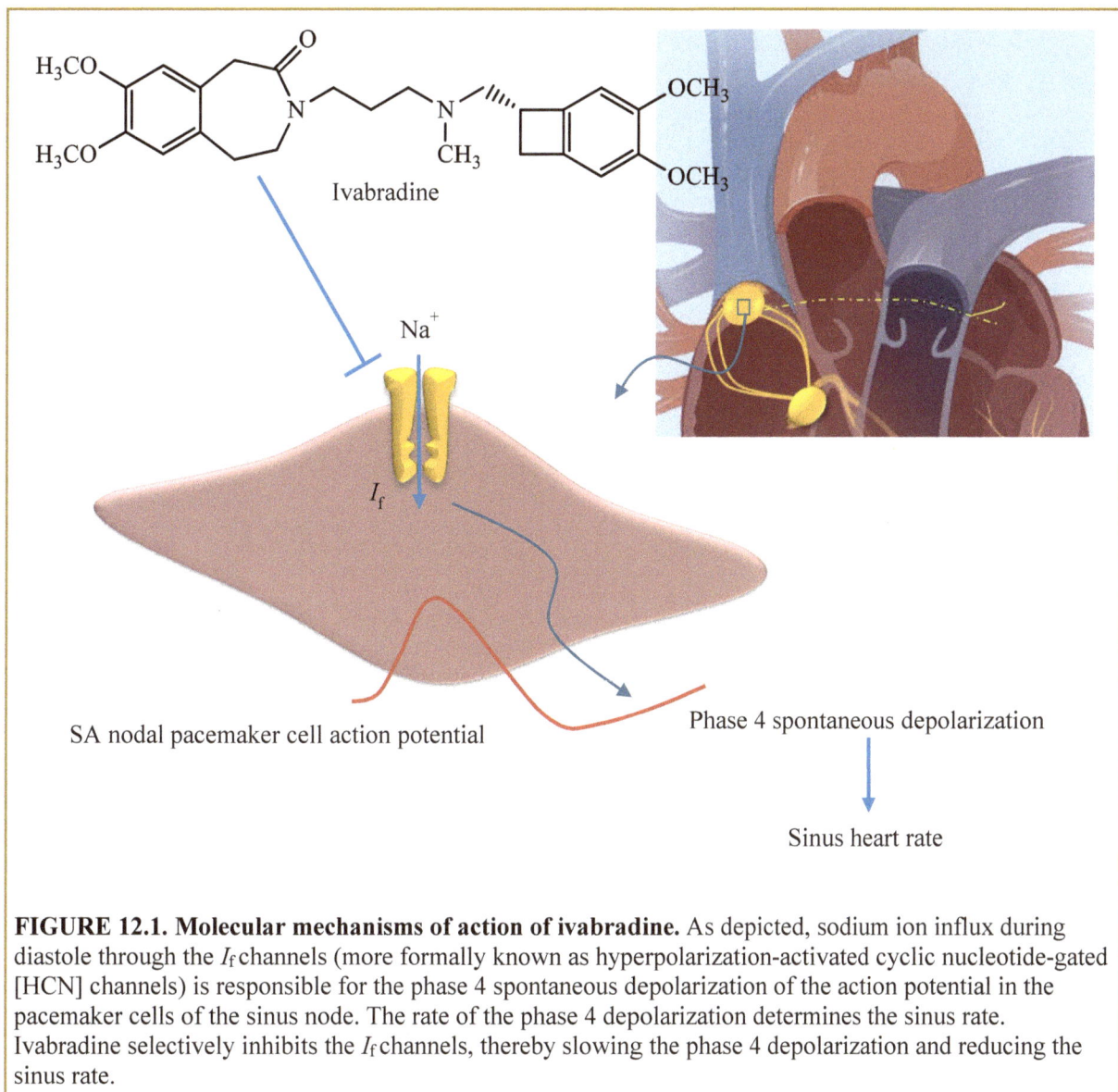

FIGURE 12.1. Molecular mechanisms of action of ivabradine. As depicted, sodium ion influx during diastole through the I_f channels (more formally known as hyperpolarization-activated cyclic nucleotide-gated [HCN] channels) is responsible for the phase 4 spontaneous depolarization of the action potential in the pacemaker cells of the sinus node. The rate of the phase 4 depolarization determines the sinus rate. Ivabradine selectively inhibits the I_f channels, thereby slowing the phase 4 depolarization and reducing the sinus rate.

with meals). Assess the patient's response after two weeks and adjust the dose to achieve a resting heart rate between 50 and 60 bpm. The maximum dose is 7.5 mg twice daily. In patients with a history of conduction defects, or other patients in whom bradycardia could lead to hemodynamic compromise, initiate therapy at 2.5 mg twice daily before increasing the dose based on heart rate.

2.6. Adverse Effects and Drug Interactions

2.6.1. Adverse Effects

The most common adverse reactions occurring in patients in the SHIFT trial [5] include bradycardia and phosphenes (see Section 2.3.2 for definition of phosphenes).

2.6.2. Drug Interactions

2.6.2.1. CYP3A4 INHIBITORS OR INDUCERS

Ivabradine is primarily metabolized by cytochrome P450 (CYP) 3A4 (see **Table 12.1**). Concomitant use of CYP3A4 inhibitors increases ivabradine plasma concentrations, and concomitant use of CYP3A4 inducers decreases them. Increased plasma concentrations of ivabradine may exacerbate bradycardia and conduction disturbances. As such, the concomitant use of strong CYP3A4 inhibitors (e.g., the azole antifungal itraconazole, the macrolide clarithromycin, the HIV protease inhibitor nelfinavir, and the antidepressant nefazodone) is contraindicated. Simultaneous use of moderate CYP3A4 inhibitors (e.g., grapefruit juice and the calcium channel blockers diltiazem and verapamil) should be avoided. Likewise, co-administration of CYP3A4 inducers (e.g., St. John's wort, rifampicin, barbiturates, and phenytoin) should also be avoided due to diminished efficacy of ivabradine.

2.6.2.2. NEGATIVE CHRONOTROPES

Many patients receiving ivabradine may also be treated with a β-blocker or other negative chronotropes (drugs that slow heart rate). The risk of bradycardia increases with concomitant administration of negative chronotropes (e.g., amiodarone [an antiarrhythmic agent], β-blockers, and digoxin), and as such, heart rate in patients taking ivabradine concomitantly with other negative chronotropes should be closely monitored.

2.6.2.3. PACEMAKERS

Ivabradine dosing is based on heart rate reduction, targeting a heart rate of 50–60 bpm. Patients with demand pacemakers set to a rate ≥60 bpm cannot achieve a target heart rate <60 bpm, and as such, ivabradine is not recommended in such patients.

2.6.3. Contraindications and FDA Pregnancy Category

- Acute decompensated heart failure
- Blood pressure <90/50 mm Hg
- Sick sinus syndrome, sinoatrial block or 3rd degree atrioventricular (AV) block, unless a functioning demand pacemaker is present
- Resting heart rate <60 bpm prior to treatment
- Severe hepatic impairment
- Pacemaker dependence (heart rate maintained exclusively by the pacemaker)
- Concomitant use of strong CYP3A4 inhibitors (also see Section 2.6.2)
- FDA pregnancy category: not classified. Based on findings in animals, ivabradine may cause fetal harm when administered to a pregnant woman. However, currently, there are no adequate and well-controlled studies of this drug in pregnant women to inform any drug-associated risks.

2.7. Comparison with Existing Members and New Development since the US FDA Approval

Ivabradine is the first-in-class and currently the only member of the I_f channel-inhibiting drug class approved by the US FDA. Extensive clinical research demonstrates that adding ivabradine to standard therapy in HFrEF with resting heart rate ≥70 bpm improves the symptoms and reduces hospital readmission [5, 9–14]. However, currently, this new drug has not been conclusively shown to reduce the mortality in HFrEF in randomized controlled trials, though a retrospective subgroup analysis of the SHIFT trial suggested a survival benefit [15, 16]. The efficacy of ivabradine has recently been evaluated in a trial involving 112 pediatric patients, and it was found to safely reduce the resting heart rate and improve LVEF with favorable trends in clinical status and quality of life in children with chronic HF and dilated cardiomyopathy [17]. In contrast to the symptom-improving efficacy in HFrEF, the role of ivabradine therapy in HFpEF remains controversial [18–20]. Moreover, among patients who had stable coronary artery disease without clinical HF, the addition of ivabradine to standard background therapy to reduce the heart rate did not improve cardiovascular outcomes (e.g., cardiovascular mortality and non-fatal myocardial infarction) [21] or angina-related quality of life [22].

The benefits of ivabradine treatment suggest the importance of heart rate reduction in the symptomatic management of HFrEF; however, the superiority of β-blockers indicates that their pleiotropic effects contribute to improved patient's outcomes and should remind practitioners to use them vigorously [8]. In this regard, the recent HF management guidelines provide a IIa recommendation stating that ivabradine can be beneficial to reduce HF hospitalization for patients with symptomatic (NYHA class II–III) stable chronic HFrEF (LVEF ≤35%) who are receiving guideline-directed evaluation and management (GDEM), including a β-blocker at maximum tolerated dose, and who are in sinus rhythm with a heart rate of ≥70 bpm at rest. The guidelines emphasize that given the well-proven mortality benefits of β-blocker therapy, it is important to initiate and up titrate these agents to target doses, as tolerated, before assessing the resting heart rate for consideration of ivabradine initiation [23, 24].

3. FIXED-DOSE COMBINATION OF SACUBITRIL AND VALSARTAN (ENTRESTO)

3.1. Overview

Abnormal activation of the RAAS contributes to the clinical progression of HF, especially HFrEF. However, despite the use of ACE inhibitors, ARBs, β-blockers, and aldosterone receptor antagonists (ARAs), patients remain at high risk of worsening HF. Such progression may be related to inadequate activation of, or a diminished response to, the compensatory actions of endogenous adaptive neurohormonal systems. In this context, the natriuretic peptide (NP) system, which includes atrial natriuretic peptide (ANP), B-type natriuretic peptide (BNP), and C-type natriuretic peptide (CNP), has an important role in cardiovascular homeostasis, promoting a number of physiological effects including diuresis, vasodilation, and inhibition of the RAAS [25]. Indeed, HF is associated with defects in NP processing and synthesis, and there is a strong relationship between NP levels and disease state. Moreover, NPs are useful biomarkers in HF, and their use in diagnosis and evaluation of prognosis is well established, particularly in patients with HFrEF [26]. There has also been interest in their use to guide disease management and therapeutic decision-making [25, 27–29]. Understanding of NPs in HF has also resulted in interest in synthetic NPs for the treatment of HF and in treatments that target neprilysin, a protease that degrades NPs. Neprilysin, a zinc-dependent endopeptidase, is ubiquitous in distribution and promiscuous in function, having >50 putative peptide substrates with varying levels of in vitro and/or in vivo evidence of functional relevance. In this regard, the role of neprilysin in degrading the cardiovascular protective NPs has received much attention in recent years. Consequently, efforts have been spent on developing pharmacological agents to inhibit neprilysin to treat HFrEF [25, 27–29].

Recently, a novel fixed-dose combination drug—the angiotensin receptor-neprilysin inhibitor (ARNI) sacubitril/valsartan (Entresto), which simultaneously inhibits neprilysin and blocks the angiotensin II type I receptor, was shown to have a favorable efficacy and safety profile in patients with HFrEF and has been approved by the US FDA. The approval of Entresto (Novartis Pharmaceuticals, Basel, Switzerland) was based on a randomized controlled trial (PARADIGM-HF) involving 8,442 patients with NYHA class II–IV HF and a LVEF of ≤40%. The trial demonstrated that Entresto was superior to enalapril in reducing the risks of all-cause mortality (by 18%), cardiovascular death (by 20%), and hospitalization (by 21%) for HF, compared with enalapril therapy [30].

3.2. Chemistry and Pharmacokinetics

Entresto tablets contain a complex of anionic forms of sacubitril and valsartan, sodium cations, and water molecules in the molar ratio of 1:1:3:2.5, respectively. Following oral administration, the complex dissociates into sacubitril (a prodrug that is further metabolized to its active metabolite, designated as LBQ657) and valsartan (an ARB commonly used for treating HF). Sacubitril is a biphenyl compound and valsartan is a valine derivative (structures shown in **Figure 12.2**). The major pharmacokinetic properties of Entresto are summarized in **Table 12.2**.

3.3. Molecular Mechanisms and Pharmacological Effects

3.3.1. Molecular Mechanisms

As noted earlier, Entresto contains a neprilysin inhibitor sacubitril, and an ARB valsartan. Entresto inhibits neprilysin via LBQ657, the active metabolite of sacubitril, and blocks the angiotensin II type 1 (AT1) receptors via valsartan (**Figure 12.2**). The cardiovascular and renal effects of Entresto in HF patients are attributed to the increased levels of peptides that are degraded by neprilysin, such as natriuretic

Angiotensin receptors

The biological effects of angiotensin molecules, including angiotensin II are mediated by their receptors known as angiotensin receptors. While angiotensin receptors as a family remain poorly understood, the G protein-coupled receptors that mediate the biological functions of angiotensin II have been extensively characterized, and they are named angiotensin II type 1 receptor (AT1 receptor) and angiotensin II type II receptor (AT2 receptor) (Karnik SS, Unal H, Kemp JR, Tirupula KC, Eguchi S, Vanderheyden PM, Thomas WG. International Union of Basic and Clinical Pharmacology. XCIX. Angiotensin receptors: interpreters of pathophysiological angiotensinergic stimuli. *Pharmacol Rev* 2015; 67:754–819). AT1 receptor signaling mediates the adverse effects of angiotensin II on the cardiovascular and renal systems, whereas AT2 receptor activation has been suggested to be cardiovascular protective. At present, clinically available angiotensin receptor blockers (ARBs) are selective for AT1 receptors, and hence, they should be called angiotensin II type 1 receptor blockers.

Table 12.2. Major pharmacokinetic properties of Entresto

Property	Description
Oral Bioavailability	≥60%
t_{max}	0.5 h (sacubitril); 2 h (LBQ657); 1.5 h (valsartan)
Effect of food	No clinically significant effect
Plasma protein binding	>90%
Vd	103 L (sacubitril); 75 L (valsartan)
Metabolism	Sacubitril is readily converted to LBQ657 by esterases; LBQ657 is not further metabolized to a significant extent; valsartan is minimally metabolized
Elimination	Sacubitril (mainly LBQ657) eliminated in both urine and feces; valsartan eliminated mainly in feces
$t_{1/2}$	1.4 h (sacubitril); 11.5 h (LBQ657); 9.9 h (valsartan)

Note: $t_{1/2}$, elimination half-life; t_{max}, the time when the maximum plasma concentration is reached; Vd, volume of distribution per 70 kg body weight.

peptides, via the action of LBQ657, and the simultaneous inhibition of the effects of angiotensin II by valsartan. Valsartan inhibits the effects of angiotensin II by selectively blocking the AT1 receptors, and also inhibits angiotensin II-dependent aldosterone release from the adrenal gland and possibly other tissues (e.g., the cardiac tissue). Both angiotensin II and aldosterone cause cardiovascular remodeling, contributing to the disease progression of HF.

3.3.2. Pharmacological/Clinical Effects

Entresto causes simultaneous neprilysin inhibition and RAAS blockage. In the PARADIGM-HF trial, Entresto decreases plasma NT-proBNP (not a neprilysin substrate) and increases plasma BNP (a neprilysin substrate) and urine cyclic guanosine monophosphate (cGMP) compared with enalapril. Entresto also causes a significant non-sustained increase in natriuresis, increased urine ANP and plasma cGMP, and decreased plasma aldosterone and endothelin-1 as well as serum uric acid [31].

Entresto blocks the AT1 receptors (via the action of valsartan) leading to increased plasma renin activity and plasma renin concentrations. It is worth mentioning that activation of the AT1 receptors by angiotensin II in the renal juxtaglomerular cells reduces renin release from these cells, thereby serving as a negative feedback mechanism to regulate renin production. Conversely, blockage of the AT1 receptors by Entresto causes increased release of renin from these cells, leading to increased plasma renin activity.

Neprilysin is one of the multiple enzymes involved in the clearance of amyloid-β (Aβ) from the brain and cerebrospinal fluid (CSF). Entresto treatment is associated with an increase in CSF Aβ1–38 in healthy human volunteers [32]. The clinical relevance of this effect

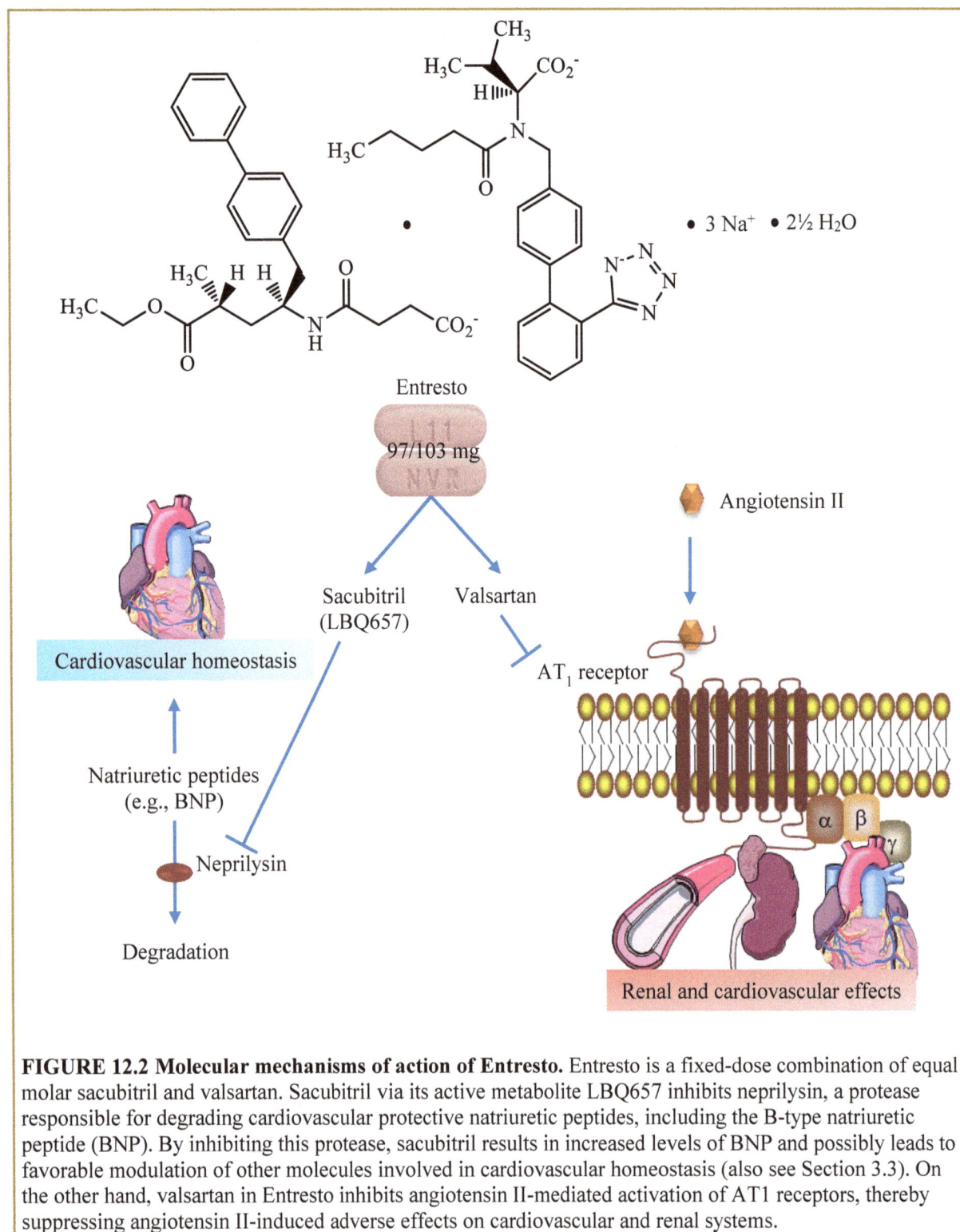

FIGURE 12.2 Molecular mechanisms of action of Entresto. Entresto is a fixed-dose combination of equal molar sacubitril and valsartan. Sacubitril via its active metabolite LBQ657 inhibits neprilysin, a protease responsible for degrading cardiovascular protective natriuretic peptides, including the B-type natriuretic peptide (BNP). By inhibiting this protease, sacubitril results in increased levels of BNP and possibly leads to favorable modulation of other molecules involved in cardiovascular homeostasis (also see Section 3.3). On the other hand, valsartan in Entresto inhibits angiotensin II-mediated activation of AT1 receptors, thereby suppressing angiotensin II-induced adverse effects on cardiovascular and renal systems.

is currently unknown though interference with Aβ homeostasis might have potential implications in Alzheimer's disease. In cynomolgus monkeys, Entresto caused a transient increase in Aβ concentrations in the central nervous system; however, no microscopic brain changes or Aβ deposition, as assessed by immunohistochemical staining, were present following treatment with Entresto (300 mg/kg) for 39 weeks [33]. A recent analysis showed no evidence that Entresto, compared with enalapril, increased dementia-related adverse events in the PARADIGM-HF study and other trials involving patients with HFrEF [34].

3.4. Clinical Uses

Entresto is indicated to reduce the risk of cardiovascular death and hospitalization for HF in patients with chronic HFrEF (NYHA Class II–IV). It is usually administered in conjunction with other HF therapies, as a replacement for an ACE inhibitor or other ARB.

3.5. Therapeutic Dosages

The dosage forms and strengths of Entresto are listed below. As noted earlier, tablets contain the equal molar sacubitril and valsartan.

- Oral: Entresto 24/26 mg (sacubitril 24 mg and valsartan 26 mg), 49/51 mg (sacubitril 49 mg and valsartan 51 mg), and 97/103 mg (sacubitril 97 mg and valsartan 103 mg) tablets

The typical dosage regimens for Entresto therapy are summarized below.

- The recommended starting dose of Entresto is 49/51 mg twice daily. Double the dose after 2–4 weeks to the target maintenance dose of 97/103 mg twice daily, as tolerated by the patient.
- Reduce the starting dose to 24/26 mg twice daily for: (1) patients not currently taking an ACE inhibitor or an ARB or previously taking a low dose of these agents; (2) patients with severe renal impairment; and (3) patients with moderate hepatic impairment. Double the dose after 2–4 weeks to the target maintenance dose of 97/103 mg twice daily, as tolerated by the patient.
- Entresto is contraindicated with concomitant use of an ACE inhibitor. If switching from an ACE inhibitor to Entresto, allow a washout period of 36 h between administration of the two drugs.

3.6. Adverse Effects and Drug Interactions

3.6.1. Adverse Effects

Common adverse effects include hypotension, hyperkalemia, cough, dizziness, and renal impairment. Angioedema, though rarely, may also occur.

3.6.2. Drug Interactions

- *Other inhibitors of the RAAS*: Concomitant use of an ACE inhibitor may increase the risk of angioedema. Concomitant use of aliskiren in diabetic patients who are on an ARB therapy (e.g., valsartan in

Entresto) may increase the risk of hyperkalemia, hypotension, and renal impairment [35].

- *Potassium-sparing diuretics*: Concomitant use of potassium-sparing diuretics (e.g., spironolactone, eplerenone, triamterene, amiloride), potassium supplements, or salt substitutes containing potassium may lead to increases in serum potassium.
- *Nonsteroidal anti-inflammatory drugs (NSAIDs)*: In patients who are elderly, volume-depleted, or with compromised renal function, concomitant use of NSAIDs, including cyclooxygenase (COX)-2 inhibitors may result in worsening of renal function, including possible acute renal failure.
- *Lithium*: Concomitant use of an ARB (e.g., valsartan in Entresto) may increase blood lithium concentrations and lithium toxicity.

3.6.3. Contraindications and FDA Pregnancy Category

- Hypersensitivity to any component of the drug product
- History of angioedema related to previous ACE inhibitor or ARB therapy
- Concomitant use with ACE inhibitors
- Concomitant use with aliskiren in patients with diabetes due to increased harm
- FDA pregnancy category: not assigned. Entresto can cause fetal harm when administered to a pregnant woman. Use of drugs that act on the RAAS during the second and third trimesters of pregnancy reduces fetal renal function and increases fetal and neonatal morbidity and death. Entresto should be discontinued as soon as possible when pregnancy is detected.

3.7. Comparison with Existing Members and New Development since the US FDA Approval

Entresto is the first-in-class and currently the only member of the ARNI drug class approved by the US FDA. Since its approval in 2015, a number of post-hoc analyses of the PARADIGM-HF trial as well as additional studies have further established the clinical efficacy of Entresto in reducing all-cause mortality, cardiovascular death, and hospital readmission in patients with HFrEF [36–39]. Moreover, the superior efficacy of Entresto over ACE inhibitor therapy extends to various patients' conditions and scenarios. These include HFrEF patients with various LVEF [40], in diverse age groups [41], among a spectrum of risk [42], with diabetes and prediabetes [43], with regard to clinical progression [27], in outpatient settings [44], and with background therapy [45], as well as cost-effectiveness and health-related quality of life outcomes [46–49]. It is estimated that Entresto therapy, as compared with ACE inhibitor therapy may result in a projected benefit of 1–2 years of increased life expectancy and survival free from HF for patients such as those in the PARADIGM-HF trial [50]. A network meta-analysis of 57 randomized controlled trials published between 1987 and 2015 suggested that the combination of ARNI + β-blocker + ARA resulted in the greatest mortality reduction in patients with HFrEF among treatments with ACE inhibitor, ARB, ARA, and ARNI, and their combinations [51].

In line with the above promising clinical findings, the "2017 ACC/AHA/HFSA focused update of the 2013 ACCF/AHA guideline for the management of heart failure" provides a class I recommendation stating that in patients with chronic symptomatic HFrEF (NYHA class II or III) who tolerate an ACE inhibitor or ARB, replacement by an ARNI is recommended to further reduce morbidity and mortality [24]. In addition to the efficacy in HFrEF, multiple randomized controlled trials also suggested a potential beneficial role for Entresto therapy (as compared to valsartan) in patients with HFpEF [52–55]. Moreover, the PARAMETER study (Prospective Comparison of Angiotensin Receptor Neprilysin Inhibitor with Angiotensin Receptor Blocker Measuring Arterial Stiffness in the Elderly), for the first time, demonstrated superiority of sacubitril/valsartan versus olmesartan in reducing clinic and ambulatory central aortic and brachial pressures in elderly patients with systolic hypertension and stiff arteries [56]. As new knowledge on Entresto accumulates via clinical trials in various patient populations, the coming years will likely witness the evolvement of Entresto into a valuable therapy in cardiovascular medicine for the management of HF as well as other cardiovascular disorders, such as resistant hypertension [57, 58].

4. SELF-ASSESSMENT QUESTIONS

5.1. A 54-year-old man is diagnosed with heart failure with reduced ejection fraction (HFrEF). A treatment regimen is designed to include a drug that inhibits both neprilysin activity and angiotensin II type 1 (AT1) receptor-mediated signaling. Which of the following is most likely the drug?

A. Bidil
B. Entresto
C. Ivabradine
D. Sacubitril
E. Valsartan

5.2. A decision is made to add a newly approved drug inhibiting the sinus nodal I_f current to the standard therapy for a patient with stable chronic heart failure and a reduced left ventricular ejection fraction (LVEF). Which of the following conditions must be met for the addition of this drug?

A. The patient must also take nefazodone
B. The patient must be of African heritage
C. The patient's heart rate must be ≤60 beats per minute
D. The patient's heart rate must be ≥70 beats per minute
E. The patient's LVEF must be ≥45%

5.3. A 62-year-old man with systolic heart failure is put on a new drug therapy to reduce his resting heart rate. Following the drug treatment, he notices a transient enhanced brightness in a limited area of his visual field, which makes him nervous. Which of the following is most likely the drug prescribed?

A. Carvedilol
B. Digoxin
C. Ivabradine
D. Metoprolol
E. Valsartan

5.4. Which of the following substances is expected to rise in the serum of a heart failure patient upon long-term treatment with a newly approved angiotensin receptor-neprilysin inhibitor (ARNI)?

A. Aldosterone
B. B-type natriuretic peptide
C. Endothelin-1
D. NT-pro B-type natriuretic peptide
E. Troponin I

5.5. A transient increase in amyloid-β levels in the cerebrospinal fluid is detected in a 59-year-old woman with systolic heart failure shortly following the addition of a new drug to her treatment regimen. Which of the following is most likely the added new drug?

A. Azilsartan
B. Bidil
C. Entresto
D. Ivabradine
E. Nebivolol

ANSWERS AND EXPLANATIONS

5.1. The correct answer is B. Among the drug listed, only Entresto is able to inhibit both neprilysin activity and AT1 receptor-mediated signaling. It is a fixed-dose combination of sacubitril (an inhibitor of neprilysin) and valsartan (an AT1 receptor blocker). Bidil is a fixed-dose combination of isosorbide dinitrate and hydralazine. Ivabradine is an I_f channel inhibitor that reduces heart rate.

5.2. The correct answer is D. The drug is ivabradine. It is approved by the US FDA for the reduction of the risk of hospitalization for worsening HF in patients with stable, symptomatic chronic heart failure with LVEF ≤35%, who are in sinus rhythm with resting heart rate ≥70 beats per minute. Concomitant use of nefazodone (a strong inhibitor of CYP3A4) is contraindicated. Ivabradine therapy is independent of ethnicity.

5.3. The correct answer is C. Although all the drugs listed except valsartan are negative chronotropes (drugs that reduce heart rate), only ivabradine therapy is associated with phosphenes.

5.4. The correct answer is B. The drug is Entresto. Based on the results of the PARADIGM-HF trial, Entresto treatment decreases plasma NT-proBNP (not a neprilysin substrate) concentrations and increases plasma BNP (a neprilysin substrate) levels. It also reduces plasma aldosterone and endothelin-1 levels. There is no evidence showing that Entresto increases the plasma levels of cardiac troponin I, a maker of cardiomyocyte damage.

5.5. The correct answer is C. Neprilysin is one of the multiple enzymes involved in the clearance of amyloid-β (Aβ) from the brain and CSF. Among the drugs listed, only Entresto treatment has been shown to be associated with an increase in CSF Aβ1–38 in healthy human volunteers.

REFERENCES

1. Owens AT, Brozena SC, Jessup M. New management strategies in heart failure. *Circ Res* 2016; 118(3):480–95.
2. Fox K, Ford I, Steg PG, Tendera M, Robertson M, Ferrari R, BEAUTIFUL Investigators. Heart rate as a prognostic risk factor in patients with coronary artery disease and left-ventricular systolic dysfunction (BEAUTIFUL): a subgroup analysis of a randomised controlled trial. *Lancet* 2008; 372(9641):817–21.
3. Bui AL, Grau-Sepulveda MV, Hernandez AF, Peterson ED, Yancy CW, Bhatt DL, Fonarow GC. Admission heart rate and in-hospital outcomes in patients hospitalized for heart failure in sinus rhythm and in atrial fibrillation. *Am Heart J* 2013; 165(4):567–74 e6.
4. Laskey WK, Alomari I, Cox M, Schulte PJ, Zhao X, Hernandez AF, Heidenreich PA, Eapen ZJ, Yancy C, Bhatt DL, Fonarow GC, AHA Get With The Guidelines–Heart Failure Program. Heart rate at hospital discharge in patients with heart failure is associated with mortality and rehospitalization. *J Am Heart Assoc* 2015; 4(4):e001626.
5. Swedberg K, Komajda M, Bohm M, Borer JS, Ford I, Dubost-Brama A, Lerebours G, Tavazzi L, SHIFT Investigators. Ivabradine and outcomes in chronic heart failure (SHIFT): a randomised placebo-controlled study. *Lancet* 2010; 376(9744):875–85.
6. DiFrancesco D. The role of the funny current in pacemaker activity. *Circ Res* 2010; 106(3):434–46.
7. Milanesi R, Baruscotti M, Gnecchi-Ruscone T, DiFrancesco D. Familial sinus bradycardia associated with a mutation in the cardiac pacemaker channel. *N Engl J Med* 2006; 354(2):151–7.
8. Psotka MA, Teerlink JR. Ivabradine: role in the chronic heart failure armamentarium.

Circulation 2016; 133(21):2066–75.
9. Fox K, Ford I, Steg PG, Tendera M, Ferrari R, BEAUTIFUL Investigators. Ivabradine for patients with stable coronary artery disease and left-ventricular systolic dysfunction (BEAUTIFUL): a randomised, double-blind, placebo-controlled trial. *Lancet* 2008; 372(9641):807–16.
10. Bohm M, Swedberg K, Komajda M, Borer JS, Ford I, Dubost-Brama A, Lerebours G, Tavazzi L, SHIFT Investigators. Heart rate as a risk factor in chronic heart failure (SHIFT): the association between heart rate and outcomes in a randomised placebo-controlled trial. *Lancet* 2010; 376(9744):886–94.
11. Cappato R, Castelvecchio S, Ricci C, Bianco E, Vitali-Serdoz L, Gnecchi-Ruscone T, Pittalis M, De Ambroggi L, Baruscotti M, Gaeta M, Furlanello F, Di Francesco D, et al. Clinical efficacy of ivabradine in patients with inappropriate sinus tachycardia: a prospective, randomized, placebo-controlled, double-blind, crossover evaluation. *J Am Coll Cardiol* 2012; 60(15):1323–9.
12. Reil JC, Tardif JC, Ford I, Lloyd SM, O'Meara E, Komajda M, Borer JS, Tavazzi L, Swedberg K, Bohm M. Selective heart rate reduction with ivabradine unloads the left ventricle in heart failure patients. *J Am Coll Cardiol* 2013; 62(21):1977–85.
13. Jamil HA, Gierula J, Paton MF, Byrom R, Lowry JE, Cubbon RM, Cairns DA, Kearney MT, Witte KK. Chronotropic incompetence does not limit exercise capacity in chronic heart failure. *J Am Coll Cardiol* 2016; 67(16):1885–96.
14. Komajda M, Tavazzi L, Swedberg K, Bohm M, Borer JS, Moyne A, Ford I, SHIFT Investigators. Chronic exposure to ivabradine reduces readmissions in the vulnerable phase after hospitalization for worsening systolic heart failure: a post-hoc analysis of SHIFT. *Eur J*

Heart Fail 2016; 18(9):1182–9.

15. Bohm M, Borer J, Ford I, Gonzalez-Juanatey JR, Komajda M, Lopez-Sendon J, Reil JC, Swedberg K, Tavazzi L. Heart rate at baseline influences the effect of ivabradine on cardiovascular outcomes in chronic heart failure: analysis from the SHIFT study. *Clin Res Cardiol* 2013; 102(1):11–22.

16. Ponikowski P, Voors AA, Anker SD, Bueno H, Cleland JG, Coats AJ, Falk V, Gonzalez-Juanatey JR, Harjola VP, Jankowska EA, Jessup M, Linde C, et al. 2016 ESC Guidelines for the diagnosis and treatment of acute and chronic heart failure: the Task Force for the diagnosis and treatment of acute and chronic heart failure of the European Society of Cardiology (ESC)Developed with the special contribution of the Heart Failure Association (HFA) of the ESC. *Eur Heart J* 2016; 37(27):2129–200.

17. Bonnet D, Berger F, Jokinen E, Kantor PF, Daubeney PEF. Ivabradine in children with dilated cardiomyopathy and symptomatic chronic heart failure. *J Am Coll Cardiol* 2017; 70(10):1262–72.

18. Kosmala W, Holland DJ, Rojek A, Wright L, Przewlocka-Kosmala M, Marwick TH. Effect of I_f-channel inhibition on hemodynamic status and exercise tolerance in heart failure with preserved ejection fraction: a randomized trial. *J Am Coll Cardiol* 2013; 62(15):1330–8.

19. Pal N, Sivaswamy N, Mahmod M, Yavari A, Rudd A, Singh S, Dawson DK, Francis JM, Dwight JS, Watkins H, Neubauer S, Frenneaux M, et al. Effect of selective heart rate slowing in heart failure with preserved ejection fraction. *Circulation* 2015; 132(18):1719–25.

20. Komajda M, Isnard R, Cohen-Solal A, Metra M, Pieske B, Ponikowski P, Voors AA, Dominjon F, Henon-Goburdhun C, Pannaux M, Bohm M, EDIFY Investigators. Effect of ivabradine in patients with heart failure with preserved ejection fraction: the EDIFY randomized placebo-controlled trial. *Eur J Heart Fail* 2017; 19(11):1495-1503.

21. Fox K, Ford I, Steg PG, Tardif JC, Tendera M, Ferrari R, SIGNIFY Investigators. Ivabradine in stable coronary artery disease without clinical heart failure. *N Engl J Med* 2014; 371(12):1091–9.

22. Tendera M, Chassany O, Ferrari R, Ford I, Steg PG, Tardif JC, Fox K, Investigators S. Quality of life with ivabradine in patients with angina pectoris: the study assessing the morbidity-mortality benefits of the I_f inhibitor ivabradine in patients with coronary artery disease quality of life substudy. *Circ Cardiovasc Qual Outcomes* 2016; 9(1):31–8.

23. Yancy CW, Jessup M, Bozkurt B, Butler J, Casey DE, Jr., Colvin MM, Drazner MH, Filippatos G, Fonarow GC, Givertz MM, Hollenberg SM, Lindenfeld J, et al. 2016 ACC/AHA/HFSA focused update on new pharmacological therapy for heart failure: an update of the 2013 ACCF/AHA guideline for the management of heart failure: a report of the American College of Cardiology/American Heart Association Task Force on Clinical Practice Guidelines and the Heart Failure Society of America. *J Am Coll Cardiol* 2016; 68(13):1476–88.

24. Yancy CW, Jessup M, Bozkurt B, Butler J, Casey DE, Jr., Colvin MM, Drazner MH, Filippatos GS, Fonarow GC, Givertz MM, Hollenberg SM, Lindenfeld J, et al. 2017 ACC/AHA/HFSA focused update of the 2013 ACCF/AHA guideline for the management of heart failure: a report of the American College of Cardiology/American Heart Association Task Force on Clinical Practice Guidelines and the Heart Failure Society of America. *Circulation* 2017; 136(6):e137–e61.

25. Rubattu S, Triposkiadis F. Resetting the neurohormonal balance in heart failure (HF): the relevance of the natriuretic peptide (NP) system to the clinical management of patients with HF. *Heart Fail Rev* 2017; 22(3):279–88.

26. Chow SL, Maisel AS, Anand I, Bozkurt B, de Boer RA, Felker GM, Fonarow GC, Greenberg B, Januzzi JL, Jr., Kiernan MS, Liu PP, Wang TJ, et al. Role of biomarkers for the prevention, assessment, and management of heart failure: a scientific statement from the American Heart Association. *Circulation* 2017; 135(22):e1054–e91.

27. Packer M, McMurray JJ, Desai AS, Gong J, Lefkowitz MP, Rizkala AR, Rouleau JL, Shi VC, Solomon SD, Swedberg K, Zile M, Andersen K, et al. Angiotensin receptor neprilysin inhibition compared with enalapril on the risk of clinical progression in surviving patients with heart failure. *Circulation* 2015; 131(1):54–61.

28. Bayes-Genis A, Barallat J, Richards AM. A test in context: neprilysin: function, inhibition, and biomarker. *J Am Coll Cardiol* 2016; 68(6):639–53.

29. Packer M, McMurray JJV. Importance of endogenous compensatory vasoactive peptides in broadening the effects of inhibitors of the renin-angiotensin system for the treatment of heart failure. *Lancet* 2017; 389(10081):1831–40.

30. McMurray JJ, Packer M, Desai AS, Gong J, Lefkowitz MP, Rizkala AR, Rouleau JL, Shi VC, Solomon SD, Swedberg K, Zile MR, PARADIGM-HF Investigators, et al. Angiotensin-neprilysin inhibition versus enalapril in heart failure. *N Engl J Med* 2014; 371(11):993–1004.

31. Mogensen UM, Kober L, Jhund PS, Desai AS, Senni M, Kristensen SL, Dukat A, Chen CH, Ramires F, Lefkowitz MP, Prescott MF, Shi VC, et al. Sacubitril/valsartan reduces serum uric acid concentration, an independent predictor of adverse outcomes in PARADIGM-HF. *Eur J Heart Fail* 2018 (in press).

32. Langenickel TH, Tsubouchi C, Ayalasomayajula S, Pal P, Valentin MA, Hinder M, Jhee S, Gevorkyan H, Rajman I. The effect of LCZ696 (sacubitril/valsartan) on amyloid-beta concentrations in cerebrospinal fluid in healthy subjects. *Br J Clin Pharmacol* 2016; 81(5):878–90.

33. Schoenfeld HA, West T, Verghese PB, Holubasch M, Shenoy N, Kagan D, Buono C, Zhou W, DeCristofaro M, Douville J, Goodrich GG, Mansfield K, et al. The effect of angiotensin receptor neprilysin inhibitor, sacubitril/valsartan, on central nervous system amyloid-beta concentrations and clearance in the cynomolgus monkey. *Toxicol Appl Pharmacol* 2017; 323:53–65.

34. Cannon JA, Shen L, Jhund PS, Kristensen SL, Kober L, Chen F, Gong J, Lefkowitz MP, Rouleau JL, Shi VC, Swedberg K, Zile MR, et al. Dementia-related adverse events in PARADIGM-HF and other trials in heart failure with reduced ejection fraction. *Eur J Heart Fail* 2017; 19(1):129–37.

35. Parving HH, Brenner BM, McMurray JJ, de Zeeuw D, Haffner SM, Solomon SD, Chaturvedi N, Persson F, Desai AS, Nicolaides M, Richard A, Xiang Z, et al. Cardiorenal end points in a trial of aliskiren for type 2 diabetes. *N Engl J Med* 2012; 367(23):2204–13.

36. Solomon SD, Claggett B, McMurray JJ, Hernandez AF, Fonarow GC. Combined neprilysin and renin-angiotensin system inhibition in heart failure with reduced ejection fraction: a meta-analysis. *Eur J Heart Fail* 2016; 18(10):1238–43.

37. Mogensen UM, Kober L, Kristensen SL, Jhund PS, Gong J, Lefkowitz MP, Rizkala AR, Rouleau JL, Shi VC, Swedberg K, Zile MR, Solomon SD, et al. The effects of sacubitril/valsartan on coronary outcomes in PARADIGM-HF. *Am Heart J* 2017; 188:35–41.

38. Campbell DJ. Long-term neprilysin inhibition: implications for ARNIs. *Nat Rev Cardiol* 2017; 14(3):171–86.

39. Desai AS, Claggett BL, Packer M, Zile MR, Rouleau JL, Swedberg K, Shi V, Lefkowitz M, Starling R, Teerlink J, McMurray JJ, Solomon SD, et al. Influence of sacubitril/valsartan (LCZ696) on 30-day readmission after heart failure hospitalization. *J Am Coll Cardiol* 2016; 68(3):241–8.

40. Solomon SD, Claggett B, Desai AS, Packer M, Zile M, Swedberg K, Rouleau JL, Shi VC, Starling RC, Kozan O, Dukat A, Lefkowitz MP, et al. Influence of ejection fraction on outcomes and efficacy of sacubitril/valsartan (LCZ696) in heart failure with reduced ejection fraction: the prospective comparison of ARNI with ACEI to determine impact on global mortality and morbidity in heart failure (PARADIGM-HF) trial. *Circ Heart Fail* 2016; 9:e002744.

41. Jhund PS, Fu M, Bayram E, Chen CH, Negrusz-Kawecka M, Rosenthal A, Desai AS, Lefkowitz MP, Rizkala AR, Rouleau JL, Shi VC, Solomon SD, et al. Efficacy and safety of LCZ696 (sacubitril-valsartan) according to age: insights from PARADIGM-HF. *Eur Heart J* 2015; 36(38):2576–84.

42. Simpson J, Jhund PS, Silva Cardoso J, Martinez F, Mosterd A, Ramires F, Rizkala AR, Senni M, Squire I, Gong J, Lefkowitz MP, Shi VC, et al. Comparing LCZ696 with enalapril according to baseline risk using the MAGGIC and EMPHASIS-HF risk scores: an analysis of mortality and morbidity in PARADIGM-HF. *J Am Coll Cardiol* 2015; 66(19):2059–71.

43. Kristensen SL, Preiss D, Jhund PS, Squire I, Cardoso JS, Merkely B, Martinez F, Starling RC, Desai AS, Lefkowitz MP, Rizkala AR, Rouleau JL, et al. Risk related to pre-diabetes mellitus and diabetes mellitus in heart failure with reduced ejection fraction: insights from Prospective Comparison of ARNI with ACEI to Determine Impact on Global Mortality and Morbidity in Heart Failure trial. *Circ Heart Fail* 2016; 9:e002560.

44. Okumura N, Jhund PS, Gong J, Lefkowitz MP,

Rizkala AR, Rouleau JL, Shi VC, Swedberg K, Zile MR, Solomon SD, Packer M, McMurray JJ, et al. Importance of clinical worsening of heart failure treated in the outpatient setting: evidence from the Prospective Comparison of ARNI with ACEI to Determine Impact on Global Mortality and Morbidity in Heart Failure trial (PARADIGM-HF). *Circulation* 2016; 133(23):2254–62.

45. Okumura N, Jhund PS, Gong J, Lefkowitz MP, Rizkala AR, Rouleau JL, Shi VC, Swedberg K, Zile MR, Solomon SD, Packer M, McMurray JJ, et al. Effects of sacubitril/valsartan in the PARADIGM-HF trial (Prospective Comparison of ARNI with ACEI to Determine Impact on Global Mortality and Morbidity in Heart Failure) according to background therapy. *Circ Heart Fail* 2016; 9:e003212.

46. Ollendorf DA, Sandhu AT, Pearson SD. Sacubitril-valsartan for the treatment of heart failure: effectiveness and value. *JAMA Intern Med* 2016; 176(2):249–50.

47. Sandhu AT, Ollendorf DA, Chapman RH, Pearson SD, Heidenreich PA. Cost-effectiveness of sacubitril-valsartan in patients with heart failure with reduced ejection fraction. *Ann Intern Med* 2016; 165(10):681–9.

48. King JB, Shah RU, Bress AP, Nelson RE, Bellows BK. Cost-effectiveness of sacubitril-valsartan combination therapy compared with enalapril for the treatment of heart failure with reduced ejection fraction. *JACC Heart Fail* 2016; 4(5):392–402.

49. Lewis EF, Claggett BL, McMurray JJV, Packer M, Lefkowitz MP, Rouleau JL, Liu J, Shi VC, Zile MR, Desai AS, Solomon SD, Swedberg K. Health-related quality of life outcomes in PARADIGM-HF. *Circ Heart Fail* 2017; 10:e003430.

50. Claggett B, Packer M, McMurray JJ, Swedberg K, Rouleau J, Zile MR, Jhund P, Lefkowitz M, Shi V, Solomon SD, PARADIGM-HF Investigators. Estimating the long-term treatment benefits of sacubitril-valsartan. *N Engl J Med* 2015; 373(23):2289–90.

51. Burnett H, Earley A, Voors AA, Senni M, McMurray JJ, Deschaseaux C, Cope S. Thirty years of evidence on the efficacy of drug treatments for chronic heart failure with reduced ejection fraction: a network meta-analysis. *Circ Heart Fail* 2017; 10:e003529.

52. Solomon SD, Zile M, Pieske B, Voors A, Shah A, Kraigher-Krainer E, Shi V, Bransford T, Takeuchi M, Gong J, Lefkowitz M, Packer M, et al. The angiotensin receptor neprilysin inhibitor LCZ696 in heart failure with preserved ejection fraction: a phase 2 double-blind randomised controlled trial. *Lancet* 2012; 380(9851):1387–95.

53. Jhund PS, Claggett B, Packer M, Zile MR, Voors AA, Pieske B, Lefkowitz M, Shi V, Bransford T, McMurray JJ, Solomon SD. Independence of the blood pressure lowering effect and efficacy of the angiotensin receptor neprilysin inhibitor, LCZ696, in patients with heart failure with preserved ejection fraction: an analysis of the PARAMOUNT trial. *Eur J Heart Fail* 2014; 16(6):671–7.

54. Voors AA, Gori M, Liu LC, Claggett B, Zile MR, Pieske B, McMurray JJ, Packer M, Shi V, Lefkowitz MP, Solomon SD, PARAMOUNT Investigators. Renal effects of the angiotensin receptor neprilysin inhibitor LCZ696 in patients with heart failure and preserved ejection fraction. *Eur J Heart Fail* 2015; 17(5):510–7.

55. Zile MR, Jhund PS, Baicu CF, Claggett BL, Pieske B, Voors AA, Prescott MF, Shi V, Lefkowitz M, McMurray JJ, Solomon SD, PARAMOUNT Investigators. Plasma biomarkers reflecting profibrotic processes in heart failure with a preserved ejection fraction: data from the Prospective Comparison of ARNI with ARB on Management of Heart Failure with Preserved Ejection Fraction study. *Circ Heart Fail* 2016; 9:e002551.

56. Williams B, Cockcroft JR, Kario K, Zappe DH, Brunel PC, Wang Q, Guo W. Effects of sacubitril/valsartan versus olmesartan on central hemodynamics in the elderly with systolic hypertension: the PARAMETER study. *Hypertension* 2017; 69(3):411–20.

57. Schmieder RE, Wagner F, Mayr M, Delles C, Ott C, Keicher C, Hrabak-Paar M, Heye T, Aichner S, Khder Y, Yates D, Albrecht D, et al. The effect of sacubitril/valsartan compared to olmesartan on cardiovascular remodelling in subjects with essential hypertension: the results of a randomized, double-blind, active-controlled study. *Eur Heart J* 2017; 38(44):3308–17.

58. Cheung DG, Aizenberg D, Gorbunov V, Hafeez K, Chen CW, Zhang J. Efficacy and safety of sacubitril/valsartan in patients with essential hypertension uncontrolled by olmesartan: a randomized, double-blind, 8-week study. *J Clin Hypertens (Greenwich)* 2018; 20(1):150–8.

INDEX

Note: *b, f,* and *t denote box, figure,* and *table, respectively.*

Cardiovascular Medicine: New Therapeutic Drugs Approved by the US FDA (2013–2017) | First Edition **247**